# Management of Dementia from the Preclinical Stage

Yuan-Han Yang
Editor

# Management of Dementia from the Preclinical Stage

## An Update

Springer

*Editor*
Yuan-Han Yang
Neuroscience Research Center
Kaohsiung Medical University
Kaohsiung, Taiwan

ISBN 978-981-95-5221-4 ISBN 978-981-95-5222-1 (eBook)
https://doi.org/10.1007/978-981-95-5222-1



This Springer imprint is published by the registered company Springer Nature Singapore Pte Ltd.
The registered company address is: 152 Beach Road, #21-01/04 Gateway East, Singapore 189721, Singapore

# Preface

The challenge of dementia is one of the defining medical and societal issues of our time. For decades, our efforts were largely concentrated on managing symptoms after significant and irreversible neurodegeneration had already occurred. Today, we stand at an inflection point. The focus has decisively shifted toward the preclinical and prodromal stages, where intervention holds the greatest promise for slowing or even preventing progression.

This book is conceived to provide a comprehensive overview of this new landscape. Our aim is to bridge the gap between established clinical knowledge and the cutting-edge innovations that are reshaping every facet of the field.

In this book, we begin by establishing the conceptual framework of the disease cascade. We then detail the essential tools for detection: from electrophysiology (EEG) and structural/functional neuroimaging to the transformative power of fluid biomarkers. A deep understanding of clinical manifestations—neuropsychiatric, vascular, and neuropathological—provides the necessary clinical context.

The latter part is dedicated to the future. We explore how machine learning algorithms harnessed to data from wearable devices can create early warning systems for behavioral symptoms. We delve into the emerging paradigms of pharmacological precision medicine and the expanding role of digital therapeutics. Finally, we reflect on the evolving face of dementia itself, providing critical historical context for the changes we see today.

We are profoundly grateful to the international team of expert authors who have contributed their invaluable insights to this volume. It is our hope that this book will serve as a valuable resource for neurologists, psychiatrists, geriatricians, researchers, and students, inspiring a more proactive, personalized, and effective approach to managing dementia from its earliest origins.

Kaohsiung, Taiwan | Yuan-Han Yang

# Contents

# Chapter 1
# The Dementia Cascade: From the Preclinical Stage

**Qin Chen, Jun Xu, Hui Gao, and Hanlin Cai**

**Abstract** Dementia is a clinical syndrome associated with declines in memory and other cognitive domains that are sufficient to impair daily function. The characteristic disease course of neurodegenerative dementia is an insidious onset that gradually progresses. A growing body of research indicates that both genetically predisposed and cognitively normal individuals may go through an extended asymptomatic phase, termed the preclinical stage of dementia. At this stage, toxic proteins gradually accumulate in the patient's brain and can be detected using molecular imaging or biofluid assays in vivo. Previous studies have demonstrated that these toxic proteins begin to accumulate decades before cognitive decline occurs. In this chapter, we focus on the pathology, genetics, biomarkers, and clinical characteristics of dementia from the preclinical stage.

**Keywords** Dementia · Alzheimer's disease · Mild cognitive impairment · Lewy body dementia · Frontotemporal lobar degeneration

## Abbreviations

| | |
|---|---|
| AD | Alzheimer's disease |
| FTLD | Frontotemporal lobar degeneration |
| LBD | Lewy body dementias |
| MCI | Mild cognitive impairment |
| PET | Positron emission tomography |

Q. Chen (✉) · H. Gao · H. Cai
Department of Neurology, West China Hospital of Sichuan University, Chengdu, Sichuan, People's Republic of China
e-mail: chen.qin@scu.edu.cn

J. Xu
Department of Neurology, Beijing Tiantan Hospital, Capital Medical University, Fengtai District, Beijing, People's Republic of China



Y.-H. Yang (ed.), *Management of Dementia from the Preclinical Stage*,
https://doi.org/10.1007/978-981-95-5222-1_1

## 1.1 Introduction

### 1.1.1 Definitions, Types, and Global Impact of Dementia

Dementia is a clinical syndrome associated with declines in memory and other cognitive domains (e.g., executive, visuospatial, language function) that are sufficient to impair daily function [1]. Dementia can be clearly differentiated from congenital intellectual disability. This definition also implies that it is a clinical syndrome that may arise from various etiologies, including neurodegenerative and non-neurodegenerative causes [1]. So far, the most widely used diagnostic criteria for dementia include the *International Classification of Disease*—11th edition and the *Diagnostic and Statistical Manual*—Version 5 [2].

Given the expected trends of aging and population growth, it is anticipated that the number of people with dementia will gradually increase. Dementia affects approximately 50 million individuals globally, and by 2050, that number is predicted to increase to 152 million [3]. It is expected to rise, especially in low- and middle-income countries (LMIC), where about two-thirds of dementia patients reside [3]. Another evidence from a global burden of disease study demonstrated an age-standardized prevalence of dementia of 694.0 per 100,000 people, in which female patients were more common, with a female-to-male ratio of 1.31 [4]. Alzheimer's disease (AD) and related dementias are the fifth leading cause of death among individuals aged 65 years and above in 2021 [5]. The age-standardized death rate of AD and related dementias is 25.2 per 100,000 people in 2021, which has increased by 1.5% in the past three decades [4]. For individuals aged 60 and above, dementia is the second most common neurological cause of disability-adjusted life-years worldwide [4]. A recent study projected that dementia costs the world around $1 trillion a year, causing a significant burden on patients with dementia, their families, and society [1].

### 1.1.2 Key Pathological Markers and Mechanisms Common to Dementia

Dementia may arise due to both neurodegenerative and non-neurodegenerative causes. Common non-neurodegenerative causes of dementia include vitamin deficiency, thyroid dysfunction, infections of the central nervous system, psychiatric disorders, and substance abuse. Since most of the dementia caused by these conditions may be reversible, these conditions should be ruled out before diagnosing neurodegenerative dementia (NDD) [6].

The term 'neurodegenerative dementia' (NDD) refers to a group of illnesses in which harmful proteins are abnormally deposited in the brain, causing neuronal death and cognitive impairment over time. Alzheimer's disease (AD), Lewy body dementia (LBD), frontotemporal lobar degeneration (FTLD), and

**Table 1.1** Association between neuropathology and neurodegenerative diseases [7]

| Proteinopathy | Pathological hallmark | Disease |
|---|---|---|
| β-amyloid | Amyloid plaque | Alzheimer's disease |
| Tau | Neurofibrillary tangle | Alzheimer's disease; primary age-related tauopathy; chronic traumatic encephalopathy; progressive supranuclear palsy; corticobasal degeneration |
| | Astroglial inclusions | Chronic traumatic encephalopathy; age-related tau astrogliopathy; progressive supranuclear palsy; corticobasal degeneration |
| | Coiled body | Progressive supranuclear palsy; corticobasal degeneration |
| | Pick body | Pick disease |
| α-synuclein | Lewy body | Lewy body disease |
| TDP-43 | TDP-43 inclusions | Limbic-predominant age-related TDP-43 encephalopathy neuropathological changes; frontotemporal lobar degeneration-TDP |

Source from: Scholz and Cobos [7]

limbic-predominant age-related transactive response DNA-binding protein 43 (TDP-43) encephalopathy (LATE) are common NDDs verified by pathological evidence [7]. The common pathogenic proteins of these illnesses are listed below (Table 1.1) [7]. Specific protein depositions may be identified in specific brain areas for each NDDs. Vascular dementia (VaD) is generally recognized as a non-neurodegenerative cause of dementia. However, due to the high prevalence of vascular pathologies in the elderly, it is also a common copathology in neurodegenerative dementias [8].

### *1.1.3 The Progressive Stages of Dementia*

The characteristic disease course of neurodegenerative dementia is an insidious onset that gradually progresses. A growing body of research indicates that both genetically predisposed and cognitively normal individuals may go through an extended asymptomatic phase, termed the preclinical stage of dementia [9]. At this stage, toxic proteins gradually accumulate in the patient's brain and can be detected using molecular imaging or biofluid assays in vivo. Previous studies have demonstrated that these toxic proteins begin to accumulate decades before cognitive decline occurs [9]. For example, β-amyloid is typically recognized as the first pathological protein deposited in patients with AD and can be detected 10–15 years before symptom onset [9]. The accumulation of β-amyloid could further trigger tau protein deposition and neuronal loss, leading to cognitive impairment, which is referred to as "the amyloid cascade hypothesis" [6, 10] (Fig. 1.1).

Following preclinical stages, patients with AD experience varying degrees of cognitive decline, which may not affect their daily life functions. This transitional phase is

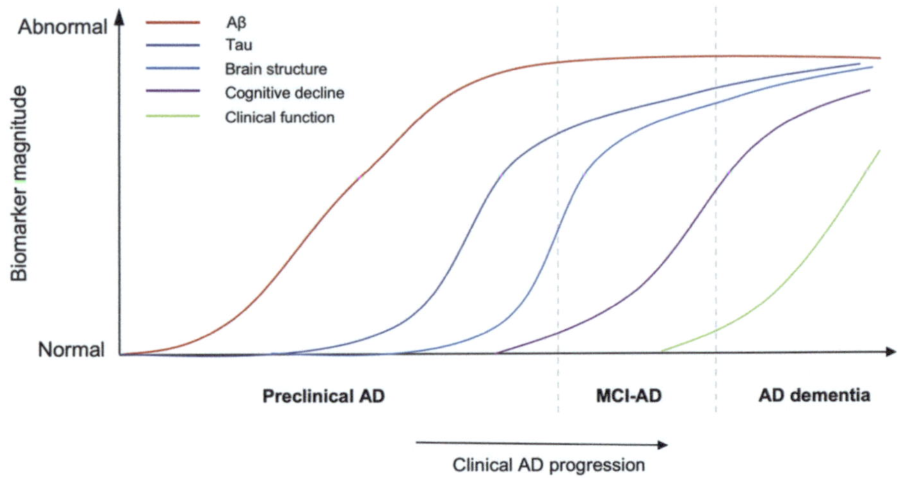


**Fig. 1.1** Proposed model of the amyloid cascade hypothesis and AD continuum. Notes: Aβ β-amyloid, MRI magnetic resonance imaging, AD Alzheimer's disease. (Source from: Jack et al. [10])

known as mild cognitive impairment (MCI) [11]. At this point, patients and their caregivers may complain about cognitive decline, which may be demonstrated in some neuropsychological tests, although their performance in activities of daily living (ADL) remains reserved. Most patients with MCI may only be affected in one cognitive domain at first, depending on which brain region is initially affected by toxic proteins [12].

Most patients with MCI may experience years of stability until their symptoms worsen and interfere with their ability to perform daily tasks, at which point they enter the dementia stage [12]. This typically occurs in conjunction with the spread of toxic proteins, neuronal death, and brain atrophy, which results in more severe impairment of more cognitive domains and daily function [12]. Patients with severe dementia may also exhibit psychiatric symptoms and lose their ability to perform daily tasks, leaving them bedridden and requiring round-the-clock care for years. NDDs are also fatal diseases, and most patients may ultimately die from complications caused by NDDs in the end [6].

### *1.1.4 Relevance of Early Detection and Intervention*

Early detection may be crucial for patients at risk for dementia in its early stages, because individuals with NDDs may experience symptoms for a long time before developing dementia. In NDDs, halting the downstream cascades of toxic proteins requires early, accurate, and targeted interventions [13]. Therefore, this chapter will focus on the basic theories and methods of early detection and intervention of the preclinical and prodromal stages of dementia.

## 1.2 The Definition of Preclinical Stage of Dementia

### *1.2.1 Definition of the Preclinical Stage: Characteristics and Diagnostic Challenges*

In the late twentieth century, the term "preclinical stage of AD" was initially used to describe cognitively unimpaired individuals who display AD brain pathology on post-mortem examination [14]. Since it is now possible to identify in vivo biomarkers of AD pathology, this definition has been modified to describe cognitively normal people with AD pathology [15]. A similar definition could also be applied to other types of dementia with supportive related biomarkers [16]. The International Working Group (IWG) has defined two different preclinical states: presymptomatic and asymptomatic at-risk state [15]. The presymptomatic state recognizes that individuals carrying autosomal dominant monogenic mutations are destined to develop clinical dementia. The asymptomatic at-risk state indicates the absence of clinical symptoms and the presence of at least one supportive biomarker [15].

However, difficulties in defining cognitive normal, cognitive decline, and determining the best biomarker for brain pathologies remain. In addition, the definition of preclinical AD would theoretically span from the appearance of the first neuropathologic changes to the onset of the first clinical symptom, while these boundaries among other disease stages are still unclear [15]. More studies are needed to accurately define the preclinical stages of dementia. Understanding this concept is important for identifying novel disease biomarkers, designing prevention trials for disease progression, and developing disease-modifying therapies.

### *1.2.2 Biomarkers of Early-Stage Pathology: Genetic, Imaging, and Biochemical Markers*

The diagnosis of preclinical stage dementia largely relies on the detection of early-stage biomarkers. Therefore, the genetic, neuroimaging, and biochemical biomarkers of common types of neurodegenerative dementia syndromes, including AD, LBD, and FTD, are discussed in this section.

#### 1.2.2.1 Alzheimer's Disease

AD is the most common type of neurodegenerative dementia, accounting for 60–70% cases of dementia in the population aged 60 years and over [5]. The pathological hallmarks of AD include extracellular aggregates of β-amyloid (Aβ) in plaques and intracellular aggregates of hyperphosphorylated tau in neurofibrillary tangles. In addition, synapse loss, neuroinflammation, and microvascular damage can also be found in affected brain regions and synergistically lead to neuronal loss [7].

#### 1.2.2.1.1 Genetics

A positive family history is the second strongest risk factor for AD [7]. Mutations in presenilin 1 (*PSEN1*), presenilin 2 (*PSEN2*), and amyloid precursor protein (*APP*) are the most common causes of autosomal dominantly inherited AD [17–20]. The pathogenesis of *PSEN1*, *PSEN2*, and *APP* mutations leads to increased production or decreased solubility of Aβ, which leads to amyloid plaque formation [17–20]. Aβ deposition could also cause increased neurofibrillary tangle formation according to "amyloid cascade hypothesis" [6]. However, sporadic AD is more common than familial AD. The most extensively researched risk gene for AD is the apolipoprotein E (APOE) ε4 allele, which is present in over half of patients with AD. Individuals with one copy of APOE ε4 have a threefold higher risk of developing AD compared to the general population, whereas homozygous APOE ε4 carriers have a 15-fold risk [7]. One of the pathogeneses of APOE ε4 is the impairment of Aβ transportation and clearance across the blood-brain barrier, ultimately resulting in amyloid deposition [21].

#### 1.2.2.1.2 Biofluid Markers

According to previous studies conducted in cognitively normal healthy individuals, cerebrospinal fluid (CSF) Aβ42 level alone, in combination with total tau (T-tau), or with phosphorylated tau (P-tau) levels, was linked to the development of prodromal AD [22–24]. In addition, cognitively normal healthy subjects with low Aβ42 levels show significant changes in cortical thickness [25]. Furthermore, a meta-analysis showed a 20-year interval between positive evidence of Aβ and the onset of dementia [26]. These data suggest that CSF Aβ42 is one of the first biomarkers of asymptomatic at-risk patients with AD [26]. The total tau level in CSF has been identified as a non-specific marker of neuronal damage. Therefore, the AD CSF biomarker panel now includes pTau181, a marker specific to AD pathophysiology [27]. A combination of low Aβ42 and high p-tau levels significantly improved preclinical AD diagnostic performance [28, 29]. In both cognitively unimpaired (CU) and MCI groups, p-Tau217 demonstrates high accuracy in distinguishing A+ from A- individuals [30, 31]. Moreover, CSF pTau217 exhibited the highest magnitude of change in symptomatic stages, in contrast to pTau231, which was predominantly associated with early Aβ alterations before clinical onset [32, 33]. Simultaneously, compared with pTau181, CSF pTau217 provided higher diagnostic accuracy for AD and exhibited stronger concordance with CSF Aβ42 and positron emission tomography (PET) signal retention of [18F] flortaucipir and [18F] flutemetamol, radiotracers indicating AD pathology [34, 35]. Furthermore, pTau217 demonstrates significant associations with established measures of cognitive function in AD, including the Mini-Mental State Examination (MMSE) and clinical dementia rating, instruments routinely employed to evaluate mental status and neuropathological burden [35–37]. Different phosphorylation sites of CSF tau biomarkers exhibit dynamic changes across the AD spectrum [32, 38]. The combination of CSF Aβ42/p-tau/t-tau biomarkers can serve as a standard tool for assessing patients with mild cognitive impairment and dementia [39, 40], while attention should be paid to the stage-specific performance of each biomarker [9] and potential influences of factors such as ethnicity [41, 42]. In addition, CSF neurofilament light chain (NfL), an intraneuronal protein that leaks into the CSF upon neuronal injury, has also been correlated with clinical progression in an asymptomatic state [43, 44].

In recent years, blood-based biomarkers have been validated for dementia in addition to conventional CSF AD biomarkers. Due to their blood-based nature, sample acquisition for detection is considerably simpler and less invasive, leading to their popularity in early diagnosis. Biomarkers in blood differ from those in CSF. For example, Aβ can also be measured in the plasma; however, it cannot provide useful diagnostic information compared to Aβ in the CSF [45]. The CSF Aβ42/Aβ40 ratio has diagnostic value in AD, with a 50% difference between patients with AD and healthy controls, whereas the plasma Aβ42/Aβ40 ratio only showed a 20% difference [45]. Thus, the plasma Aβ42/Aβ40 ratio has shown restricted sensitivity and specificity relative to CSF and PET Aβ findings, which has constrained its extensive application in AD diagnosis [45]. In contrast to plasma Aβ42/40, plasma p-tau can be consistently quantified using immunoassays, highlighting its potential for routine clinical use. Among the p-tau isoforms, pTau217 shows the greatest fold-change between AD and non-AD conditions and is most closely associated with disease progression [46–49]. Plasma pTau181 and pTau217 reliably forecasted future progression from MCI to AD [50, 51]. Both immunoassay and mass spectrometry analyses of pTau181, pTau217, and pTau231 can robustly separate A+ from A− individuals in numerous studies [52]. Plasma p-tau levels markedly rise in parallel with extracellular Aβ plaque accumulation, a pattern observed throughout the AD spectrum [52]. Evidence indicates that pTau181 and pTau217 can effectively distinguish amyloid-PET or tau-PET positive individuals from negative ones [50]. p-Tau231 is considered the earliest known biomarker of AD, showing a two- to threefold increase in plasma and serum, with even higher levels observed in CSF [53].

Glial fibrillary acidic protein (GFAP) is among the most extensively studied glial markers and is probably released in response to Aβ pathology in AD [54]. Plasma GFAP exhibits a closer relationship with cerebral Aβ deposition than CSF GFAP, which may reflect its instability in CSF [55]. Plasma GFAP was observed to reduce in response to amyloid-clearing therapy (lecanemab) in a phase 3 clinical study [56]. In addition, S100B correlates with brain atrophy and shows a negative relationship with MMSE performance in AD patients [57, 58], yet its expression in non-neuronal cells necessitates caution when evaluating serum concentrations [59]. YKL-40, chitinase 3-L1, and CHI3L1 show promise as biomarkers for the early detection of MCI-AD and AD-related dementia, due to their nonspecific nature [56].

Synaptic dysfunction is also considered to be one of the pathophysiological processes of AD, and the discovery of synaptic biomarkers is still in progress. Elevated neurogranin (Ng) in AD is linked to t-tau and p-tau concentrations, although plasma Ng does not reflect levels measured in CSF [60, 61]. Accordingly, plasma Ng is unlikely to provide a useful blood-based indicator for AD. Elevated β-synuclein in CSF and blood is linked to brain atrophy in AD, providing a means to distinguish it from other neurodegenerative disorders such as frontotemporal lobar degeneration

[62, 63]. Its role in preclinical AD and interactions with amyloid and tau pathologies remain to be clarified through further investigation. As an essential presynaptic protein involved in vesicular release, SNAP-25 contributes significantly to cognition [64]. High-precision mass spectrometry using anti-Aβ antibodies has enabled detailed characterization of CSF Aβ peptides [64]. Additionally, using the IP-MS approach, higher CSF levels of SNAP-25 and synaptotagmin-1 (SYT1) were observed in patients with AD dementia and those in the prodromal stage [64, 65].

In research on peripheral blood biomarkers for AD, blood cell-derived biomarkers have demonstrated considerable potential. Single-cell RNA sequencing analyses have shown that peripheral blood mononuclear cells are involved in various neurodegenerative processes, with their gene expression profiles potentially reflecting the neurodegenerative mechanisms of AD, thereby providing novel insights into AD pathology [66]. Platelets share certain biochemical characteristics with neurons, such as amyloid precursor protein metabolic pathways, making them a useful surrogate model for studying AD pathology. Although the literature does not directly address platelets, it emphasizes the importance of peripheral blood biomarkers in validating Aβ pathology [67, 68]. Additionally, while red blood cell-associated molecules have not been specifically reported, several studies have indicated that changes in peripheral blood Aβ42 levels are closely related to AD [68, 69]. Blood-based biomarkers can reflect brain pathological features, including Aβ deposition and tau phosphorylation [70, 71]. Nevertheless, the clinical application of blood biomarkers remains limited by technical and validation challenges.

##### 1.2.2.1.3 Imaging Markers

Amyloid PET can directly label Aβ plaques in the brain, and is thus undisputed as an AD core imaging marker. It was positive in 8–44% of cognitively unimpaired individuals; this percentage may be altered according to APOE ε4 status [26, 72]. The positivity rate of amyloid PET is also significantly associated with aging in cognitively normal individuals [26]. Moreover, those without cognitive impairment who exhibit positive amyloid PET imaging are two to three times more predisposed to developing MCI or dementia [73]. Tau-PET can detect tau accumulation in the brain and is another core imaging biomarker of AD pathology. Approximately 12% of preclinical AD patients demonstrate both amyloid-PET and Tau-PET positivity [74]. The staging system proposed by Braak et al. is based on the anatomical localization of tau neurofibrillary tangles. This hierarchical system stages AD according to tau aggregation in the transentorhinal cortex (stage I), entorhinal cortex and hippocampus (stage II), inferior temporal neocortex (stage III), association cortices (stages IV and V), and primary sensory cortices (stage VI) [75]. Tau deposition on Tau-PET is significantly correlated with the Braak stage in postmortem studies [76, 77]. The medial temporal lobe (entorhinal cortex, hippocampus, and amygdala) in patients with preclinical AD showed the earliest and largest annual increase in Tau PET SUVR [74, 78], which occurs approximately 10 years after amyloid PET positivity [79]. Increased tau accumulation is also related to local atrophy in the entorhinal cortex, Brodmann area 35, hippocampus, and worse memory performance [80]. Compared with amyloid-PET and structural MRI, baseline Tau-PET accumulation may be a better marker of longitudinal cognitive decline in patients with preclinical AD [81]. Thus, tau-PET imaging is superior to amyloid-PET imaging in risk stratification and prognostic prediction.

As downstream consequences of Aβ and Tau accumulation, topographical biomarkers of AD could be detected by structural MRI, mainly changes in brain volume (hippocampal atrophy, cortical thickness, etc.). Brain dysfunction can be shown as hypometabolism of neocortical regions and thus be determined by fluorodeoxyglucose (FDG)-PET [15]. Since these changes typically occur later in the AD continuum in accordance with the "amyloid cascade hypothesis" and are not unique to AD pathology, these topographical markers by themselves are not sufficient to diagnose preclinical AD.

Breakthroughs in the development of biofluids and neuroimaging biomarkers have transformed the definition of AD from a clinical syndrome to a clinical-biological construct. Aβ (A)/Tau (T)/Neurodegeneration (N) is the proposed framework for the diagnosis of AD. To include other possible disease mechanisms, an A/T/(X)/N system was created by adding X as new candidate biomarkers to this framework [82]. In light of these discoveries, a novel set of criteria for AD diagnosis and staging has recently been proposed: the 2024 AA Criteria for Diagnosis and Staging of Alzheimer's Disease [83], integrating significant biomarkers for diagnosis, risk stratification, and prognostic prediction in relation to disease-modifying medications (Table 1.2).

**Table 1.2** Categorization of common AD biomarkers [83]

| Biomarker category | CSF or plasma biomarkers | Imaging biomarkers |
|---|---|---|
| *Core biomarkers* | | |
| Core 1 | | |
| *A* (Aβ proteinopathy) | Aβ42 | Amyloid PET |
| $T_1$ (phosphorylated and secreted AD tau) | p-tau217, p-tau181, p-tau231 | |
| Core 2 | | |
| $T_2$ (AD tau proteinopathy) | MTBR-tau243, other phosphorylated tau forms, nonphosphorylated mid-region tau fragments | Tau PET |
| *Biomarkers of nonspecific processes involved in AD pathophysiology* | | |
| *N* (injury, dysfunction, or degeneration of neuropil) | NfL | Anatomic MRI, FDG PET |
| *I* (inflammation) | GFAP | |
| *Biomarkers of non-AD copathology* | | |
| *V* (vascular brain injury) | | Infarction on MRI or CT, WMH |
| *S* (α-synuclein) | αSyn-SAA | |

Source from: Jack et al. [83]

#### 1.2.2.2 Lewy Body Dementia

Lewy body dementia (LBD) is the second most prevalent etiology of neurodegenerative dementia. The term LBD encompasses Parkinson's disease dementia (PDD) and dementia with Lewy bodies (DLB), both characterized by the pathological hallmark of α-synuclein aggregation as Lewy bodies [84].

DLB can be clinically distinguished from AD based on four core symptom features: (1) parkinsonism, (2) cognitive fluctuations, (3) rapid eye movement (REM) sleep behavioral disorder (RBD), and (4) visual hallucinations [84]. These core features are common in both DLB and PDD; thus, it is difficult to distinguish between them. The existing clinical criteria differentiate DLB from PDD only based on the "1-year rule," which stipulates that dementia presents more than 1 year after the onset of parkinsonism. However, the aforementioned clinical symptoms exhibit insufficient sensitivity and specificity in differentiating DLB from other neurodegenerative dementias; hence, more suggestive biomarkers have been recommended under current consensus standards [85].

##### 1.2.2.2.1 Genetics

LBD typically occurs sporadically, with an onset in later life. While most cases are not inherited, a small number of familial occurrences have been reported. Furthermore, specific mutations within the *SNCA* gene, responsible for producing the α-synuclein protein, are infrequently identified as the origin of autosomal dominant forms of Parkinson's disease. However, the clinical manifestation of *SCNA* variant carriers often has nonmotor symptoms, such as cognitive problems, which is consistent with LBD [7]. Another noteworthy finding in the genetics of LBD is that mutations in *GBA*, which encodes the lysosomal enzyme β-glucocerebrosidase, are strongly correlated with an elevated risk of LBD. Homozygous *GBA* mutations have been demonstrated to elevate the risk of Parkinson's disease and dementia with Lewy bodies by around fivefold [7].

##### 1.2.2.2.2 Biofluid Markers

Typically, CSF α-synuclein is reduced in patients with LBD and increased in patients with AD, although mixed findings have also been reported [84]. These findings potentially reflect two contrasting processes: the aggregation of α-synuclein into Lewy bodies and its concurrent release from degenerating synaptic terminals. A significant limitation of earlier α-synuclein immunoassays is their quantification of total protein levels, failing to distinguish pathological forms specific to Lewy bodies. This lack of specificity has obstructed the translation of biofluid α-synuclein into a clinically useful diagnostic marker for LBD. More recently, the real-time quaking-induced conversion (RT-QuIC) technique has emerged as a highly sensitive tool for identifying misfolded α-synuclein in LBD patients, with its diagnostic accuracy confirmed through postmortem examination [86]. Besides, this assay also provides a novel approach in diagnosing prodromal synucleinopathies, such as REM sleep behavior disorder (RBD) and asymptomatic PD gene carriers [87].

##### 1.2.2.2.3 Imaging Markers

Recent diagnostic criteria for DLB categorize imaging findings into suggestive and supportive biomarkers based on their specificity for Lewy body disease, which can also assist in diagnosing PDD [85]. The diagnostic framework proposes three indicative biomarkers: (1) diminished dopamine transporter uptake within the basal ganglia, visualized via PET or single photon emission computed tomography (SPECT); (2) decreased retention observed on metaiodobenzylguanidine (MIBG) myocardial scintigraphy; and (3) polysomnography (PSG)-verified REM sleep without atonia. Additional supportive biomarkers can also aid in the diagnostic assessment, although they lack definitive diagnostic specificity. These include: (1) comparatively intact medial temporal lobe architecture on structural MRI; (2) diffuse hypo-perfusion or hypometabolism on SPECT/PECT imaging, characterized by reduced occipital lobe activity and the presence of the cingulate island sign on fluorodeoxyglucose-PET (FDG-PET); and (3) electroencephalography findings showing prominent posterior-dominant slow waves accompanied by periodic fluctuations within the pre-alpha/theta range [85]. Each biomarker serves as an indirect indicator of DLB, and their integration with core features enhances the diagnostic precision of DLB; however, the existence of an aberrant biomarker in isolation, devoid of core clinical signs, is insufficient for DLB diagnosis [85].

#### 1.2.2.3 Frontotemporal Dementia

Frontotemporal dementia (FTD) is a neurodegenerative clinical syndrome characterized by progressive deficits in behavior, executive function, and language [88]. FTD is the second most common cause of dementia in individuals younger than 65 years. The three major FTD syndromes include behavioral variant FTD (bvFTD), nonfluent variant primary progressive aphasia (PPA), and semantic variant PPA [88]. Frontotemporal lobar degeneration (FTLD) usually refers to a varied series of underlying pathological changes that may be associated with FTD. FTLD is characterized by neuronal loss, gliosis, and microvascular changes in the frontal and temporal lobes. The subtypes of FTLD are associated with different patterns of pathological protein deposition. The microtubule-associated protein tau (MAPT), TAR DNA-binding protein with a molecular weight of 43 kDa (TDP-43), and fused-in-sarcoma (FUS) protein account for nearly all cases of FTLD. Therefore, the main pathological subtypes of FTLD are divided into FTLD-tau, FTLD-TDP, and FTLD-FUS, respectively [7, 89].

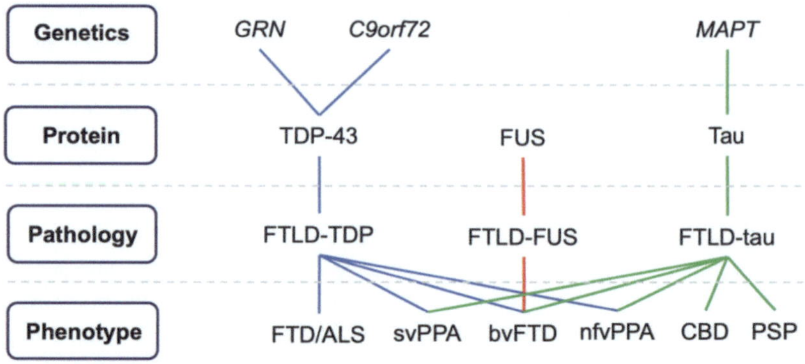


**Fig. 1.2** Genetics, neuropathology, and clinical relevance of frontotemporal lobar degeneration. Notes: FTLD frontotemporal lobar degeneration, TDP-43 transactive response DNA-binding protein 43, FUS RNA-binding protein FUS, ALS amyotrophic lateral sclerosis, bvFTD behavioral variant FTD, CBD corticobasal degeneration, nfvPPA nonfluent variant primary progressive aphasia, PSP progressive supranuclear palsy, svPPA semantic variant primary progressive aphasia. (Source from: Seelaar et al. [91])

#### 1.2.2.3.1 Genetics

FTLD is distinguished from Alzheimer's or Lewy body diseases by its substantial genetic component. An autosomal dominant inheritance pattern is observed in an estimated 30–50% of cases, primarily associated with pathogenic variants in three genes: the microtubule-associated protein tau (*MAPT*), progranulin (*GRN*), and chromosome 9 open reading frame 72 (*C9orf72*), the latter involving hexanucleotide repeat expansions. Importantly, these mutations associated with hereditary FTLD can initiate neurodegenerative processes many years prior to the emergence of clinical symptoms. Patients with various mutations typically have unique histological and clinical characteristics, even during asymptomatic phases (Fig. 1.2) [90, 91].

The most common genetic abnormality and cause of familial bvFTD and amyotrophic lateral sclerosis (ALS) is the pathogenic $[GGGGCC]_n$-hexanuleotide repeat expansion in *C9orf72*, which results in abnormal inclusions containing TDP-43. *C9orf72* repeat expansion accounts for 25% of familial and 6% of sporadic FTD cases [7]. Common clinical presentations of *C9orf72* repeat expansion carriers include bvFTD, FTD-motor neuron disease, ALS, late-onset psychosis, and parkinsonism [89].

*GRN* mutations are associated with haploinsufficiency, with a loss of two-thirds of the functional progranulin concentrations in the serum and CSF. Progranulin is a secreted protein involved in cell cycle regulation, axonal growth, and modulation of inflammation. Variations in the *GRN* gene also result in TDP-43 pathology. The most common clinical presentations are bvFTD and nonfluent variant PPA, while some patients may also exhibit Parkinsonism and corticobasal syndrome (CBS) [89].

Mutations in *MAPT* were the first identified genetic cause of familial FTLD. *MAPT* mutations change microtubule stabilization and increase the propensity for tau aggregation, causing neurodegeneration years before the onset of clinical symptoms. Distinct pathological tauopathies are linked to specific types of *MAPT* mutations. Pathogenic variants located within exon 10 predominantly lead to the accumulation of tau protein with four microtubule-binding repeats (4R-tau), in contrast to the three-repeat (3R-tau) isoform. Conversely, mutations occurring outside of this exon typically result in a mixed pathological profile containing both 3R and 4R tau isoforms. *MAPT* mutation carriers usually become symptomatic earlier than those with *GRN* mutation or *C9orf72* repeat expansion. Common clinical presentations of *MAPT* mutation carriers include bvFTD and parkinsonism [89, 90].

#### 1.2.2.3.2 Biofluid Markers

Current fluid biomarkers for FTD remain restricted and vague. NfL levels in the blood and cerebrospinal fluid may indicate neuroaxonal degeneration in neurodegenerative disorders. Increased NfL levels signify poorer prognosis in patients with FTD and AD, although they are unable to differentiate between the two disorders. Plasma NfL levels are abnormal in asymptomatic familial FTD [88]. *C9orf72* repeat expansion carriers demonstrate increased plasma NfL levels approximately 30 years prior to symptom onset, whereas GRN mutation carriers show aberrant plasma NfL levels 15 years before symptom onset, with a more pronounced increase compared to other genetic variants [88].

#### 1.2.2.3.3 Imaging Markers

Structural MRI can capture cortical atrophy with a mutation-specific neurodegenerative pattern in asymptomatic familial FTD mutation carriers. Asymptomatic *GRN* mutation carriers often exhibit asymmetrical and widespread cortical atrophy, predominantly involving the frontal, temporal, and parietal cortices, which may be reflected in the clinical presentation [90]. For *MAPT* and *C9orf72* repeat expansion carriers, cortical atrophy was more symmetric relative to *GRN* mutation carriers, with *MAPT* being associated with greater temporal lobe atrophy and *C9orf72* being associated with greater frontal lobe atrophy. Besides, the early involvement of subcortical regions is a specific atrophy pattern in asymptomatic *C9orf72* repeat expansion carriers, which is estimated to occur about 25 years before symptom onset [88, 90, 92].

PET imaging has also been suggested as a useful biomarker for cortical metabolism in asymptomatic familial FTD. Distinct metabolic patterns are observed across the major genetic subtypes. Carriers of *MAPT* mutations typically display glucose hypometabolism in anterior regions, including the cingulate, frontal, parietal, and anteromesial temporal lobes on FDG-PET. However, findings from tau-PET imaging in these individuals are inconsistent. Elevated tracer uptake is often seen in cases with mixed 3R/4R tau pathology, while negative scans are common in those with pure 4R tauopathies, a discrepancy potentially attributable to the limited binding affinity of first-generation tau-PET ligands. In contrast, presymptomatic carriers of the *C9orf72* repeat expansion exhibit widespread FDG-PET hypometabolism a decade before symptom emergence, affecting temporal, orbitofrontal, parietal, and posterior cingulate cortices, as well as the insula, caudate, and thalamus. Similarly, *GRN* mutation carriers demonstrate reduced metabolism in the frontal, temporal, and parietal lobes, alongside the anterior cingulate and insular regions. To date, a PET tracer for the in vivo detection of TDP-43 pathology does not exist [88, 90, 92].

## 1.3 Natural History of Dementia Cascade and Its Influencing Factors

### *1.3.1 Transitioning from Preclinical to Symptomatic: Understanding the Definition of Mild Cognitive Impairment (MCI)*

Mild cognitive impairment (MCI) is a transitional phase in which patients exhibit cognitive decline in one or more cognitive domains, but have preserved independence in functional abilities [93]. The first clinical criteria were proposed by investigators from the Mayo Clinic in 1999 [94]. The original criteria required the presence of self- or informant-reported memory complaints, objective memory impairment, and preserved independence in functional ability. These criteria emphasize memory loss, which is thought to be one of the primary clinical signs of AD. The need for a more comprehensive description of MCI is highlighted by the fact that not all cases of MCI develop into AD dementia, and that MCI can be caused by multiple underlying etiologies. Therefore, rather than concentrating only on memory impairment, a revised set of core clinical criteria was established in 2003, which now includes impairments in other cognitive domains. In 2011, the National Institute on Aging-Alzheimer's Association workgroup (NIA-AA) included biofluid and neuroimaging markers to support the diagnosis of MCI due to AD based on these fundamental clinical criteria of MCI [93, 95]. Furthermore, diagnostic criteria for MCI due to Lewy bodies were also proposed for research purposes [96].

According to the recent core clinical criteria for MCI, this concept can be classified into two categories: amnestic MCI (aMCI) and non-amnestic MCI (naMCI), based on whether patients exhibit poor episodic memory function or impairment in other cognitive domains, such as executive, language, or visuospatial functions. Additionally, cognitive impairment can be restricted to only one cognitive domain (MCI single domain) or multiple domains (MCI multiple domains). Therefore, the definition of MCI includes four clinical subtypes: aMCI-single domain, naMCI-single domain, aMCI-multiple domains, and naMCI-multiple domains [93].

Determining the MCI stage requires objective assessment of cognitive decline. Neuropsychological testing is the best method to objectively determine the level of cognitive impairment. Typically, individuals with 1 to 1.5 standard deviations below the normative mean scores on cognitive tests for age- and education-matched peers define an MCI stage [93]. Impairment of episodic memory is regarded as a characteristic symptom in patients with MCI, who are highly likely to progress to AD dementia. Neuropsychological tests assessing episodic memory performance often include a learning process, followed by intermediate and delayed recall. Common tests are the Rey Auditory Verbal Learning Test, the California Verbal Learning Test, the Free and Cued Selective Reminding Test, and Logical Memory I and II of the Wechsler Memory Scale Revised. In addition, patients with MCI could exhibit various degrees of impairment in other cognitive domains, which could be objectively measured using corresponding neuropsychological batteries, such as the Trail Making Test (attention and executive function); Boston Naming Test (language); and Clock-drawing Test (visuospatial function) [93]. Additionally, some neuropsychological batteries, such as the Mini-Mental State Examination and Montreal Cognitive Assessment, measure the general cognitive function of an individual. Clinicians should determine which cognitive domains are predominantly impaired based on a full set of neuropsychological batteries [95].

Maintaining independence in functional capacity is another requirement of MCI. When performing tasks such as driving, cooking, or paying bills, patients with MCI may be less effective or make more mistakes than they were before. Nonetheless, individuals frequently continue to be independent in their day-to-day tasks, without the help of others. Defining these criteria is challenging. A quick, standardized tool called the Functional Activities Questionnaire (FAQ) is used by clinicians to obtain information on instrumental activities of daily living from informants. A cut-off value of $\geq$6 points on the FAQ was found to distinguish MCI from dementia with an accuracy of 85% [95, 97].

### 1.3.2 *Etiology of the MCI: Transitions from Clinical into Biological Definition of MCI*

Dementia can result from various underlying causes, which is the same for patients with MCI. It is important to rule out non-neurodegenerative causes of cognitive impairment, such as vascular, depressive, and infectious diseases. Therefore, comprehensive medical history taking, neuropsychological assessments, laboratory tests, and neuroimaging are critical for clinicians to elucidate the primary causes of MCI [93].

Two primary questions were intended to be addressed using biomarkers for MCI patients: (1) To look for evidence of the underlying cause of cognitive impairment, which could help choose the best course of treatment, particularly for disease-modifying treatments (2). To ascertain whether and at what point a person with MCI develops dementia. The concept of "MCI due to AD (MCI-AD)" was defined in

2011 and mainly incorporates AD biomarkers based on MCI diagnosis. According to the 2011 NIA-AA criteria, AD biomarkers were divided into Aβ biomarkers (CSF or PET Aβ) and neuronal injury biomarkers (mainly CSF tau, structural MRI, and FDG-PET). Patients with MCI can also be classified as "MCI due to AD-high likelihood," "MCI due to AD-intermediate likelihood," and "MCI-unlikely due to AD," based on their AD biomarker profiles [95]. However, these concepts have further evolved because of the huge progress in AD biomarker research and the proposal of the A/T/(X)/N framework [83].

On the other hand, MCI due to Lewy bodies (MCI-LB) may exhibit different clinical presentations than MCI-AD. Cognitive impairment in MCI-LB typically includes disproportionate attention/executive and visual processing deficits and relatively preserved memory. Parkinsonism often develops during the predementia stage, and RBD may occur years or decades before the onset of dementia or parkinsonism. In patients with MCI, both parkinsonism and RBD strongly predict the transition to DLB rather than AD. Since the underlying pathology of MCI-LB is primarily α-synuclein aggregation in the form of Lewy bodies, the proposed biomarkers for MCI-LB were the same as DLB, which included (1) reduced dopamine transporter uptake in the basal ganglia as demonstrated by PET or SPECT, (2) reduced uptake on MIBG myocardial scintigraphy, and (3) PSG confirmation of REM sleep without atonia. According to recent criteria, probable MCI-LB can be diagnosed if two or more core clinical features of DLB are present, with or without a proposed biomarker, or only one core clinical feature, but with one or more proposed biomarkers [96].

### *1.3.3 Epidemiology, Risk Factors, and Prognosis of the MCI*

According to a recent report, MCI prevalence was 6.7% for ages 60–64, 8.4% for 65–69, 10.1% for 70–74, 14.8% for 75–79, and 25.2% for 80–84. These data demonstrated that aging is a risk factor for MCI. Additionally, ApoE ε4 carriers and a positive family history are unmodifiable risk factors for MCI, while modifiable risk factors include low educational level, vascular risk factors such as hypertension and diabetes, diet, and lifestyle factors. Therefore, clinicians should prioritize primary prevention strategies for patients with MCI. A prior meta-analysis concluded that physical activity and the management of vascular risk factors could significantly reduce the risk of cognitive decline. A healthy diet and lifelong learning also provide strong evidence to reduce the risk of cognitive decline [98, 99].

The prognosis of patients with MCI varies among individuals. Since patients with MCI can improve, remain stable, or progress to dementia, they must be monitored over time to change diagnosis and treatment strategies [12]. The reported annual rate of MCI conversion to dementia ranges from <5% to 20%, while 40–70% of MCI may not progress even after 10 years. Risk factors for MCI progression include older age, low education level, history of stroke, diabetes, and the amnestic

MCI subtype. A systematic review summarized possible predictors of MCI conversion to AD dementia; older age, female gender, depression, diabetes, hypertension, and at least one ApoE ε4 allele are risk factors for MCI progression [93, 97]. Other predictors, including a lower MMSE score, higher ADAS-cog score, hippocampal and medial temporal lobe atrophy, abnormal CSF pTau, tTau, and tau/Aβ42 ratio at baseline, have also been found [100].

However, the fact that some individuals with AD pathologies remain cognitively normal and that lifestyle, genetic, and brain factors may slow down cognitive decline raises the hypothesis of cognitive reserve. Cognitive reserve refers to the capacity of cognitive processes to help explain the differential susceptibility of cognitive functions to brain pathologies. The cognitive reserve is not fixed. It can be influenced by innate individual differences and lifetime exposures, such as early life cognitive ability, education, occupation, physical exercise, or social engagement [101]. Cognitive reserve may modify the relationship between clinical and biological AD stages, which has been proposed in the latest staging criteria for AD [83].

## 1.4 Therapeutic Interventions and Management Across the Cascade

### *1.4.1 Nonpharmacological Interventions: Cognitive Training, Physical Exercise, Diet, and Social Engagement*

Clinical syndromes of dementia are complex because they often occur in the elderly who are comorbid with various copathologies, leading to memory loss, behavioral changes, motor symptoms, psychiatric symptoms, and loss of independence. Although recent advances in disease-modifying therapies for AD have made significant progress, medications for dementia treatment remain limited. Therefore, nonpharmacological interventions such as cognitive training, physical exercise, and diet management are crucial, especially for patients in preclinical stages [13, 102].

Computerized cognitive training was developed to engage in certain cognitive processes through standardized activities that can focus on one or more cognitive domains and adjust task difficulty based on individual performance. Computerized cognitive training is effective in enhancing global cognition, memory, working memory, attention, and alleviating depressive symptoms in individuals with MCI [103].

Vitamin B supplementation is also associated with the slowing of cognitive decline, especially in those who received early intervention [104]. Furthermore, adherence to a Mediterranean-style dietary pattern has been correlated with a deceleration in age-related cognitive deterioration and a lower incidence of Alzheimer's disease. This traditional eating pattern is distinguished by a diverse nutritional composition, featuring an abundance of plant-based foods such as fruits, vegetables, whole grains, and legumes. It is further defined by a low intake of saturated fats, with olive oil serving as the principal lipid source. The diet also includes moderate fish consumption, limited dairy and red meat products, and a modest amount of alcohol, typically consumed with meals [105]. Physical exercise, especially aerobic exercise, also improves global cognitive function in patients with MCI [106]. A previous randomized controlled trial demonstrated that a multidomain intervention including diet, exercise, cognitive training, and vascular risk monitoring could improve or maintain cognitive functioning in at-risk elderly people [107].

## *1.4.2 Pharmacological Treatments: Current Medications and Research on Disease-Modifying Therapies*

### 1.4.2.1 Disease-Modifying Therapies

Rapid progress in the in vivo detection of amyloid and tau pathologies has paved a new avenue for disease-modifying treatments (DMTs) in Alzheimer's disease and associated dementias. Advances in molecular imaging, particularly the creation of PET ligands for Aβ and tau, now enable the precise detection of Alzheimer's disease pathology. These imaging techniques provide objective proof that DMTs can facilitate the clearance of these pathogenic proteins. Despite this promising diagnostic capability, many initial clinical trials investigating anti-amyloid immunotherapies failed to demonstrate clinical efficacy and were associated with significant adverse events. Amyloid-related imaging abnormalities (ARIA) are one of the most significant adverse effects of anti-amyloid immunotherapies, occurring in approximately 10–30% of patients treated in anti-amyloid clinical trials [108]. ARIA can manifest as edema or effusion (ARIA-E), microhemorrhage, or superficial siderosis (ARIA-H). Most ARIA events are asymptomatic (74–97%) and can be detected using MRI [108]. ARIA often occurs in the early course of immunotherapy, but it may also lead to the discontinuation of immunotherapy or other severe consequences, including death. APOE ε4 carriers are associated with a higher risk of ARIA than non-carriers. Despite these controversies, several anti-amyloid immunotherapies still obtained approval by the US Food and Drug Administration (FDA), since they exhibited significant reductions in brain amyloid levels and improved overall cognitive function compared to placebos [102].

In June 2021, the U.S. FDA granted initial approval for aducanumab. This regulatory decision was predicated on findings from Phase 3 clinical trials that demonstrated a substantial decrease in cerebral amyloid plaque burden in subjects diagnosed with MCI due to Alzheimer's disease or mild AD dementia [109]. Although its two Phase 3 trials, EMERGE and ENGAGE, were designed similarly, they did not show similar effectiveness in clinical cognitive outcome measurements. Therefore, this drug was discontinued by the manufacturer in 2024 [102].

The second FDA-approved antiamyloid drug for MCI due to AD or mild AD dementia was Lecanemab in January 2023. Phase 3 clinical trials of Lecanemab demonstrated that intravenous administration of Lecanemab 10 mg/kg every 2 weeks for 18 months is associated with slowing of cognitive decline in patients with MCI due to AD or mild AD dementia compared to placebo controls in multiple clinical endpoints, with a magnitude of 25–35%. Amyloid PET revealed a more than 70% reduction of cerebral amyloid over 18 months of therapy. Common adverse effects, including acute infusion reactions (26%), ARIA-E (12.6%), and ARIA-H (17.3%), were reported in Phase 3 trials [102, 110].

In July 2024, another anti-amyloid drug—donanemab was approved by the FDA for patients with MCI due to AD or mild AD dementia. According to Phase 3 clinical trial of donanemab, a 22–36% slowing of cognitive decline compared to the placebo group was observed after 18 months of administration of donanemab. The effectiveness of donanemab was affected by tau-PET burden at baseline; those with low to medium tau burden may exhibit greater slowing of progression than those with high tau burden. Donanemab could be discontinued based on the assessment of amyloid burden, often achievable within one to one and a half years. Notably, ARIA was reported in 36.8% of the intervention group, ARIA-E in 24%, and ARIA-H in 19.7% of participants after donanemab administration [102, 111].

To date, over 164 clinical trials of 127 agents in AD have been conducted, and 80% of these drugs are disease-modifying therapies. More trials of agents targeting amyloid, tau, α-synuclein, and other proteinopathies are required [102, 112].

#### 1.4.2.2 Symptomatic Treatment

Although disease-modifying therapies have entered clinical practice, they have only been approved for patients with MCI due to AD or mild AD dementia. As dementia clinical syndromes advance, alterations in cognition, behavior, and functionality will become evident. Symptomatic treatment is essential in the management of these disorders [13].

Acetylcholinesterase inhibitors (AChEIs) and N-methyl-D-aspartate (NMDA) antagonists have been approved by the FDA for treating mild-to-moderate dementia due to AD, and are frequently used off-label for dementia with Lewy bodies and vascular dementia. Typically, treatment for cognitive symptoms starts with AChEI. Common AChEIs include donepezil, rivastigmine, and galantamine. According to the results of randomized, double-blind, placebo-controlled trials of AChEIs among patients with mild-to-moderate symptomatic AD dementia, AChEIs exhibit consistent benefits on cognitive endpoints up to 24 months [113]. However, no consistent benefit was found for AChEIs on cognition or function in patients with MCI [102]. Adverse events of AChEIs include gastrointestinal disturbances, bradycardia, and vivid dreams, while gradually titrating the AChEI dose may reduce these adverse effects. To date, no clinical trial of AChEI has targeted participants with biomarker-confirmed AD. Thus, its efficacy in cognitive measurements compared to that of the approved DMT is unclear.

Memantine is an NMDA antagonist used to treat patients with moderate-to-severe AD dementia. Treatment with memantine 20 mg daily resulted in the slowing of cognitive decline over 28 weeks in a double-blind placebo-controlled clinical trial in patients with moderate to severe symptomatic AD dementia. Memantine was well tolerated. The adverse effects in the memantine group were not significantly higher than those in the placebo groups [114]. However, the evidence of memantine in treating mild AD dementia is less robust, and no clinical trials have reported the benefits of memantine treatment in patients with MCI [102].

Behavioral and psychological symptoms of dementia (BPSD) are common in the later stages of dementia. Mood disturbances such as anxiety or depression may require additional therapy such as selective serotonin reuptake inhibitors (SSRI) or other mood stabilizers. In patients with significant agitation or psychosis, low-dose antipsychotics could be used cautiously because these medications have an FDA boxed warning of increasing the risk of stroke and death in patients with dementia [13].

## 1.5 Conclusion

Dementia is a clinical syndrome associated with a decline in memory and other cognitive domains, which are sufficient to impair daily functioning. Alzheimer's, Lewy body dementia, and frontotemporal dementia are the three most prevalent neurodegenerative causes of dementia. Patients with neurodegenerative dementia would experience a long interval between the occurrence of brain pathology, cognitive decline, and functional impairment. Early in vivo detection of brain pathology is possible by recent developments in genetics and biomarker research, which also leads to early diagnosis and intervention for dementia. More trials on disease-modifying therapies will become available in the foreseeable future.

## References

1. Livingston G, Huntley J, Sommerlad A, et al. Dementia prevention, intervention, and care: 2020 report of the Lancet Commission. Lancet. 2020;396(10248):413–46. https://doi.org/10.1016/S0140-6736(20)30367-6.
2. Wetterberg H, Najar J, Rydberg Sterner T, Kern S, Skoog I. The effect of diagnostic criteria on dementia prevalence - a population-based study from Gothenburg, Sweden. Am J Geriatr Psychiatry. 2024;32(2):230–43. https://doi.org/10.1016/j.jagp.2023.08.018.
3. Collaborators GBDDF. Estimation of the global prevalence of dementia in 2019 and forecasted prevalence in 2050: an analysis for the Global Burden of Disease Study 2019. Lancet Public Health. 2022;7(2):e105–25. https://doi.org/10.1016/S2468-2667(21)00249-8.
4. Collaborators GBDNSD. Global, regional, and national burden of disorders affecting the nervous system, 1990–2021: a systematic analysis for the Global Burden of Disease Study 2021. Lancet Neurol. 2024;23(4):344–81. https://doi.org/10.1016/S1474-4422(24)00038-3.
5. 2024 Alzheimer's disease facts and figures. Alzheimers Dement. 2024;20(5):3708–21. https://doi.org/10.1002/alz.13809.

6. Day GS. Diagnosing Alzheimer disease. Continuum (Minneap Minn). 2024;30(6):1584–613. https://doi.org/10.1212/con.0000000000001507.
7. Scholz SW, Cobos I. Genetics and neuropathology of neurodegenerative dementias. Continuum (Minneap Minn). 2024;30(6):1801–22. https://doi.org/10.1212/con.0000000000001505.
8. Silbert LC. Vascular cognitive impairment. Continuum (Minneap Minn). 2024;30(6):1699–725. https://doi.org/10.1212/con.0000000000001508.
9. Sperling RA, Aisen PS, Beckett LA, et al. Toward defining the preclinical stages of Alzheimer's disease: recommendations from the National Institute on Aging-Alzheimer's Association workgroups on diagnostic guidelines for Alzheimer's disease. Alzheimers Dement. 2011;7(3):280–92. https://doi.org/10.1016/j.jalz.2011.03.003.
10. Jack CR Jr, Knopman DS, Jagust WJ, et al. Hypothetical model of dynamic biomarkers of the Alzheimer's pathological cascade. Lancet Neurol. 2010;9(1):119–28. https://doi.org/10.1016/S1474-4422(09)70299-6.
11. Petersen RC. Mild cognitive impairment as a diagnostic entity. J Intern Med. 2004;256(3):183–94. https://doi.org/10.1111/j.1365-2796.2004.01388.x.
12. Petersen RC, Lopez O, Armstrong MJ, et al. Practice guideline update summary: mild cognitive impairment: Report of the Guideline Development, Dissemination, and Implementation Subcommittee of the American Academy of Neurology. Neurology. 2018;90(3):126–35. https://doi.org/10.1212/wnl.0000000000004826.
13. Carlsson CM. Management of Dementia. Continuum (Minneap Minn). 2022;28(3):885–900. https://doi.org/10.1212/con.0000000000001132.
14. Hubbard BM, Fenton GW, Anderson JM. A quantitative histological study of early clinical and preclinical Alzheimer's disease. Neuropathol Appl Neurobiol. 1990;16(2):111–21. https://doi.org/10.1111/j.1365-2990.1990.tb00940.x.
15. Dubois B, Hampel H, Feldman HH, et al. Preclinical Alzheimer's disease: Definition, natural history, and diagnostic criteria. Alzheimers Dement. 2016;12(3):292–323. https://doi.org/10.1016/j.jalz.2016.02.002.
16. Hughes JC, Ingram TA, Jarvis A, Denton E, Lampshire Z, Wernham C. Consent for the diagnosis of preclinical dementia states: a review. Maturitas. 2017;98:30–4. https://doi.org/10.1016/j.maturitas.2017.01.008.
17. Sherrington R, Rogaev EI, Liang Y, et al. Cloning of a gene bearing missense mutations in early-onset familial Alzheimer's disease. Nature. 1995;375(6534):754–60. https://doi.org/10.1038/375754a0.
18. Levy-Lahad E, Wasco W, Poorkaj P, et al. Candidate gene for the chromosome 1 familial Alzheimer's disease locus. Science. 1995;269(5226):973–7. https://doi.org/10.1126/science.7638622.
19. Rogaev EI, Sherrington R, Rogaeva EA, et al. Familial Alzheimer's disease in kindreds with missense mutations in a gene on chromosome 1 related to the Alzheimer's disease type 3 gene. Nature. 1995;376(6543):775–8. https://doi.org/10.1038/376775a0.
20. Goate A, Chartier-Harlin MC, Mullan M, et al. Segregation of a missense mutation in the amyloid precursor protein gene with familial Alzheimer's disease. Nature. 1991;349(6311):704–6. https://doi.org/10.1038/349704a0.
21. Ulrich JD, Ulland TK, Mahan TE, et al. ApoE facilitates the microglial response to amyloid plaque pathology. J Exp Med. 2018;215(4):1047–58. https://doi.org/10.1084/jem.20171265.
22. Gustafson DR, Skoog I, Rosengren L, Zetterberg H, Blennow K. Cerebrospinal fluid beta-amyloid 1–42 concentration may predict cognitive decline in older women. J Neurol Neurosurg Psychiatry. 2007;78(5):461–4. https://doi.org/10.1136/jnnp.2006.100529.
23. Fagan AM, Roe CM, Xiong C, Mintun MA, Morris JC, Holtzman DM. Cerebrospinal fluid tau/beta-amyloid(42) ratio as a prediction of cognitive decline in nondemented older adults. Arch Neurol. 2007;64(3):343–9. https://doi.org/10.1001/archneur.64.3.noc60123.
24. Stomrud E, Hansson O, Blennow K, Minthon L, Londos E. Cerebrospinal fluid biomarkers predict decline in subjective cognitive function over 3 years in healthy elderly. Dement Geriatr Cogn Disord. 2007;24(2):118–24. https://doi.org/10.1159/000105017.

25. Fortea J, Sala-Llonch R, Bartrés-Faz D, et al. Cognitively preserved subjects with transitional cerebrospinal fluid ß-amyloid 1-42 values have thicker cortex in Alzheimer's disease vulnerable areas. Biol Psychiatry. 2011;70(2):183–90. https://doi.org/10.1016/j.biopsych.2011.02.017.
26. Jansen WJ, Ossenkoppele R, Knol DL, et al. Prevalence of cerebral amyloid pathology in persons without dementia: a meta-analysis. JAMA. 2015;313(19):1924–38. https://doi.org/10.1001/jama.2015.4668.
27. Hampel H, Buerger K, Zinkowski R, et al. Measurement of phosphorylated tau epitopes in the differential diagnosis of Alzheimer disease: a comparative cerebrospinal fluid study. Arch Gen Psychiatry. 2004;61(1):95–102. https://doi.org/10.1001/archpsyc.61.1.95.
28. Duits FH, Teunissen CE, Bouwman FH, et al. The cerebrospinal fluid "Alzheimer profile": easily said, but what does it mean? Alzheimers Dement. 2014;10(6):713–723.e2. https://doi.org/10.1016/j.jalz.2013.12.023.
29. Ewers M, Mattsson N, Minthon L, et al. CSF biomarkers for the differential diagnosis of Alzheimer's disease: a large-scale international multicenter study. Alzheimers Dement. 2015;11(11):1306–15. https://doi.org/10.1016/j.jalz.2014.12.006.
30. Janelidze S, Bali D, Ashton NJ, et al. Head-to-head comparison of 10 plasma phospho-tau assays in prodromal Alzheimer's disease. Brain J Neurol. 2023;146(4):1592–601. https://doi.org/10.1093/brain/awac333.
31. Zhong X, Wang Q, Yang M, et al. Plasma p-tau217 and p-tau217/Abeta1-42 are effective biomarkers for identifying CSF- and PET imaging-diagnosed Alzheimer's disease: Insights for research and clinical practice. Alzheimer's Dement. 2025;21(2):e14536. https://doi.org/10.1002/alz.14536.
32. Ashton NJ, Benedet AL, Pascoal TA, et al. Cerebrospinal fluid p-tau231 as an early indicator of emerging pathology in Alzheimer's disease. EBioMedicine. 2022;76:103836. https://doi.org/10.1016/j.ebiom.2022.103836.
33. Mila-Aloma M, Ashton NJ, Shekari M, et al. Plasma p-tau231 and p-tau217 as state markers of amyloid-beta pathology in preclinical Alzheimer's disease. Nat Med. 2022;28(9):1797–801. https://doi.org/10.1038/s41591-022-01925-w.
34. Leuzy A, Janelidze S, Mattsson-Carlgren N, et al. Comparing the clinical utility and diagnostic performance of CSF P-Tau181, P-Tau217, and P-Tau231 assays. Neurology. 2021;97(17):e1681–94. https://doi.org/10.1212/wnl.0000000000012727.
35. Dresse MT, Ferreira PCL, Prasadan A, et al. Plasma biomarkers identify brain ATN abnormalities in a dementia-free population-based cohort. Alzheimer's Res Ther. 2025;17(1):173. https://doi.org/10.1186/s13195-025-01803-w.
36. Mattsson-Carlgren N, Salvado G, Ashton NJ, et al. Prediction of longitudinal cognitive decline in preclinical Alzheimer disease using plasma biomarkers. JAMA Neurol. 2023;80(4):360–9. https://doi.org/10.1001/jamaneurol.2022.5272.
37. Selma-Gonzalez J, Rubio-Guerra S, Garcia-Castro J, et al. Association of Plasma Phosphorylated Tau 217 with clinical deterioration across Alzheimer disease stages. Neurology. 2025;105(1):e213769. https://doi.org/10.1212/wnl.0000000000213769.
38. Lantero-Rodriguez J, Snellman A, Benedet AL, et al. P-tau235: a novel biomarker for staging preclinical Alzheimer's disease. EMBO Mol Med. 2021;13(12):e15098. https://doi.org/10.15252/emmm.202115098.
39. Fan DY, Jian JM, Huang S, et al. Establishment of combined diagnostic models of Alzheimer's disease in a Chinese cohort: the Chongqing Ageing & Dementia Study (CADS). Transl Psychiatry. 2022;12(1):252. https://doi.org/10.1038/s41398-022-02016-7.
40. Rodriguez-Santiago MA, Wojna V, Miranda-Valentin E, Arnold S, Sepulveda-Rivera V. Diagnosing Alzheimer's disease: Which dementia screening test to use in elderly Puerto Ricans with mild cognitive impairment and early Alzheimer's disease? Alzheimer's Dement (Amsterdam, Netherlands). 2024;16(1):e12554. https://doi.org/10.1002/dad2.12554.
41. Wang ZB, Tan L, Wang HF, et al. Differences between ante mortem Alzheimer's disease biomarkers in predicting neuropathology at autopsy. Alzheimer's Dement. 2023;19(8):3613–24. https://doi.org/10.1002/alz.12997.

42. Nayyar A, Li ML, Sotelo V, et al. Influence of cognitive impairment and race on plasma p-Tau(217) in two diverse cohorts. Alzheimer's Dement. 2025;21(2):e14585. https://doi.org/10.1002/alz.14585.
43. Dhiman K, Villemagne VL, Fowler C, et al. Cerebrospinal fluid neurofilament light predicts risk of dementia onset in cognitively healthy individuals and rate of cognitive decline in mild cognitive impairment: a prospective longitudinal study. Biomedicines. 2022;10(5). https://doi.org/10.3390/biomedicines10051045.
44. Svenningsson AL, Stomrud E, Palmqvist S, Hansson O, Ossenkoppele R. Axonal degeneration and amyloid pathology predict cognitive decline beyond cortical atrophy. Alzheimer's Res Ther. 2022;14(1):144. https://doi.org/10.1186/s13195-022-01081-w.
45. Brand AL, Lawler PE, Bollinger JG, et al. The performance of plasma amyloid beta measurements in identifying amyloid plaques in Alzheimer's disease: a literature review. Alzheimer's Res Ther. 2022;14(1):195. https://doi.org/10.1186/s13195-022-01117-1.
46. Yu L, Boyle PA, Janelidze S, et al. Plasma p-tau181 and p-tau217 in discriminating PART, AD and other key neuropathologies in older adults. Acta Neuropathol. 2023;146(1):1–11. https://doi.org/10.1007/s00401-023-02570-4.
47. Ashton NJ, Brum WS, Di Molfetta G, et al. Diagnostic accuracy of a plasma phosphorylated tau 217 immunoassay for Alzheimer disease pathology. JAMA Neurol. 2024;81(3):255–63. https://doi.org/10.1001/jamaneurol.2023.5319.
48. Feizpour A, Doecke JD, Dore V, et al. Detection and staging of Alzheimer's disease by plasma pTau217 on a high throughput immunoassay platform. EBioMedicine. 2024;109:105405. https://doi.org/10.1016/j.ebiom.2024.105405.
49. Ashton NJ, Keshavan A, Brum WS, et al. The Alzheimer's Association Global Biomarker Standardization Consortium (GBSC) plasma phospho-tau Round Robin study. Alzheimer's Dement. 2025;21(2):e14508. https://doi.org/10.1002/alz.14508.
50. Lehmann S, Schraen-Maschke S, Vidal JS, et al. Clinical value of plasma ALZpath pTau217 immunoassay for assessing mild cognitive impairment. J Neurol Neurosurg Psychiatry. 2024;95(11):1046–53. https://doi.org/10.1136/jnnp-2024-333467.
51. Devanarayan V, Llano DA, Hu YH, et al. Plasma pTau181 enhances the prediction of future clinical decline in amyloid-positive mild cognitive impairment. Alzheimer's Dement (Amsterdam, Netherlands). 2024;16(3):e12621. https://doi.org/10.1002/dad2.12621.
52. Bluma M, Chiotis K, Bucci M, et al. Disentangling relationships between Alzheimer's disease plasma biomarkers and established biomarkers in patients of tertiary memory clinics. EBioMedicine. 2025;112:105504. https://doi.org/10.1016/j.ebiom.2024.105504.
53. Kac PR, Gonzalez-Ortiz F, Simren J, et al. Diagnostic value of serum versus plasma phospho-tau for Alzheimer's disease. Alzheimer's Res Ther. 2022;14(1):65. https://doi.org/10.1186/s13195-022-01011-w.
54. Pereira JB, Janelidze S, Smith R, et al. Plasma GFAP is an early marker of amyloid-beta but not tau pathology in Alzheimer's disease. Brain J Neurol. 2021;144(11):3505–16. https://doi.org/10.1093/brain/awab223.
55. Benedet AL, Mila-Aloma M, Vrillon A, et al. Differences between plasma and cerebrospinal fluid glial fibrillary acidic protein levels across the Alzheimer disease continuum. JAMA Neurol. 2021;78(12):1471–83. https://doi.org/10.1001/jamaneurol.2021.3671.
56. Arslan B, Zetterberg H, Ashton NJ. Blood-based biomarkers in Alzheimer's disease - moving towards a new era of diagnostics. Clin Chem Lab Med. 2024;62(6):1063–9. https://doi.org/10.1515/cclm-2023-1434.
57. Nehra G, Maloney BJ, Smith RR, et al. Plasma S100beta is a predictor for pathology and cognitive decline in Alzheimer's disease. Fluids Barriers CNS. 2025;22(1):4. https://doi.org/10.1186/s12987-024-00615-8.
58. Pappas C, Bauer CE, Zachariou V, et al. Synergistic effects of plasma S100B and MRI measures of cerebrovascular disease on cognition in older adults. GeroScience. 2025;47(3):3131–46. https://doi.org/10.1007/s11357-024-01498-1.
59. Murcko R, Marchi N, Bailey D, Janigro D. Diagnostic biomarker kinetics: how brain-derived biomarkers distribute through the human body, and how this affects their diagnostic sig-

nificance: the case of S100B. Fluids Barriers CNS. 2022;19(1):32. https://doi.org/10.1186/s12987-022-00329-9.

60. Ohrfelt A, Dumurgier J, Zetterberg H, et al. Full-length and C-terminal neurogranin in Alzheimer's disease cerebrospinal fluid analyzed by novel ultrasensitive immunoassays. Alzheimer's Res Ther. 2020;12(1):168. https://doi.org/10.1186/s13195-020-00748-6.
61. Dittrich A, Ashton NJ, Zetterberg H, et al. Plasma and CSF NfL are differentially associated with biomarker evidence of neurodegeneration in a community-based sample of 70-year-olds. Alzheimer's Dement (Amsterdam, Netherlands). 2022;14(1):e12295. https://doi.org/10.1002/dad2.12295.
62. Oeckl P, Anderl-Straub S, Danek A, et al. Relationship of serum beta-synuclein with blood biomarkers and brain atrophy. Alzheimer's Dement. 2023;19(4):1358–71. https://doi.org/10.1002/alz.12790.
63. Mohaupt P, Pons ML, Vialaret J, Delaby C, Hirtz C, Lehmann S. beta-Synuclein as a candidate blood biomarker for synaptic degeneration in Alzheimer's disease. Alzheimer's Res Ther. 2022;14(1):179. https://doi.org/10.1186/s13195-022-01125-1.
64. Nilsson J, Ashton NJ, Benedet AL, et al. Quantification of SNAP-25 with mass spectrometry and Simoa: a method comparison in Alzheimer's disease. Alzheimer's Res Ther. 2022;14(1):78. https://doi.org/10.1186/s13195-022-01021-8.
65. Mila-Aloma M, Brinkmalm A, Ashton NJ, et al. CSF synaptic biomarkers in the preclinical stage of Alzheimer disease and their association with MRI and PET: a cross-sectional Study. Neurology. 2021;97(21):e2065–78. https://doi.org/10.1212/wnl.0000000000012853.
66. Xiong LL, Xue LL, Du RL, et al. Single-cell RNA sequencing reveals B cell-related molecular biomarkers for Alzheimer's disease. Exp Mol Med. 2021;53(12):1888–901. https://doi.org/10.1038/s12276-021-00714-8.
67. Scholl M, Verberk IMW, Del Campo M, et al. Challenges in the practical implementation of blood biomarkers for Alzheimer's disease. Lancet Healthy Longev. 2024;5(10):100630. https://doi.org/10.1016/j.lanhl.2024.07.013.
68. Ferretti G, Serafini S, Angiolillo A, Monterosso P, Di Costanzo A, Matrone C. Advances in peripheral blood biomarkers of patients with Alzheimer's disease: Moving closer to personalized therapies. Biomed Pharmacother. 2023;165:115094. https://doi.org/10.1016/j.biopha.2023.115094.
69. Sekiya M, Sakakibara Y, Hirota Y, et al. Decreased plasma nicotinamide and altered NAD(+) metabolism in glial cells surrounding Abeta plaques in a mouse model of Alzheimer's disease. Neurobiol Dis. 2024;202:106694. https://doi.org/10.1016/j.nbd.2024.106694.
70. Ossenkoppele R, van der Kant R, Hansson O. Tau biomarkers in Alzheimer's disease: towards implementation in clinical practice and trials. Lancet Neurol. 2022;21(8):726–34. https://doi.org/10.1016/s1474-4422(22)00168-5.
71. Ashton NJ, Janelidze S, Mattsson-Carlgren N, et al. Differential roles of Abeta42/40, p-tau231 and p-tau217 for Alzheimer's trial selection and disease monitoring. Nat Med. 2022;28(12):2555–62. https://doi.org/10.1038/s41591-022-02074-w.
72. Therriault J, Pascoal TA, Benedet AL, et al. Frequency of biologically defined Alzheimer disease in relation to age, sex, APOE ε4, and cognitive impairment. Neurology. 2021;96(7):e975–85. https://doi.org/10.1212/wnl.0000000000011416.
73. Donohue MC, Sperling RA, Petersen R, Sun CK, Weiner MW, Aisen PS. Association between elevated brain amyloid and subsequent cognitive decline among cognitively normal persons. JAMA. 2017;317(22):2305–16. https://doi.org/10.1001/jama.2017.6669.
74. St-Onge F, Chapleau M, Breitner JCS, Villeneuve S, Pichet Binette A, Initiative ftAsDN. Tau accumulation and its spatial progression across the Alzheimer's disease spectrum. Brain Commun. 2024;6(1) https://doi.org/10.1093/braincomms/fcae031.
75. Therriault J, Pascoal TA, Lussier FZ, et al. Biomarker modeling of Alzheimer's disease using PET-based Braak staging. Nat Aging. 2022;2(6):526–35. https://doi.org/10.1038/s43587-022-00204-0.
76. Marquié M, Siao Tick Chong M, Antón-Fernández A, et al. [F-18]-AV-1451 binding correlates with postmortem neurofibrillary tangle Braak staging. Acta Neuropathol. 2017;134(4):619–28. https://doi.org/10.1007/s00401-017-1740-8.

77. Fleisher AS, Pontecorvo MJ, Devous MD Sr, et al. Positron emission tomography imaging with [18F]flortaucipir and postmortem assessment of Alzheimer disease neuropathologic changes. JAMA Neurol. 2020;77(7):829–39. https://doi.org/10.1001/jamaneurol.2020.0528.
78. Braak H, Braak E. Neuropathological stageing of Alzheimer-related changes. Acta Neuropathol. 1991;82(4):239–59. https://doi.org/10.1007/bf00308809.
79. Cody KA, Langhough RE, Zammit MD, et al. Characterizing brain tau and cognitive decline along the amyloid timeline in Alzheimer's disease. Brain. 2024; https://doi.org/10.1093/brain/awae116.
80. Berron D, Vogel JW, Insel PS, et al. Early stages of tau pathology and its associations with functional connectivity, atrophy and memory. Brain. 2021;144(9):2771–83. https://doi.org/10.1093/brain/awab114.
81. Ossenkoppele R, Smith R, Mattsson-Carlgren N, et al. Accuracy of tau positron emission tomography as a prognostic marker in preclinical and prodromal Alzheimer disease: a head-to-head comparison against amyloid positron emission tomography and magnetic resonance imaging. JAMA Neurol. 2021;78(8):961–71. https://doi.org/10.1001/jamaneurol.2021.1858.
82. Hampel H, Cummings J, Blennow K, Gao P, Jack CR Jr, Vergallo A. Developing the ATX(N) classification for use across the Alzheimer disease continuum. Nat Rev Neurol. 2021;17(9):580–9. https://doi.org/10.1038/s41582-021-00520-w.
83. Jack CR Jr, Andrews JS, Beach TG, et al. Revised criteria for diagnosis and staging of Alzheimer's disease: Alzheimer's Association Workgroup. Alzheimers Dement. 2024;20(8):5143–69. https://doi.org/10.1002/alz.13859.
84. Galvin JE. Lewy Body Dementia. Continuum (Minneap Minn). 2024;30(6):1673–98. https://doi.org/10.1212/con.0000000000001496.
85. McKeith IG, Boeve BF, Dickson DW, et al. Diagnosis and management of dementia with Lewy bodies: fourth consensus report of the DLB Consortium. Neurology. 2017;89(1):88–100. https://doi.org/10.1212/wnl.0000000000004058.
86. Arnold MR, Coughlin DG, Brumbach BH, et al. α-synuclein seed amplification in CSF and brain from patients with different brain distributions of pathological α-synuclein in the context of co-pathology and non-LBD diagnoses. Ann Neurol. 2022;92(4):650–62. https://doi.org/10.1002/ana.26453.
87. Siderowf A, Concha-Marambio L, Lafontant DE, et al. Assessment of heterogeneity among participants in the Parkinson's Progression Markers Initiative cohort using α-synuclein seed amplification: a cross-sectional study. Lancet Neurol. 2023;22(5):407–17. https://doi.org/10.1016/s1474-4422(23)00109-6.
88. Clark DG. Frontotemporal Dementia. Continuum (Minneap Minn). 2024;30(6):1642–72. https://doi.org/10.1212/con.0000000000001506.
89. Bang J, Spina S, Miller BL. Frontotemporal dementia. Lancet. 2015;386(10004):1672–82. https://doi.org/10.1016/s0140-6736(15)00461-4.
90. Chen Q, Kantarci K. Imaging biomarkers for neurodegeneration in presymptomatic familial frontotemporal lobar degeneration. Front Neurol. 2020;11:80. https://doi.org/10.3389/fneur.2020.00080.
91. Seelaar H, Rohrer JD, Pijnenburg YA, Fox NC, van Swieten JC. Clinical, genetic and pathological heterogeneity of frontotemporal dementia: a review. J Neurol Neurosurg Psychiatry. 2011;82(5):476–86. https://doi.org/10.1136/jnnp.2010.212225.
92. Risacher SL. Neuroimaging in Dementia. Continuum (Minneap Minn). 2024;30(6):1761–89. https://doi.org/10.1212/con.0000000000001509.
93. Petersen RC, Caracciolo B, Brayne C, Gauthier S, Jelic V, Fratiglioni L. Mild cognitive impairment: a concept in evolution. J Intern Med. 2014;275(3):214–28. https://doi.org/10.1111/joim.12190.
94. Petersen RC, Smith GE, Waring SC, Ivnik RJ, Tangalos EG, Kokmen E. Mild cognitive impairment: clinical characterization and outcome. Arch Neurol. 1999;56(3):303–8. https://doi.org/10.1001/archneur.56.3.303.
95. Albert MS, DeKosky ST, Dickson D, et al. The diagnosis of mild cognitive impairment due to Alzheimer's disease: recommendations from the National Institute on Aging-Alzheimer's

Association workgroups on diagnostic guidelines for Alzheimer's disease. Alzheimers Dement. 2011;7(3):270–9. https://doi.org/10.1016/j.jalz.2011.03.008.
96. McKeith IG, Ferman TJ, Thomas AJ, et al. Research criteria for the diagnosis of prodromal dementia with Lewy bodies. Neurology. 2020;94(17):743–55. https://doi.org/10.1212/wnl.0000000000009323.
97. Langa KM, Levine DA. The diagnosis and management of mild cognitive impairment: a clinical review. JAMA. 2014;312(23):2551–61. https://doi.org/10.1001/jama.2014.13806.
98. Jia L, Du Y, Chu L, et al. Prevalence, risk factors, and management of dementia and mild cognitive impairment in adults aged 60 years or older in China: a cross-sectional study. Lancet Public Health. 2020;5(12):e661–71. https://doi.org/10.1016/s2468-2667(20)30185-7.
99. Baumgart M, Snyder HM, Carrillo MC, Fazio S, Kim H, Johns H. Summary of the evidence on modifiable risk factors for cognitive decline and dementia: a population-based perspective. Alzheimers Dement. 2015;11(6):718–26. https://doi.org/10.1016/j.jalz.2015.05.016.
100. Li JQ, Tan L, Wang HF, et al. Risk factors for predicting progression from mild cognitive impairment to Alzheimer's disease: a systematic review and meta-analysis of cohort studies. J Neurol Neurosurg Psychiatry. 2016;87(5):476–84. https://doi.org/10.1136/jnnp-2014-310095.
101. Stern Y, Arenaza-Urquijo EM, Bartrés-Faz D, et al. Whitepaper: defining and investigating cognitive reserve, brain reserve, and brain maintenance. Alzheimers Dement. 2020;16(9):1305–11. https://doi.org/10.1016/j.jalz.2018.07.219.
102. Geldmacher DS. Treatment of Alzheimer disease. Continuum (Minneap Minn). 2024;30(6):1823–44. https://doi.org/10.1212/con.0000000000001503.
103. Hill NT, Mowszowski L, Naismith SL, Chadwick VL, Valenzuela M, Lampit A. Computerized cognitive training in older adults with mild cognitive impairment or dementia: a systematic review and meta-analysis. Am J Psychiatry. 2017;174(4):329–40. https://doi.org/10.1176/appi.ajp.2016.16030360.
104. Wang Z, Zhu W, Xing Y, Jia J, Tang Y. B vitamins and prevention of cognitive decline and incident dementia: a systematic review and meta-analysis. Nutr Rev. 2022;80(4):931–49. https://doi.org/10.1093/nutrit/nuab057.
105. Lourida I, Soni M, Thompson-Coon J, et al. Mediterranean diet, cognitive function, and dementia: a systematic review. Epidemiology. 2013;24(4):479–89. https://doi.org/10.1097/EDE.0b013e3182944410.
106. Song D, Yu DSF, Li PWC, Lei Y. The effectiveness of physical exercise on cognitive and psychological outcomes in individuals with mild cognitive impairment: a systematic review and meta-analysis. Int J Nurs Stud. 2018;79:155–64. https://doi.org/10.1016/j.ijnurstu.2018.01.002.
107. Ngandu T, Lehtisalo J, Solomon A, et al. A 2 year multidomain intervention of diet, exercise, cognitive training, and vascular risk monitoring versus control to prevent cognitive decline in at-risk elderly people (FINGER): a randomised controlled trial. Lancet. 2015;385(9984):2255–63. https://doi.org/10.1016/s0140-6736(15)60461-5.
108. Cogswell PM, Andrews TJ, Barakos JA, et al. Alzheimer disease anti-amyloid immunotherapies: imaging recommendations and practice considerations for monitoring of amyloid-related imaging abnormalities. AJNR Am J Neuroradiol. 2025; https://doi.org/10.3174/ajnr.A8469.
109. Sevigny J, Chiao P, Bussière T, et al. The antibody aducanumab reduces Aβ plaques in Alzheimer's disease. Nature. 2016;537(7618):50–6. https://doi.org/10.1038/nature19323.
110. van Dyck CH, Swanson CJ, Aisen P, et al. Lecanemab in Early Alzheimer's Disease. N Engl J Med. 2023;388(1):9–21. https://doi.org/10.1056/NEJMoa2212948.
111. Sims JR, Zimmer JA, Evans CD, et al. Donanemab in Early Symptomatic Alzheimer Disease: the TRAILBLAZER-ALZ 2 randomized clinical trial. JAMA. 2023;330(6):512–27. https://doi.org/10.1001/jama.2023.13239.

112. Cummings J, Zhou Y, Lee G, Zhong K, Fonseca J, Cheng F. Alzheimer's disease drug development pipeline: 2024. Alzheimers Dement (N Y). 2024;10(2):e12465. https://doi.org/10.1002/trc2.12465.
113. Birks J. Cholinesterase inhibitors for Alzheimer's disease. Cochrane Database Syst Rev. 2006;2006(1):Cd005593. https://doi.org/10.1002/14651858.Cd005593.
114. Reisberg B, Doody R, Stöffler A, Schmitt F, Ferris S, Möbius HJ. Memantine in moderate-to-severe Alzheimer's disease. N Engl J Med. 2003;348(14):1333–41. https://doi.org/10.1056/NEJMoa013128.

# Chapter 2
# Using Electroencephalography in Dementia Practice From Diagnostic to Clinical Outcomes

**Wei-Pin Hong and Chin-Wei Huang**

**Abstract** Electroencephalography (EEG) is a non-invasive, cost-effective neurophysiological tool with high temporal resolution, widely used in the study and clinical evaluation of dementia. EEG reflects abnormal neuronal activity and loss of functional connectivity during neurodegeneration. Quantitative EEG (qEEG) and coherence analysis can aid in distinguishing various types of dementia, such as Alzheimer's disease (AD), dementia with Lewy bodies (DLB), frontotemporal lobar degeneration (FTLD), and vascular dementia (VaD). In AD, EEG typically shows generalized slowing, reduced alpha activity, and subclinical epileptiform discharges (SEDs), which have been associated with faster cognitive decline and more pronounced behavioral and psychological symptoms (BPSD). Epileptic activity is also more frequent in AD, potentially triggered by amyloid-β and tau-related hyperexcitability. In DLB, prominent slow-wave activity with periodic fluctuations in the pre-alpha/theta frequency range is considered a supportive biomarker. In Creutzfeldt-Jakob disease (CJD), periodic sharp wave complexes (PSWCs) are characteristic, especially in the middle to late stages of the disease. The integration of EEG with other biomarkers—enhanced by artificial intelligence and deep learning—has shown promise in improving the accuracy of early diagnosis, monitoring disease progression, and tailoring individualized therapeutic interventions in dementia care.

**Keywords** EEG, Quantitative EEG, Dementia syndromes, Alzheimer's disease, Dementia with Lewy bodies, Frontotemporal dementia, Vascular cognitive impairment, Subclinical epileptiform discharges

---

W.-P. Hong · C.-W. Huang (✉)
Department of Neurology, National Cheng Kung University Hospital, College of Medicine, National Cheng Kung University, Tainan, Taiwan
e-mail: huangcw@mail.ncku.edu.tw



Y.-H. Yang (ed.), *Management of Dementia from the Preclinical Stage*,
https://doi.org/10.1007/978-981-95-5222-1_2

## 2.1 Introduction

### *2.1.1 EEG: A Noninvasive and Widely Available Tool*

Richard Caton is credited with first discovering the electrical properties of the brain and recording the electrical activity [1]. Hans Berger recorded the first human electroencephalography (EEG) in 1924 [1], making routine scalp EEG a noninvasive and widely available tool for neurophysiologic activities. Dementia syndromes, characterized by the disturbance of brain function, reduced brain connectivity, and neuronal loss, can be studied using EEG. EEG measures the interaction and summation of excitatory or inhibitory postsynaptic potentials of pyramidal cells underlying the cerebral cortex [2]. Compared with other modern technologies for brain activities, EEG is cost-effective, and there is no concern of radiation. It is primarily used for diagnosing and localizing epileptic disorders, and other conditions like consciousness dysfunction, sleep disorder, metabolic encephalopathy, encephalitis, and dementia. The standard electrode position refers to the international 10–20 electrode system proposed by International Federation of Clinical Neurophysiology, including 19 electrodes, and later extended to 25 electrodes covering inferior-basal and anterior temporal region [3, 4]. There is almost no contraindication for EEG, except for rare cases of skin allergy to metal electrodes or craniotomy while placing the electrodes and some specific conditions during hyperventilation or photic stimulation.

EEG provided high temporal resolution, capturing actual neuronal activity within milliseconds, surpassing functional magnetic resonance imaging (MRI) in this regard [5, 6]. Recently, one study suggested that combined resting-state EEG and evoked potentials by auditory stimulation may be better than mini-mental status examination (MMSE) to predict dementia, especially through the observation of slowing and asymmetry of prefrontal EEG activities [7]. Combining with other spatial neuroimaging, it will provide good information of brain activity. Network science and graph theory are used to map functional brain neuronal connectivity and further understand the cognitive process [8]. Using multimodal approach integrating EEG, MRI, and transcranial magnetic stimulation (TMS) is now regarded as a powerful way to study brain connectivity and further develop the visualization of brain activity [9]. The visualization of brain connectivity can be categorized into heat maps, data statistics, and head maps [10]. It helps us to understand the coherence and the response to external stimuli. The rapid progress of machine learning brings the better understanding of neural network [10]. The application has already been studied in diagnosing conditions like Alzheimer's disease (AD), Parkinson disease dementia (PDD), depression, emotion, and attention deficit hyperactivity disorder, and applications such as emotion and gait analysis, and even lie detection [10, 11].

EEG records electrical activities from cortex, which is mainly the interaction of postsynaptic potentials from pyramidal cells. Recording EEG requires electrodes, accurate electrodes placement, and amplification, all of which can affect the quality of EEG. EEG is highly sensitive to many artifacts, such as environmental artifacts and physiologic artifacts. Accurately recognizing these artifacts during visual analysis is crucial to avoid misinterpretation. Besides, using calibration, sensitivity modification, and filters (high, low-frequency, and notch) influences the quality of EEG. The EEG processing involves signal acquisition, denoising, feature extraction, and classification [5]. The common methods of EEG denoising include independent component analysis and wavelet transform analysis. The frequently used methods of feature extraction include linear technique and spectral analysis. EEG coherence quantifies the function of cortical connection and synchronization, and nonlinear dynamic methods like fractal dimension and zero-crossing interval are effective for dementia detection [5].

### *2.1.2 Quantitative Analysis and EEG Coherence*

EEG is a widely used technique in the research of brain function and dementia. Visual EEG analysis is commonly used in clinical diagnosis. However, digital signal processing methods are needed to differentiate patterns and subtypes of dementia syndromes. The most common way is quantitative EEG (qEEG) [12]. With assistance from other new technologies such as low-resolution brain electromagnetic tomography, it allows the accurate 3-dimensional localization of EEG from domains of time and frequency [12].

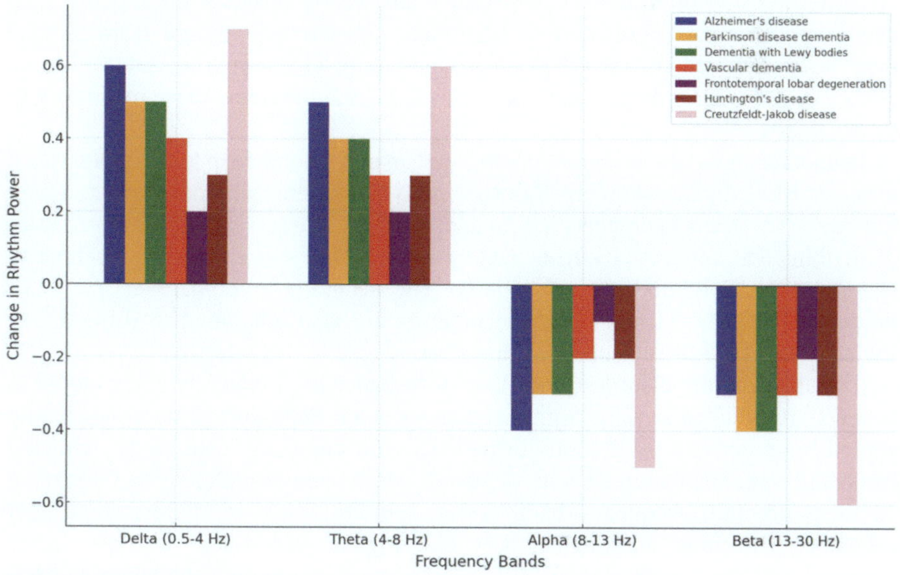


**Fig. 2.1** This bar chart displays the changes in dominant rhythm power across various neurodegenerative diseases

QEEG can identify different types of dementia and is compatible with the process of neurodegeneration [13]. The power of delta and theta bands was increased in AD [13]. However, similar power increases are found in PDD and cognitive decline and may be used to predict further development of dementia [14]. The mean dominant rhythm of AD was 7.5–8.8 Hz, and dementia with Lewy bodies (DLB) was 6.7–7.5 Hz [15, 16]. Combining neuropsychological tests with quantitative EEG can differentiate between AD, frontotemporal lobar degeneration (FTLD), and normal aging [13] (Fig. 2.1).

EEG coherence also provides information about brain connectivity. In AD, disrupted intrahemispheric and midline low-frequency band coherence is observed, compared to mild cognitive impairment (MCI) and Healthy control [17]. Interestingly, midline frontal and temporal theta coherence is increased in MCI, compared to healthy control [17]. This finding is similar to the hippocampal hypertrophy seen in MCI or asymptomatic AD [18, 19].

### *2.1.3 EEG Analysis (Engineering)*

Recently, researchers have used wearable EEG recordings and multifractal detrended fluctuation analysis incorporated with machine learning to differentiate MCI and normal with good accuracy [20]. Another review discussed the current application of artificial intelligence in early detection of dementia, highlighting computerized cognitive test, movement test, speech and conversation and language test, and computer-assisted interpretation of brain scans. Using artificial intelligence (AI) may decrease errors compared to traditional subjective judgment from clinical interviews of clinicians or psychologists. Combining AI and multimodal test is seen as the future for early diagnosis of dementia [21]. Standardizing these methods will be necessary.

In another study, the researchers proposed an end-to-end deep learning approach to screen EEG signals, showing high specificity for patients with dementia and high sensitivity for normal subjects [22]. In another study, the researchers used variables of rhythms and connectivity from resting EEG with a support vector machine to classify AD, DLB, and normal elderly. The accuracy was 94.79–99.7% [23]. Wearable EEG and virtual reality technology are also integrated to differentiate subjects with MCI from healthy control [24].

Circadian rhythm disorders and sleep disturbance are frequently encountered in patients with dementia [25]. Some studies focus on EEG during sleep, analyzing altered brain activity oscillations in patients with dementia. One study extracted EEG data from 8044 subjects with dementia, MCI, and normal cognition, focusing on sleep structure, frequency band power, spindles, slow oscillations, and EEG coherence. Machine learning models like logistic regression, support vector machine, and random forest can differentiate participants with dementia or MCI from normal subjects [26].

Current reviews indicate that AI and deep learning techniques can effectively differentiate normal cognition from cognitive impairment. More research is needed to distinguish further subtypes of dementia syndromes.

## 2.2 EEG in MCI-AD or AD

According to the diagnostic criteria for dementia or MCI due to AD, EEG is not included as supportive evidence [27, 28]. The core features in the diagnosis of AD focus on the clinical deficits of cognitive domains and biomarkers which reflect amyloid deposition and neuron damage. EEG hallmarks in AD include a power spectrum shift to lower frequencies, slower mean frequency, and decreased coherence of fast rhythms in cortical regions [29]. Recently, the Electrophysiology Professional Interest Area and Global Brain Consortium have endorsed recommendations on candidate EEG measures for AD clinical trials [30]. Compared to cognitive normal elderly, AD patients showed decreased amplitude and frequency of the posterior dominant rhythm and increased theta and delta rhythms, reflecting disconnection in thalamocortico-corticothalamic signals [30] (Fig. 2.1).

Despite not being included in diagnostic criteria, EEG is still used to assist in AD diagnosis [29]. EEG abnormalities in cortical dementia syndromes are more prominent than in subcortical dementia [5, 29]. In AD, EEG typically shows generalized slowing, reduced alpha activity, and increased theta and delta frequencies. Occasionally, sharp or spike waves without clinical seizure manifestations, known as subclinical epileptiform discharges, may be observed.

### 2.2.1 *Slow Waves*

The alpha rhythm in resting EEG is modulated by the interaction of cortex and thalamus [31]. Previous studies have already revealed that the decrease of alpha rhythm is correlated with declines in memory and attention. In one recent study, median frequency, peak frequency, and alpha-to-theta ratio of resting-state EEG were used as a regression model to predict the total score of MMSE with moderate to good predictability [31]. The common features of patients with AD are a shift of power spectrum to lower frequencies, a decrease in coherence of fast rhythms, and reduced EEG-complexity [29, 32]. The qEEG findings of AD are decreased alpha and beta power, increased delta and theta power. The coherence and connectivity also change in AD [33] (Table 2.1) (Fig. 2.1).

**Table 2.1** The remarks of EEG findings in common types of dementia syndromes

| | | |
|---|---|---|
| AD | EEG | Generalized slowing of the EEG, theta, and delta frequency increased<br>Reduced alpha activity |
| | qEEG | Increased delta and theta power<br>Decreased alpha and beta power<br>Reduced coherence in the alpha band, particularly in posterior regions<br>Altered connectivity patterns, especially reduced functional connectivity in alpha and beta bands |
| | SED | SEDs are relatively uncommon but can occur, particularly in the later stages of the disease<br>Often seen as sharp waves or spikes, predominantly in the temporal regions |
| PDD | EEG | Mild to moderate slowing of background rhythm<br>Increased theta and delta activity<br>Diffuse slow-wave activity in more advanced stages |
| | qEEG | Increased slow-wave (theta and delta) activity<br>Reduced alpha and beta power<br>Enhanced theta/delta ratio<br>Abnormalities in frontal and central regions |
| | SED | SEDs are not typically prominent<br>EEG abnormalities are more often related to generalized slowing rather than epileptiform activity |
| DLB | EEG | Prominent diffuse slow-wave activity<br>Lower alpha power compared to controls<br>Prominent posterior slow-wave activities with periodic fluctuation in the pre-alpha/theta ranges<br>FIRDA (frontal intermittent rhythmic delta activities) |
| | qEEG | Prominent increase in delta and theta power<br>Significant decrease in alpha and beta power<br>Lower coherence in alpha and beta bands, especially in occipital regions<br>Fluctuating EEG patterns |
| | SED | Less common than in AD<br>When present, they may appear as isolated spikes, often in the occipital or temporal regions, may be more frequent at night |
| VaD | EEG | Focal or generalized slowing, depending on the extent of vascular lesions<br>Higher incidence of focal slowing in regions corresponding to vascular injury<br>Reduced alpha activity, especially in regions affected by strokes |
| | qEEG | Increased delta and theta activity, often focal depending on lesion locations<br>Decreased alpha power<br>Increased alpha/theta ratio in some regions<br>Reduced coherence in the affected regions |
| | SED | SEDs are not commonly seen, but focal sharp waves or spikes can occur, corresponding to regions of vascular injury<br>The presence of SEDs may vary depending on the extent and location of vascular lesions |

(continued)

**Table 2.1** (continued)

| | | |
|---|---|---|
| FTLD | EEG | Generally, less pronounced slowing compared to AD<br>Frontal or frontotemporal slowing may be observed<br>Preservation of posterior alpha rhythm at early stage |
| | qEEG | Mild to moderate slowing in frontal regions<br>Increased delta and theta activity in frontotemporal regions<br>Relative preservation of posterior alpha rhythm<br>Changes in coherence and connectivity, particularly in frontal lobes |
| | SED | SEDs are infrequent in FTLD<br>EEG abnormalities are more often related to focal slowing in frontal or frontotemporal regions rather than epileptiform discharges |
| HD | EEG | Early stages show generalized low voltage, normal or slightly reduced alpha activity<br>Progression leads to increased theta and delta activity |
| | qEEG | Early stages may show normal or slightly decreased alpha activity<br>Progressive increase in theta and delta power<br>Changes in coherence, especially in frontotemporal regions |
| | SED | SEDs are relatively rare<br>More frequent in juvenile HD |
| CJD | EEG | Periodic sharp wave complexes (PSWCs) are characteristic and may appear in later stages<br>Generalized slowing with periodic bursts of high-amplitude slow waves (intermittent rhythmic delta activities)<br>EEG changes evolve as the disease progresses |
| | qEEG | Marked increase in delta and theta activity<br>Periodic sharp wave complexes (PSWCs), particularly in later stages<br>Generalized slowing with bursts of high-amplitude slow waves<br>Rapidly evolving EEG abnormalities |
| | SED | SEDs are a prominent feature in CJD, with periodic sharp wave complexes (PSWCs) being highly characteristic<br>These periodic discharges are often seen throughout the EEG and are considered a hallmark of the disease |

*AD* Alzheimer's disease, *PDD* Parkinson's disease dementia, *DLB* dementia with Lewy bodies, VaD vascular dementia, *FTLD* frontotemporal lobar degeneration, *HD* Huntington's disease, *CJD* Creutzfeldt-Jakob disease, *SED* subclinical epileptiform discharge, *EEG* electroencephalography, *qEEG* quantitative electroencephalography

## 2.2.2 Subclinical Epileptiform Discharge

Epileptic seizures are frequently associated with AD [34]. Epilepsy occurs not only in the later stages of AD, but also in the early stages. Younger patients are more frequently comorbid with epilepsy [35]. According to different studies, the prevalence of unprovoked epilepsy in AD ranges from 10% to 64%. AD with epilepsy experiences a fast decline in cognition. Adequate treatment with anticonvulsants may slow down the deterioration [34] (Table 2.1).

Isolated epileptic discharges without clinical seizures may play an important role in dementia. These discharges are called subclinical epileptiform discharge (SED) [36]. SED is common in normal controls. However, SED may also have a negative impact on cognition. SED is also common in AD. In an exploratory study, overnight high-density EEG found that spikes appeared on 46% patients with amnestic MCI [37]. Another study found that with normal routine resting EEG, the frequency of subclinical epileptiform discharge was 19.8% in patients with AD [38]. The researchers also found that frequency increased with the severity of dementia. Cognition declined faster in those AD patients with epileptiform discharges [38].

In a study involving 1674 patients with AD, MCI, and other dementias, epileptiform discharges were found in 3% of the patients, of which 40% suffered from clinical seizures. These epileptiform discharges were predominantly located in the temporal region. There was no difference in seizure occurrence among neurodegenerative diseases [35]. However, another study found that no significant difference in SED during sleep among patients with AD, MCI, or normal controls [39]. This study enrolled 50 patients with probable AD, 50 patients with MCI due to AD, and 50 normal subjects and underwent full-night video PSG. None of the subjects had a clinical seizure history. SED were found in 6.38% of the AD group, 11.63% of the MCI group, and 4.54% of the normal group. There was no statistically significant difference between these three groups. However, there might be substantial differences if the authors combined AD and MCI groups and compared them with the normal group.

Recently, a study in Taiwan involving 263 patients with AD found that 17.1% of patients ($n = 45$) with SED on routine 13-min 10–20 system scalp EEG. Comparing behavioral and psychological symptoms of dementia using the neuropsychiatric inventory in patients with or without subclinical epileptiform discharge, irritability and lability were more frequently seen in the group with SED [40].

### 2.2.3 AD and Epilepsy

Older age is a risk factor for both dementia and epilepsy [41]. The most common causes of epilepsy in older age are cerebrovascular disease, brain tumor, traumatic brain injury, and neurodegenerative disease [41].

Patients with dementia are more prone to seizures than patients without dementia, especially AD. In one case report, a patient diagnosed with AD presented with frequent transient unresponsiveness during follow-up periods. The EEG showed epileptiform discharges from the bilateral temporal regions. The patient's cognition mildly improved after using antiseizure medications [42].

### 2.2.4 Predictors of Dementia Progression

In community-dwelling elderly individuals, the median frequency, peak frequency, and alpha-to-theta ratio of prefrontal region of resting EEG were correlated with MMSE scores in early stage of cognitive decline [31].

Combining EEG indicators including coherence and alpha amplitude, there was a high correlation with scores of MMSE in patients with AD [43]. In one study examining 38 patients with AD, the more severe the AD, the greater the amount of slow activity in visual assessment on EEG. While examining with EEG spectral analysis, the parameters in all EEG derivations were all correlated with dementia severity, MMSE, and Instrumental Activities of Daily Living scores. However, when examining the EEG coherence with intrahemispheric or interhemispheric, only the alpha frequency correlated with dementia severity and MMSE score. The authors used multiple regression and found seven EEG variables to predict MMSE scores with a high correlation [43]. The variables were the coherence between frontopolar, frontal, parietal, central, and occipital leads and alpha band, coherence between occipital leads and delta band, amplitude between temporal leads and alpha band.

## 2.3 VaD and Vascular Cognitive Impairment (VCI)

The EEG findings on vascular cognitive impairment (VCI) included slower frequency, disrupted interhemispheric and intrahemispheric connectivity [44]. Spectral analysis indicated elevated delta/theta activity and reduced alpha/beta activity [44]. There was no significant difference between EEG findings in VCI and AD. The connectivity within and between hemispheres was decreased in VCI. The EEG of VCI may show focal or generalized slowing, depending on the vascular lesions. The alpha activity was reduced, especially in regions affected by vascular damage [45].

## 2.4 EEG in DLB or PDD

EEG is already incorporated into the diagnostic criteria for DLB. In the revised criteria for clinical diagnosis of probable and possible DLB, prominent posterior slow-wave activities on EEG with periodic fluctuation in the pre-alpha/theta ranges are one of the supportive biomarkers [46]. Besides, interictal epileptiform discharge was also reported in patients with DLB. The frequency of spike was higher than normal control by using continuous EEG recording for 48 h (80% in DLB vs. 46.7% in normal control) [47].

Using EEG variability by mean frequency analysis and compressed spectral arrays, it was found that dominant alpha bands were present in patients with AD, with slower background activity in DLB and PDD. The dominant rhythm in DLB was $7.4 \pm 1.6$ Hz, compared to AD $8.3 \pm 0.6$ Hz [48]. Dominant frequency variability was different in AD and DLB. Interestingly, in four patients diagnosed as AD initially who later developed fluctuation and rapid eye movement (REM) sleep behavior disorders, their initial EEG was similar to other DLB groups. The authors concluded that EEG may help differentiate between AD and DLB at an early stage before the appearance of core clinical features [48]. Another study used qEEG to predict MCI for the further development of DLB [49]. Dominant frequency <8 Hz and dominant frequency variability ≥1.5 Hz in MCI state turn to be DLB after 3 years of follow-up with nearly 100% sensitivity and specificity [49] (Table 2.1) (Fig. 2.1).

In a previous study, patients with DLB showed a loss of alpha background and had more temporal transient slow activities compared with patients with AD, which may help in differential diagnosis between DLB and AD [50]. Other studies found that FIRDA and Grand total EEG score may differentiate DLB and AD [51–53]. The grand total EEG score is a semiquantitative scale from 0 to 54, including items of frequency, distribution, reactivity, and asymmetry of background activity, prevalence and reactivity of diffuse slow wave activity, paroxysmal activity, prevalence, reactivity, and location of focal slow waves, and epileptiform discharge [54]. It is evaluated via visual analysis and can be used to differentiate idiopathic PD and atypical parkinsonism with a cutoff value of 9. Quantitative EEG slowing and dominant frequency variability are now potential biomarkers of MCI-LB in recent research criteria of prodromal DLB [55]. Recently, a group analyzed resting-state EEG with only 8 electrodes and proposed a Linear Predictive Coding EEG Algorithm for Parkinson's Disease which correlates with cognition measured by Montreal cognitive assessment (MoCA) in patients with Parkinson's disease (PD) [56] (Table 2.1).

The EEG findings on PDD are nonspecific, typically showing mild to moderate background slowing with increased theta and delta activities [57]. These slow activities become more generalized in advanced stages. The interhemispheric coherence may be better in PDD than in PD [57]. There are no reports of SED on PDD. However, the frequency of epileptiform discharge in the temporal lobe is higher in patients with PD with visual hallucinations, compared to those without visual hallucinations [58].

In one study using qEEG to differentiate Lewy body dementia (LBD, including DLB and PDD) with non-LBD (AD and PD), it was found that LBD had significantly reduced dominant frequency, dominant frequency variability, and dominant frequency prevalence. There was no difference in EEG variables between DLB and PDD [59].

Another study used qEEG to compare the patients of PD with normal cognition, PD with MCI, PD with dementia, and normal controls. It found that the abnormalities of qEEG with increasing posterior theta or delta amplitude were associated with MCI or dementia in PD [60]. There was no difference between PD with normal cognition and normal controls. EEG can be used in subjects with PD and further follow-up if cognitive impairment develops.

## 2.5 EEG in FTLD or Other Dementias

Using cortical EEG and neuropsychological tests may help differentiate patients with AD and FTLD. In one study, researchers compared 19 subjects with FTLD and 16 subjects with AD using qEEG and neuropsychological tests (including digit symbol, trail making test, block design, clock reading, and free recall from 12 wordlists). They found that delta waves, theta waves activities, visuospatial abilities, and episodic memory were the best predictive factors to differentiate AD and FTLD with high accuracy. Patients with FTLD exhibited better visuospatial abilities and episodic memory, and their delta waves and theta waves activities did not decrease as seen in patients with AD [61]. In another study, researchers used 25 qEEG features including relative band powers, spectral ratios, center frequency, auto-mutual information, cross-mutual information, coherences, phase coherences, partial coherences, Granger causality (GC), and conditional GC to compare patients with AD, DLB/PD, and behavioral variant frontotemporal lobar degeneration (bvFTLD). There were 23 features which resulted in significant differences. For example, Granger causality could differentiate AD and DLB/PD at parietal leads and AD and bvFTLD at temporal leads. Relative band power at the right parietal lead could also differentiate bvFTLD and DLB/PD [62].

Neural networks also help differentiate between AD and FTLD. Based on frequency-based multilayer resting-state EEG networks, some extracted features can differentiate AD and FTLD with an accuracy of 81.1%. The multivariable linear regression model can also be used to predict the MMSE scale [63]. In general, at the early stage of FTLD, EEG shows less significant slowing compared to AD [61]. Neither fast activities nor slow activities changes in qEEG of FTLD [61] (Table 2.1).

In sporadic Creutzfeldt-Jakob disease (CJD), periodic sharp waves complexes (PSWC) are the supported criteria for diagnosis. EEG may reveal the typical appearance in the later stage of CJD. The typical EEG changes of CJD is diffuse slowing of background or frontal intermittent rhythmic delta activities in early stages, and then later to typical periodic sharp wave complex in middle or late stage. In the terminal stage, EEG transitions into a coma response pattern [64]. About two-third of the patients with CJD exhibit PSWC. Interestingly, epileptic seizures are uncommon in sporadic CJD [64–67]. Incorporating structural imaging and CSF biomarkers can enhance the diagnosis sensitivity [68]. PSWC is uncommon in genetic CJD and absent in patients with variant CJD [64]. The PSWC may disappear in the terminal stage of CJD [69] (Table 2.1) (Fig. 2.1).

In Huntington's disease (HD), EEG revealed generalized low voltage, especially at the frontal lobes [70]. With EEG global state and microstate analysis, reduced connectivity and increased dimensionality as the severity of HD increases [71]. Using exact LOw REsolution Tomography (eLORETA) and analysis of wake and sleep in patients with HD, delta bands were found to be increased in Brodmann areas compared to the normal controls during wakefulness. Theta and beta bands also decrease while alpha bands increase in the Brodmann area in non-REM sleep state [72]. In a case report of a young child with HD, bilateral posterior quadrant epileptiform discharges and occipital intermittent rhythmic delta activity were observed [73]. Additionally, a case report and review mentioned that epilepsy in HD is more frequent in the juvenile form [74] (Table 2.1) (Fig. 2.1).

A recent small study used portable EEG monitoring in patients to compare those with severe dementia and comorbid with chronic skeletal pain to those without pain. Patients with pain exhibited higher detrended fluctuation analysis of EEG signals.

Detrended fluctuation analysis is a method to reflex the neuronal oscillation for patients with AD and neurofeedback management [75]. However, this study was a feasibility study with only five subjects. EEG therefore could potentially assist in pain evaluation in patients with severe dementia who cannot communicate verbally. Another study focused on feasibility and potential for diagnosing patients with delirium on dementia with the bedside mini-EEG. They found that the delta and theta power ratio proves useful in distinguishing delirium on dementia and dementia alone [76], potentially serving as a marker of recovery or deterioration of delirium in patients with dementia.

## 2.6 Conclusions

Combining EEG with other new biomarkers can help clinicians differentiate dementia syndromes. Deep learning technique applied to EEG features, combined with clinical cognitive evaluation, biochemical data, and neuroimaging, can increase the accuracy of diagnosing dementia syndromes and develop adequate and efficient care plans.

## References

1. Britton JW, Frey LC, Hopp JL, Korb P, Koubeissi MZ, Lievens WE, et al. Electroencephalography (EEG): an introductory text and atlas of normal and abnormal findings in adults, children, and infants. Chicago: American Epilepsy Society; 2016.
2. Biasiucci A, Franceschiello B, Murray MM. Electroencephalography. Curr Biol. 2019;29(3):R80–5.
3. Klem GH, Lüders HO, Jasper HH, Elger C. The ten-twenty electrode system of the international federation. The International Federation of Clinical Neurophysiology. Electroencephalogr Clin Neurophysiol Suppl. 1999;52:3–6.
4. Seeck M, Koessler L, Bast T, Leijten F, Michel C, Baumgartner C, et al. The standardized EEG electrode array of the IFCN. Clin Neurophysiol. 2017;128(10):2070–7.
5. Al-Qazzaz NK, Ali SHBM, Ahmad SA, Chellappan K, Islam MS, Escudero J. Role of EEG as biomarker in the early detection and classification of dementia. Sci World J. 2014;2014
6. Lystad RP, Pollard H. Functional neuroimaging: a brief overview and feasibility for use in chiropractic research. J Can Chiropr Assoc. 2009;53(1):59–72.
7. Doan DNT, Ku B, Choi J, Oh M, Kim K, Cha W, et al. Predicting dementia with prefrontal electroencephalography and event-related potential. Front Aging Neurosci. 2021;13:659817.
8. Miraglia F, Vecchio F, Rossini PM. Searching for signs of aging and dementia in EEG through network analysis. Behav Brain Res. 2017;317:292–300.
9. Esposito R, Bortoletto M, Miniussi C. Integrating TMS, EEG, and MRI as an approach for studying brain connectivity. Neuroscientist. 2020;26(5–6):471–86.
10. Cao J, Zhao Y, Shan X, Wei HL, Guo Y, Chen L, et al. Brain functional and effective connectivity based on electroencephalography recordings: a review. Hum Brain Mapp. 2022;43(2):860–79.
11. Gao J, Gu L, Min X, Lin P, Li C, Zhang Q, et al. Brain fingerprinting and lie detection: a study of dynamic functional connectivity patterns of deception using EEG phase synchrony analysis. IEEE J Biomed Health Inform. 2022;26(2):600–13.

12. Nardone R, Sebastianelli L, Versace V, Saltuari L, Lochner P, Frey V, et al. Usefulness of EEG techniques in distinguishing frontotemporal dementia from Alzheimer's disease and other dementias. Dis Markers. 2018;2018:6581490.
13. Tomasello L, Carlucci L, Laganà A, Galletta S, Marinelli CV, Raffaele M, et al. Neuropsychological evaluation and quantitative EEG in patients with frontotemporal dementia, Alzheimer's disease, and mild cognitive impairment. Brain Sci. 2023;13(6)
14. Cozac VV, Gschwandtner U, Hatz F, Hardmeier M, Rüegg S, Fuhr P. Quantitative EEG and cognitive decline in Parkinson's disease. Parkinson's Dis. 2016;2016:9060649.
15. Iannaccone S, Houdayer E, Spina A, Nocera G, Alemanno F. Quantitative EEG for early differential diagnosis of dementia with Lewy bodies. Front Psychol. 2023;14:1150540.
16. Law ZK, Todd C, Mehraram R, Schumacher J, Baker MR, LeBeau FEN, et al. The role of EEG in the diagnosis, prognosis and clinical correlations of dementia with Lewy bodies-A systematic review. Diagnostics (Basel). 2020;10(9)
17. Fide E, Yerlikaya D, Güntekin B, Babiloni C, Yener GG. Coherence in event-related EEG oscillations in patients with Alzheimer's disease dementia and amnestic mild cognitive impairment. Cogn Neurodyn. 2023;17(6):1621–35.
18. Riudavets MA, Iacono D, Resnick SM, O'Brien R, Zonderman AB, Martin LJ, et al. Resistance to Alzheimer's pathology is associated with nuclear hypertrophy in neurons. Neurobiol Aging. 2007;28(10):1484–92.
19. Mak E, Gabel S, Su L, Williams GB, Arnold R, Passamonti L, et al. Multi-modal MRI investigation of volumetric and microstructural changes in the hippocampus and its subfields in mild cognitive impairment, Alzheimer's disease, and dementia with Lewy bodies. Int Psychogeriatr. 2017;29(4):545–55.
20. Rutkowski TM, Abe MS, Otake-Matsuura M. Neurotechnology and AI approach for early dementia onset biomarker from EEG in emotional stimulus evaluation task. Ann Int Conf IEEE Eng Med Biol Soc. 2021;2021:6675–8.
21. Li R, Wang X, Lawler K, Garg S, Bai Q, Alty J. Applications of artificial intelligence to aid early detection of dementia: a scoping review on current capabilities and future directions. J Biomed Inform. 2022;127:104030.
22. Kim MJ, Youn YC, Paik J. Deep learning-based EEG analysis to classify normal, mild cognitive impairment, and dementia: algorithms and dataset. NeuroImage. 2023;272:120054.
23. San-Martin R, Fraga FJ, Del Percio C, Lizio R, Noce G, Nobili F, et al. Classification of patients with Alzheimer's disease and dementia with Lewy bodies using resting EEG selected features at sensor and source levels: a proof-of-concept study. Curr Alzheimer Res. 2021;18(12):956–69.
24. Lee B, Lee T, Jeon H, Lee S, Kim K, Cho W, et al. Synergy through integration of wearable EEG and virtual reality for mild cognitive impairment and mild dementia screening. IEEE J Biomed Health Inform. 2022;26(7):2909–19.
25. Ju YE, Lucey BP, Holtzman DM. Sleep and Alzheimer disease pathology–a bidirectional relationship. Nat Rev Neurol. 2014;10(2):115–9.
26. Ye EM, Sun H, Krishnamurthy PV, Adra N, Ganglberger W, Thomas RJ, et al. Dementia detection from brain activity during sleep. Sleep. 2023;46(3):zsac286.
27. Albert MS, DeKosky ST, Dickson D, Dubois B, Feldman HH, Fox NC, et al. The diagnosis of mild cognitive impairment due to Alzheimer's disease: recommendations from the National Institute on Aging-Alzheimer's Association workgroups on diagnostic guidelines for Alzheimer's disease. Alzheimers Dement. 2011;7(3):270–9.
28. McKhann GM, Knopman DS, Chertkow H, Hyman BT, Jack CR Jr, Kawas CH, et al. The diagnosis of dementia due to Alzheimer's disease: recommendations from the National Institute on Aging-Alzheimer's Association workgroups on diagnostic guidelines for Alzheimer's disease. Alzheimers Dement. 2011;7(3):263–9.
29. Jeong J. EEG dynamics in patients with Alzheimer's disease. Clin Neurophysiol. 2004;115(7):1490–505.

30. Babiloni C, Arakaki X, Azami H, Bennys K, Blinowska K, Bonanni L, et al. Measures of resting state EEG rhythms for clinical trials in Alzheimer's disease: recommendations of an expert panel. Alzheimers Dement. 2021;17(9):1528–53.
31. Choi J, Ku B, You YG, Jo M, Kwon M, Choi Y, et al. Resting-state prefrontal EEG biomarkers in correlation with MMSE scores in elderly individuals. Sci Rep. 2019;9(1):10468.
32. Tsolaki A, Kazis D, Kompatsiaris I, Kosmidou V, Tsolaki M. Electroencephalogram and Alzheimer's disease: clinical and research approaches. Int J Alzheimers Dis. 2014;2014:349249.
33. Dauwels J, Vialatte F, Cichocki A. Diagnosis of Alzheimer's disease from EEG signals: where are we standing? Curr Alzheimer Res. 2010;7(6):487–505.
34. Vossel KA, Tartaglia MC, Nygaard HB, Zeman AZ, Miller BL. Epileptic activity in Alzheimer's disease: causes and clinical relevance. Lancet Neurol. 2017;16(4):311–22.
35. Liedorp M, Stam CJ, Van Der Flier WM, Pijnenburg YA, Scheltens P. Prevalence and clinical significance of epileptiform EEG discharges in a large memory clinic cohort. Dement Geriatr Cogn Disord. 2010;29(5):432–7.
36. Csernus EA, Werber T, Kamondi A, Horvath AA. The significance of subclinical Epileptiform activity in Alzheimer's disease: a review. Front Neurol. 2022;13:856500.
37. Ciliento R, Gjini K, Dabbs K, Hermann B, Riedner B, Jones S, et al. Prevalence and localization of nocturnal epileptiform discharges in mild cognitive impairment. Brain Commun. 2023;5(6):fcad302.
38. Yeh WC, Hsu CY, Li KY, Chien CF, Huang LC, Yang YH. Association between subclinical Epileptiform discharge and the severity of cognitive decline in Alzheimer's disease: a longitudinal cohort study. J Alzheimer's Dis. 2022;90(1):305–12.
39. Brunetti V, D'Atri A, Della Marca G, Vollono C, Marra C, Vita MG, et al. Subclinical epileptiform activity during sleep in Alzheimer's disease and mild cognitive impairment. Clin Neurophysiol. 2020;131(5):1011–8.
40. Yeh WC, Hsu CY, Li KY, Chien CF, Huang LC, Yang YH. Association between subclinical epileptiform discharge and the behavioral and psychological symptoms in patients with Alzheimer's dementia. Int J Geriatr Psychiatry. 2023;38(10):e6013.
41. Neri S, Mastroianni G, Gardella E, Aguglia U, Rubboli G. Epilepsy in neurodegenerative diseases. Epileptic Disord. 2022;24(2):249–73.
42. Chen YS, Chen TS, Huang CW. Dementia with non-convulsive seizures: a case report. J Int Med Res. 2021;49(12):3000605211062453.
43. Brunovsky M, Matousek M, Edman A, Cervena K, Krajca V. Objective assessment of the degree of dementia by means of EEG. Neuropsychobiology. 2003;48(1):19–26.
44. Torres-Simón L, Doval S, Nebreda A, Llinas SJ, Marsh EB, Maestú F. Understanding brain function in vascular cognitive impairment and dementia with EEG and MEG: a systematic review. NeuroImage Clin. 2022;35:103040.
45. Moretti D, Zanetti O, Binetti G, Frisoni G. Quantitative EEG markers in mild cognitive impairment: degenerative versus vascular brain impairment. Int J Alzheimers Dis. 2012;2012(1):917537.
46. McKeith IG, Boeve BF, Dickson DW, Halliday G, Taylor JP, Weintraub D, et al. Diagnosis and management of dementia with Lewy bodies: fourth consensus report of the DLB consortium. Neurology. 2017;89(1):88–100.
47. Musaeus CS, Kjaer TW, Cacic Hribljan M, Andersen BB, Høgh P, Kidmose P, et al. Subclinical Epileptiform activity in dementia with Lewy bodies. Mov Disord. 2023;38(10):1861–70.
48. Bonanni L, Thomas A, Tiraboschi P, Perfetti B, Varanese S, Onofrj M. EEG comparisons in early Alzheimer's disease, dementia with Lewy bodies and Parkinson's disease with dementia patients with a 2-year follow-up. Brain. 2008;131(3):690–705.
49. Bonanni L, Perfetti B, Bifolchetti S, Taylor J-P, Franciotti R, Parnetti L, et al. Quantitative electroencephalogram utility in predicting conversion of mild cognitive impairment to dementia with Lewy bodies. Neurobiol Aging. 2015;36(1):434–45.
50. Briel RC, McKeith I, Barker WA, Hewitt Y, Perry R, Ince P, et al. EEG findings in dementia with Lewy bodies and Alzheimer's disease. J Neurol Neurosurg Psychiatry. 1999;66(3):401–3.

51. Lee H, Brekelmans GJ, Roks G. The EEG as a diagnostic tool in distinguishing between dementia with Lewy bodies and Alzheimer's disease. Clin Neurophysiol. 2015;126(9):1735–9.
52. Roks G, Korf E, Van Der Flier W, Scheltens P, Stam C. The use of EEG in the diagnosis of dementia with Lewy bodies. J Neurol Neurosurg Psychiatry. 2008;79(4):377–80.
53. Zinno L, Negrotti A, Falzoi C, Messa G, Goldoni M, Calzetti S. Generalized Rhythmic Delta activity frontally predominant differentiates dementia with Lewy bodies from Alzheimer's disease and Parkinson's disease dementia: a conventional electroencephalography visual analysis. Clin EEG Neurosci. 2022;53(5):426–34.
54. Barcelon EA, Mukaino T, Yokoyama J, Uehara T, Ogata K, Kira J-i, et al. Grand Total EEG score can differentiate Parkinson's disease from Parkinson-related disorders. Front Neurol. 2019;10:413853.
55. McKeith IG, Ferman TJ, Thomas AJ, Blanc F, Boeve BF, Fujishiro H, et al. Research criteria for the diagnosis of prodromal dementia with Lewy bodies. Neurology. 2020;94(17):743–55.
56. Anjum MF, Espinoza AI, Cole RC, Singh A, May P, Uc EY, et al. Resting-state EEG measures cognitive impairment in Parkinson's disease. NPJ Parkinsons Dis. 2024;10(1):6.
57. Fonseca LC, Tedrus GM, Carvas PN, Machado EC. Comparison of quantitative EEG between patients with Alzheimer's disease and those with Parkinson's disease dementia. Clin Neurophysiol. 2013;124(10):1970–4.
58. Fry A, Singh D, Manganas L, Gordon ML, Christodoulou C, Leung H-C, et al. Parkinson's disease with visual hallucinations is associated with Epileptiform activity on EEG. Front Neurol. 2022;12:788632.
59. Jin L, Nawaz H, Ono K, Nowell J, Haley E, Berman BD, et al. One minute of EEG data provides sufficient and reliable data for identifying Lewy body dementia. Alzheimer Dis Assoc Disord. 2023;37(1):66–72.
60. Fonseca L, Tedrus G, Letro G, Bossoni A. Dementia, mild cognitive impairment and quantitative EEG in patients with Parkinson's disease. Clin EEG Neurosci. 2009;40(3):168–72.
61. Lindau M, Jelic V, Johansson S-E, Andersen C, Wahlund L-O, Almkvist O. Quantitative EEG abnormalities and cognitive dysfunctions in frontotemporal dementia and Alzheimer's disease. Dement Geriatr Cogn Disord. 2003;15(2):106–14.
62. Garn H, Coronel C, Waser M, Caravias G, Ransmayr G. Differential diagnosis between patients with probable Alzheimer's disease, Parkinson's disease dementia, or dementia with Lewy bodies and frontotemporal dementia, behavioral variant, using quantitative electroencephalographic features. J Neural Transm (Vienna, Austria: 1996). 2017;124(5):569–81.
63. Si Y, He R, Jiang L, Yao D, Zhang H, Xu P, et al. Differentiating between Alzheimer's disease and frontotemporal dementia based on the resting-state multilayer EEG network. IEEE Trans Neural Syst Rehabil Eng. 2023;31:4521–7.
64. Wieser HG, Schindler K, Zumsteg D. EEG in Creutzfeldt–Jakob disease. Clin Neurophysiol. 2006;117(5):935–51.
65. Neufeld MY, Talianski-Aronov A, Soffer D, Korczyn AD. Generalized convulsive status epilepticus in Creutzfeldt–Jakob disease. Seizure. 2003;12(6):403–5.
66. Miyake K, Hara T, Oshima E, Kawada K, Ishizu H, Yamauchi Y, et al. Creutzfeldt-Jakob disease with Alzheimer pathology, presenting with status epilepticus following repeated partial seizures: a case report and literature review. BMC Neurol. 2018;18:1–5.
67. Hsiao PS, Lee YM, Chu FS, Lee CL, Liu FC, Tsai PH. Probable sporadic Creutzfeldt-Jakob disease mimicking focal epilepsy. Epilepsy Behav Case Rep. 2019;11:77–80.
68. Zerr I, Kallenberg K, Summers DM, Romero C, Taratuto A, Heinemann U, et al. Updated clinical diagnostic criteria for sporadic Creutzfeldt-Jakob disease. Brain. 2009;132(10):2659–68.
69. Aguglia U, Gambardella A, Le Piane E, Messina D, Farnarier G, Oliveri R, et al. Disappearance of periodic sharp wave complexes in Creutzfeldt-Jakob disease. Neurophysiologie Clinique/Clin Neurophysiol. 1997;27(4):277–82.
70. Scott D, Heathfield K, Toone B, Margerison J. The EEG in Huntington's chorea: a clinical and neuropathological study. J Neurol Neurosurg Psychiatry. 1972;35(1):97–102.

71. Faber PL, Milz P, Reininghaus EZ, Mörkl S, Holl AK, Kapfhammer HP, et al. Fundamentally altered global- and microstate EEG characteristics in Huntington's disease. Clin Neurophysiol. 2021;132(1):13–22.
72. Piano C, Mazzucchi E, Bentivoglio AR, Losurdo A, Calandra Buonaura G, Imperatori C, et al. Wake and sleep EEG in patients with Huntington disease: an eLORETA study and review of the literature. Clin EEG Neurosci. 2017;48(1):60–71.
73. Ullrich NJ. Electroencephalographic correlate of juvenile Huntington's disease. J Child Neurol. 2004;19(7)
74. Landau ME, Cannard KR. EEG characteristics in juvenile Huntington's disease: a case report and review of the literature. Epileptic Disord. 2003;5(3):145–8.
75. Pu L, Lion KM, Todorovic M, Moyle W. Portable EEG monitoring for older adults with dementia and chronic pain – A feasibility study. Geriatr Nurs. 2021;42(1):124–8.
76. Wijnen VJM, Oudewortel L, van Luijtelaar G, Witlox J, Slooter AJC, van Gool WA. Feasibility and potential of a bedside mini-EEG for diagnosing delirium superimposed on dementia. Clin Neurophysiol. 2022;142:181–9.

# Chapter 3
# Frontiers of Molecular Neuroimaging: A Transformative Paradigm in Alzheimer's Disease Diagnosis and Research

**Hiroshi Matsuda**

**Abstract** Molecular neuroimaging has transformed the landscape of Alzheimer's disease (AD) research and diagnosis by enabling in vivo visualization of its core molecular hallmarks—amyloid-β plaques and tau neurofibrillary tangles. This transition has fundamentally reshaped AD as a biological continuum rather than a purely clinical syndrome, anchoring diagnosis in quantifiable biomarkers that precede cognitive decline by years or even decades. The integration among amyloid and tau positron emission tomography (PET) with magnetic resonance imaging provides complementary insights into both molecular pathology and structural or functional brain alterations, facilitating precise staging of disease progression and differential diagnosis among neurodegenerative disorders. Recent advances in tracer chemistry, digital photon detection, and artificial intelligence-driven analytics are propelling molecular imaging into the era of data-driven precision neurology. Molecular PET now functions as a diagnostic gatekeeper for disease-modifying therapies and a pharmacodynamic biomarker for evaluating treatment response in clinical trials. Yet these breakthroughs raise ethical, clinical, and social challenges, including equitable access to imaging technologies, data governance for large-scale neuroimaging repositories, and the psychological implications of disclosing preclinical biomarker status to cognitively normal individuals. Looking ahead, the convergence of molecular imaging, multimodal data integration, and computational modeling promises to establish a comprehensive model for individualized disease prediction, prevention, and therapeutic monitoring. In this emerging paradigm, molecular neuroimaging will not only illuminate the pathophysiological cascade of AD but also serve as a cornerstone of precision medicine across the broader spectrum of neurodegenerative diseases.

**Keywords** Alzheimer's disease · Molecular neuroimaging · Amyloid PET · tau PET · Quantitative imaging

H. Matsuda (✉)
Department of Biofunctional Neuroimaging, Fukushima Medical University, Fukushima City, Japan



Y.-H. Yang (ed.), *Management of Dementia from the Preclinical Stage*,
https://doi.org/10.1007/978-981-95-5222-1_3

## 3.1 Historical Overview and Transition

Over the past three decades, the conceptual and methodological landscape of dementia diagnosis has undergone a profound transformation. Historically, the clinical characterization of Alzheimer's disease (AD) relied almost entirely on observable cognitive and behavioral syndromes—particularly progressive memory loss, aphasia, apraxia, and executive dysfunction—confirmed postmortem through neuropathological visualization of amyloid plaques and neurofibrillary tangles. This paradigm, which emphasized symptomatology and late-stage pathological confirmation, reflected the technological limitations and conceptual model of the late twentieth century, when AD was regarded primarily as a clinical syndrome rather than a distinct biological entity.

The emergence of molecular neuroimaging redefined this trajectory. By enabling visualization of the core biochemical processes of AD in vivo, molecular imaging dissolved the temporal gap between pathological onset and clinical manifestation. It shifted the focus from end-stage confirmation to early detection and intervention, transforming both diagnostic reasoning and therapeutic strategy. This shift exemplifies a broader epistemological evolution in neuroscience and psychiatry—from descriptive, symptom-based classification toward a biologically anchored taxonomy grounded in measurable pathophysiology.

In Japan and globally, this transformation was catalyzed by the recognition that conventional imaging modalities such as magnetic resonance imaging (MRI) and brain perfusion single-photon emission computed tomography (SPECT), though invaluable for ruling out secondary causes of dementia, lacked molecular specificity. These modalities could delineate structural atrophy and perfusion deficits but could not reveal the underlying pathophysiology that distinguishes AD from other neurodegenerative disorders. The introduction of positron emission tomography (PET) tracers targeting amyloid-β and, later, tau proteins filled this diagnostic gap, enabling clinicians and researchers to map disease progression with unprecedented precision.

Our multicenter studies in Japan further underscored the diagnostic challenges of AD in the absence of amyloid PET. The positivity rate of amyloid PET among patients with clinically suspected AD was only 65% at the mild dementia stage [1] and 52% at the mild cognitive impairment (MCI) [2–4] stage [5]. These relatively low rates highlight the limitations of brain perfusion SPECT and MRI in detecting AD-specific pathophysiological patterns during early disease stages, when overlapping features of other disorders can mimic AD-related imaging changes (Fig. 3.1a, b).

Subsequent refinements in tracer chemistry, image quantification, and multicenter standardization have transformed amyloid and tau PET from research curiosities into clinical cornerstones. This progress culminated in the National Institute on Aging and Alzheimer's Association research model, which introduced the now canonical A/T/N classification [6]. Within this schema, "A" marks amyloid pathology, "T" tau pathology, and "N" neurodegeneration or neuronal injury. The A/T/N system formalized a biological definition of AD, decoupled from clinical

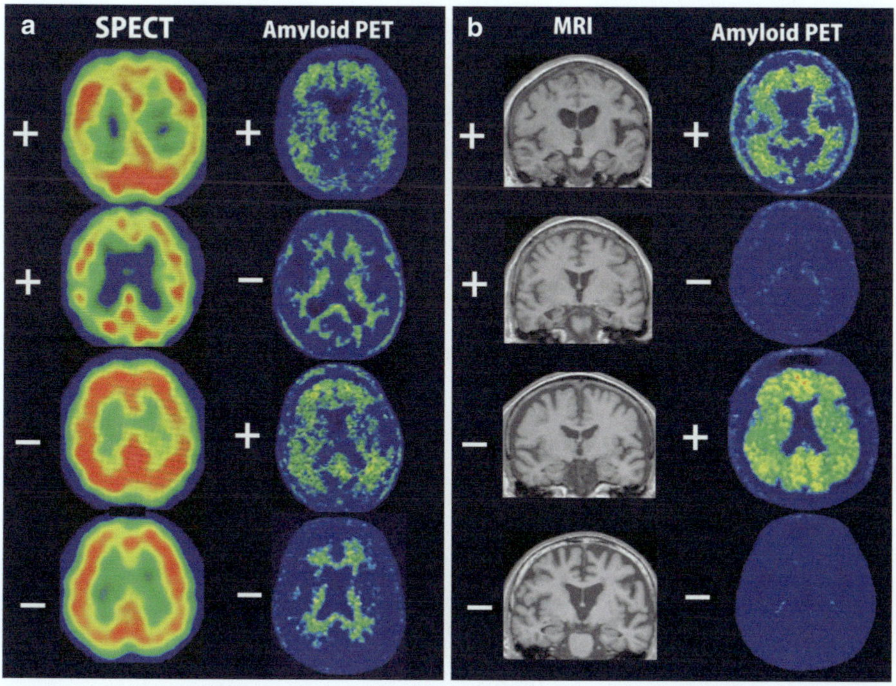


**Fig. 3.1** Comparison of brain perfusion SPECT and MRI with amyloid PET. (**a**) Comparison of brain perfusion SPECT with amyloid PET. Amyloid PET–positive (+) or –negative (−) findings are shown in relation to the presence (+) or absence (−) of parietal lobe hypoperfusion, a characteristic feature of Alzheimer's disease (AD). (**b**) Comparison of structural MRI with amyloid PET. Amyloid PET–positive (+) or –negative (−) findings are shown with (+) or without (−) medial temporal lobe atrophy, another hallmark of AD

symptoms, and laid the foundation for a biomarker-based continuum model of disease progression.

This transition also carries profound ethical, clinical, and philosophical implications. Detecting molecular pathology in cognitively normal individuals challenges traditional notions of disease onset, prognosis, and identity. The ability to visualize preclinical pathology compels a reconsideration of when disease truly begins and whether asymptomatic individuals should be informed of their biomarker status. These questions reside at the intersection of neuroscience, ethics, and public policy, demanding new models for communication, informed consent, and psychological support.

In Japan, where the integration among molecular imaging into clinical workflows has accelerated rapidly, this transition has influenced medical education, insurance policy, and public awareness. Early detection programs increasingly rely on biomarker confirmation to stratify risk and guide preventive strategies. The field's trajectory—from symptom- to biomarker-based diagnosis—underscores the dynamic interplay among technological innovation, clinical necessity, and societal readiness.

As molecular neuroimaging continues to evolve, it not only refines diagnostic precision but also redefines the very boundaries of disease. Emerging tracers, hybrid imaging technologies, and artificial intelligence (AI)-driven analytics are expanding the reach of molecular imaging beyond AD to encompass other tauopathies, α-synucleinopathies, and TDP-43 proteinopathies. The convergence of these modalities heralds a future in which dementia diagnosis, prognosis, and therapeutic monitoring are unified within a truly biological model—marking the advent of precision neurology in both research and clinical practice.

## 3.2 Evolution of Neuroimaging in Dementia Research

The evolution of neuroimaging in dementia research marks a sequential expansion of our ability to observe the brain—from macroscopic structure to microscopic molecular function. Prior to the advent of molecular imaging, structural and functional modalities such as computed tomography (CT), MRI, and brain perfusion SPECT formed the backbone of diagnostic evaluation. Each technological advance progressively narrowed the gap between morphology and pathology, ultimately preparing the ground for molecular PET.

### *3.2.1 From CT to MRI*

In the 1970s and 1980s, CT revolutionized clinical neurology by enabling noninvasive visualization of intracranial structures. CT could detect mass lesions, hemorrhage, infarction, and hydrocephalus, providing essential information for the differential diagnosis of dementia syndromes. However, its limited soft-tissue contrast and insensitivity to cortical atrophy patterns restricted its capacity to identify neurodegenerative diseases.

MRI subsequently supplanted CT as the gold standard for structural brain evaluation, owing to its superior gray–white matter contrast, multiplanar capability, and absence of ionizing radiation. MRI allowed visualization of the medial temporal lobe and hippocampus—regions critically affected in AD—with a level of precision unattainable by CT [7]. Early qualitative assessments of hippocampal atrophy were soon complemented by quantitative morphometric techniques, including voxel-based morphometry (VBM) and surface-based morphometry [8–14]. These computational methods provided objective, reproducible measures of gray matter density and cortical thickness across the entire brain, enabling correlation with cognitive and behavioral metrics. The convergence of these methodologies transformed MRI from a descriptive imaging tool into a quantitative biomarker platform, supporting both clinical diagnosis and longitudinal research.

### *3.2.2 Quantitative Imaging and Regional Analysis in Japan*

In Japan, quantitative neuroimaging has been widely incorporated into clinical workflows through the development of automated analysis software such as the Voxel-based Specific Regional Analysis System for Alzheimer's Disease (VSRAD®) [15, 16]. VSRAD® computes Z-scores by comparing a patient's MRI data with an age-matched normative database, identifying subtle hippocampal and entorhinal atrophy even in individuals with MCI. The widespread adoption of VSRAD® in clinical practice marks a major milestone in the standardization of MRI-based dementia diagnosis in Japan.

An in-vivo VBM study [17] of patients with neuropathologically confirmed AD identified three atrophy subtypes based on the distribution of neurofibrillary tangles: typical AD, hippocampal-sparing AD, and limbic-predominant AD. A fourth subtype, minimal-atrophy AD, has also been reported in several neuroimaging studies [18] (Fig. 3.2). Compared with typical AD, hippocampal-sparing AD exhibits more extensive cortical neurofibrillary tangles and atrophy with relative preservation of the hippocampus, whereas the opposite pattern characterizes limbic-predominant AD. Age at onset also differs: hippocampal-sparing AD typically presents at a younger age, while limbic-predominant AD tends to occur later in life. These distinctions help explain why early-onset AD frequently manifests as atypical clinical

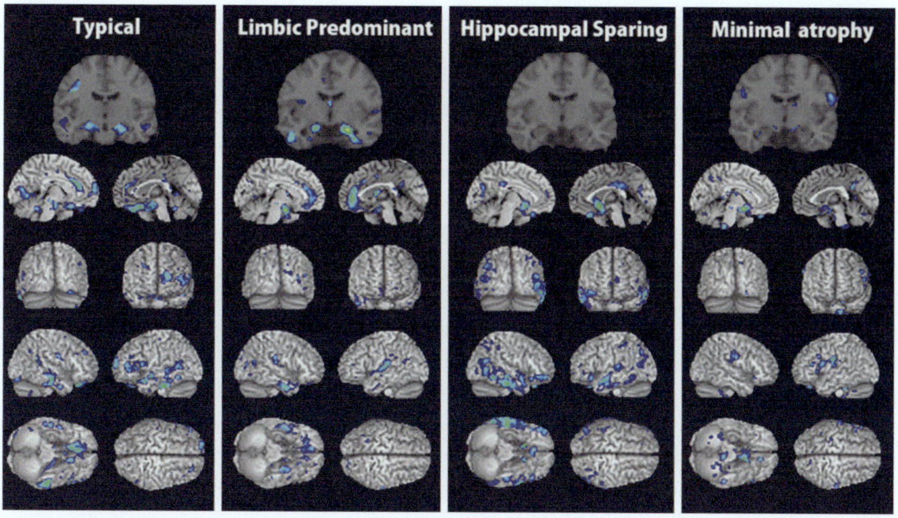


**Fig. 3.2** Subtypes of brain atrophy revealed by voxel-based morphometry in AD. Voxel-based morphometry (VBM) demonstrates four major subtypes of brain atrophy in AD: the typical subtype, showing atrophy of both the medial temporal lobe and temporoparietal cortex; the limbic-predominant subtype, showing atrophy confined to the medial temporal lobe; the hippocampal-sparing subtype, showing atrophy limited to the temporoparietal cortex; and the minimal-atrophy subtype, showing little or no atrophy. Colored Z-score maps are overlaid on tomographic sections and 3D surface renderings of a standardized brain using VSRAD® software

syndromes involving higher-order association cortices. Consistently, several studies have demonstrated topographical differences in gray matter involvement between early- and late-onset AD [19, 20].

These advancements have facilitated earlier detection and more accurate staging of AD in Japan's rapidly aging population. Integration with electronic health records and multicenter neuroimaging networks now enables population level surveillance of atrophic patterns, supporting both large-scale epidemiological research and individualized clinical decision-making. In research settings, MRI-based morphometry functions as a critical "N" component within the A/T/N biomarker model, complementing amyloid and tau PET as a quantitative measure of neurodegeneration.

### *3.2.3 Functional Imaging*

While MRI provides structural information, functional imaging techniques reveal dynamic physiological processes such as metabolism and perfusion. Brain perfusion SPECT was historically the most accessible modality for functional assessment. Using tracers such as $^{99m}$Tc-ECD or $^{123}$I-IMP, SPECT measures brain perfusion, which correlates with neuronal activity. Although its spatial resolution is modest compared with fluorodeoxyglucose (FDG)-PET [21], perfusion SPECT has remained widely used due to its relatively low cost, broad availability, and long-established clinical validation in dementia care.

Methodological advances such as three-dimensional stereotactic surface projection (3D-SSP) [22] and the easy Z-score Imaging System (eZIS) [23] transformed SPECT interpretation from subjective visual inspection into a statistically grounded process. These systems project perfusion data onto standardized brain templates, enabling voxel-wise comparison with normal databases. Characteristic AD-related patterns—posterior cingulate and precuneus hypoperfusion or hypometabolism with relative sparing of the primary sensorimotor cortex—have been consistently validated as early markers of AD and predictors of cognitive decline [24–27].

In Japan, the combination of 3D-SSP or eZIS and VSRAD® marks a dual-axis diagnostic paradigm: the former quantifies functional decline, while the latter quantifies structural atrophy. Together, they offer a multidimensional characterization of disease progression and provide essential context for interpreting subsequent PET findings. This integrative imaging strategy has become a cornerstone of dementia screening programs and academic research consortia, including large-scale multicenter initiatives.

### 3.2.4 *Quantitative Transition and Technological Convergence*

The refinement of quantitative imaging pipelines—spanning MRI morphometry, perfusion SPECT, and FDG-PET—has been instrumental in standardizing diagnostic thresholds and improving inter-rater reliability. The shift from qualitative to quantitative paradigms parallels broader trends in evidence-based medicine, emphasizing reproducibility, transparency, and objective measurement.

The emergence of hybrid scanners—including SPECT/CT, PET/CT, and PET/MR—has further blurred the boundaries between modalities, enabling simultaneous structural and functional assessment within a single session. These technologies not only enhance coregistration accuracy but also streamline workflow efficiency, reduce patient burden, and improve diagnostic confidence through integrated multimodal datasets.

The integration among these tools into routine clinical workflows paved the way for molecular imaging to assume a central role. By providing a macroscopic model within which molecular abnormalities could be localized and contextualized, structural and functional imaging served as the indispensable foundation for the molecular revolution that followed.

In this continuum, CT and MRI established the anatomical scaffold, SPECT and FDG-PET provided the functional mapping, and amyloid and tau PET ultimately supplied the molecular specificity necessary to define AD as a biologically measurable entity. Together, these technologies represent the cumulative evolution from morphology to molecular pathology—a trajectory that continues to shape the future of precision neuroimaging in dementia research.

## 3.3 Molecular PET Revolution

The emergence of molecular PET is among the most transformative advances in the history of dementia diagnostics. By moving beyond structural and functional correlates to directly image the molecular hallmarks of AD, molecular PET has reshaped what it means to visualize pathology in vivo. This revolution has connected between neuropathology and clinical manifestation, offering a means to detect disease at its biological origin rather than its symptomatic expression. Molecular PET now underpins a biologically grounded reclassification of AD, serving as a diagnostic and therapeutic cornerstone in the precision medicine era.

### 3.3.1 Amyloid PET: Establishing the Biological Signature of AD

The first major breakthrough came with the development of amyloid PET, which enabled visualization of fibrillar amyloid-β deposition—the defining molecular lesion of AD. Prior to this innovation, the existence and distribution of amyloid plaques could only be confirmed postmortem. The pioneering compound $^{11}$C-Pittsburgh Compound B ($^{11}$C-PiB), developed by Klunk and colleagues in the early 2000s [28–31], demonstrated for the first time that amyloid burden could be quantified in living humans, revolutionizing the study of preclinical and prodromal AD.

However, the short half-life of carbon-11 (approximately 20 minutes) limited PiB's use to research centers equipped with an on-site cyclotron. To overcome this logistical constraint, a new generation of fluorine-18–labeled tracers—including flutemetamol, florbetapir, and florbetaben [32–34]—was developed. With a longer half-life of approximately 110 minutes, these tracers could be centrally manufactured and distributed to clinical facilities without dedicated radiochemistry infrastructure. Their subsequent regulatory approvals by the U.S. Food and Drug Administration (FDA), the European Medicines Agency, and the Pharmaceuticals and Medical Devices Agency (PMDA) in Japan catalyzed the global clinical adoption of amyloid PET as a practical diagnostic tool.

Amyloid-negative scans typically demonstrate preserved gray–white matter contrast, whereas amyloid-positive scans show diffuse cortical uptake that blurs this distinction. This binary interpretation of amyloid status has substantial clinical implications—particularly for patient selection in antiamyloid immunotherapy trials and for assessing therapeutic response.

Beyond qualitative assessment, the introduction of quantitative models, most notably the Centiloid scale [35], revolutionized cross-study and cross-tracer comparability. By normalizing amyloid burden on a 0–100 scale anchored to $^{11}$C-PiB standards, the Centiloid system provides a universal metric for comparing amyloid levels across tracers, scanners, and institutions (Fig. 3.3). This standardization has enabled longitudinal monitoring, meta-analytic data pooling, and the definition of quantitative thresholds for "amyloid positivity," establishing amyloid PET as the first truly biological signature of AD.

Numerous studies have proposed Centiloid thresholds to define amyloid positivity. Most converge around 20 Centiloids, although variability persists across methodologies [36]. Salvadó et al. [37] proposed an optimal cutoff of 12 Centiloids based on cerebrospinal fluid (CSF) Aβ42 levels and 29 Centiloids based on phosphorylated tau/Aβ42 ratios, indicating established AD pathology. Jack et al. [38] reported a single threshold of 19 Centiloids in a longitudinal cohort. In antemortem PET–postmortem neuropathology comparisons, 20.1 Centiloids best detected moderate-to-high neuritic plaque burden per Consortium to Establish a Registry for Alzheimer's Disease (CERAD) criteria, whereas values ≤10 Centiloids optimally excluded plaques [39]. La Joie et al. [40] identified thresholds of 12.2 Centiloids for

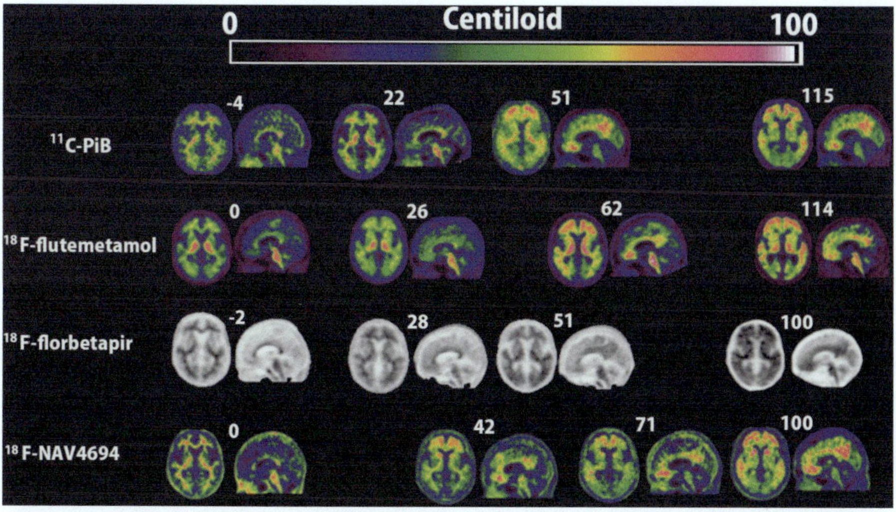


**Fig. 3.3** Amyloid PET images with different tracers scaled by Centiloids. Different PET tracers can quantify equivalent levels of amyloid-β deposition when standardized on the Centiloid scale. Representative images acquired with $^{11}$C-PiB, $^{18}$F-florbetapir, $^{18}$F-flutemetamol, and $^{18}$F-NAV4694 are shown, each scaled in Centiloid units

moderate-to-frequent neuritic plaques and 24.4 Centiloids for intermediate-to-high AD neuropathology. Visual interpretations become highly consistent at ≥26 Centiloids [5, 39], while the range of 12–30 Centiloids is often referred to as a "gray zone" [41, 42]. Collectively, these findings suggest that confident visual classification is generally achieved at 26–29 Centiloids or higher.

Several software packages have been developed for amyloid PET quantification. Semiquantitative metrics such as Standardized Uptake Value Ratio (SUVR) and Centiloid values can complement visual reads, aid longitudinal tracking of amyloid accumulation, and support the evaluation of disease-modifying therapies [43]. In addition to global Centiloid reporting, many platforms can generate voxel-wise Z-score maps by comparing a patient's amyloid PET data with a reference database derived from amyloid-negative individuals under age 50—an age group with minimal likelihood of preclinical AD [44–47]. These Z-score maps provide powerful visual and statistical support for interpretation, highlighting cortical regions of abnormal uptake (Fig. 3.4a, b).

Together, these advancements have transformed amyloid PET from a research tool into a standardized quantitative biomarker that links molecular pathology with clinical diagnosis, enabling reproducible measurement of disease burden across time, sites, and therapeutic contexts.

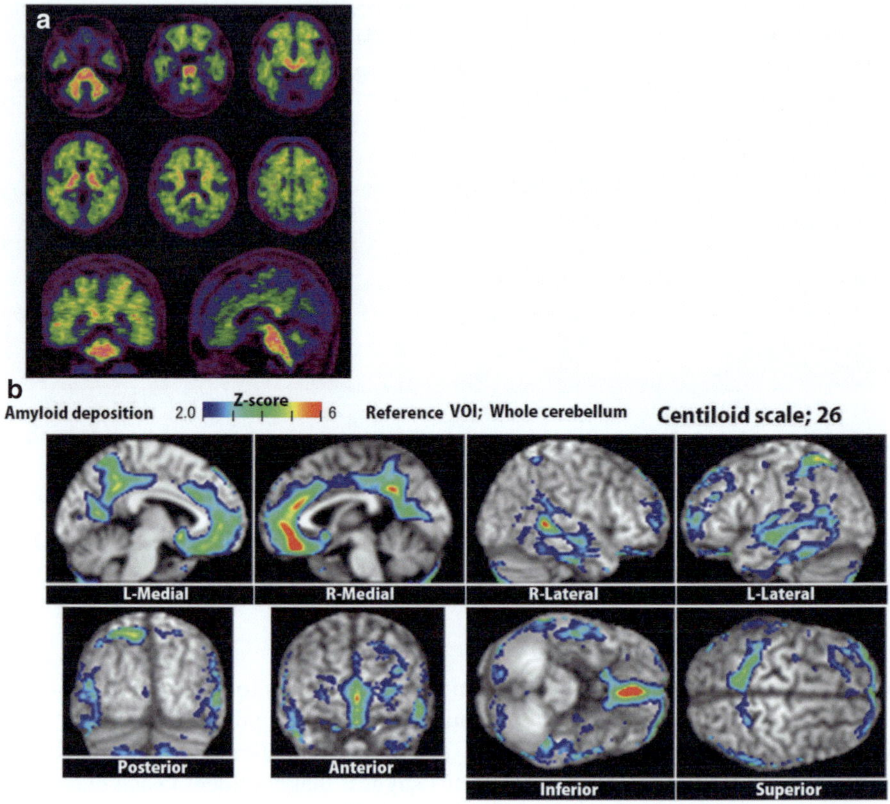


**Fig. 3.4** Usefulness of Z-score mapping in determining positive amyloid PET results. (**a**) A visually equivocal case of $^{18}$F-flutemetamol amyloid PET. (**b**) Z-score mapping demonstrates significantly increased amyloid deposition in the medial frontal lobe, posterior cingulate gyrus, and precuneus (Centiloid scale = 26)

## *3.3.2 Tau PET: Imaging the Downstream Pathology*

Following amyloid PET, this field's attention shifted toward imaging the intraneuronal tau aggregates that more closely correlate with neurodegeneration and clinical symptom severity. The first-generation tracer $^{18}$F-flortaucipir (AV-1451) [48–50] provided proof of concept for visualizing neurofibrillary tangles in vivo. Its regional binding patterns corresponded closely with the Braak staging system—beginning in the transentorhinal cortex, then spreading sequentially to limbic and neocortical regions [51]. These findings validated the long-standing hypothesis that the hierarchical propagation of tau pathology underlies the clinical progression of AD.

Despite its success, flortaucipir exhibited notable off-target binding in the choroid plexus, basal ganglia, and midbrain—likely due to interactions with monoamine oxidase-A/B and melanin-containing cells. This limitation spurred the development of second-generation tracers, including $^{18}$F-MK6240, $^{18}$F-RO948, and

$^{18}$F-GTP1, which demonstrate markedly higher selectivity, improved signal-to-noise ratio, and minimal off-target interference [52–61]. These newer compounds now enable precise quantification of regional tau deposition across the full Braak spectrum (stages I–VI) [48–65] (Fig. 3.5).

Shuping et al. [65] proposed four visual read categories for $^{18}$F-MK6240:

- "No uptake": No elevated signal in medial temporal lobe (MTL) or neocortex, and no off-target region exceeding retinal signal.
- "MTL only": Uptake confined to any MTL structure (transentorhinal, entorhinal, subiculum, hippocampus, parahippocampus, or amygdala) without neocortical uptake, corresponding to Braak I–II. This pattern may also be seen in primary age-related tauopathy [66, 67]. A sagittal PET slice in AD often shows a "hook-like" uptake from amygdala and entorhinal to parahippocampus, with weaker hippocampal uptake [68] (Fig. 3.6).
- "MTL AND": Uptake in MTL plus at least one additional neocortical region (lateral temporal, fusiform, frontal, parietal, occipital, or cingulate), corresponding to Braak III or higher. This reflects NFT spread associated with AD progression and is relevant for monitoring treatment response.
- "Outside MTL": Uptake in neocortical or subcortical regions other than MTL exceeding retinal signal. Some scans show focal uptake in areas with atypical clinical phenotypes (e.g., occipital or frontal) or medial temporal preservation

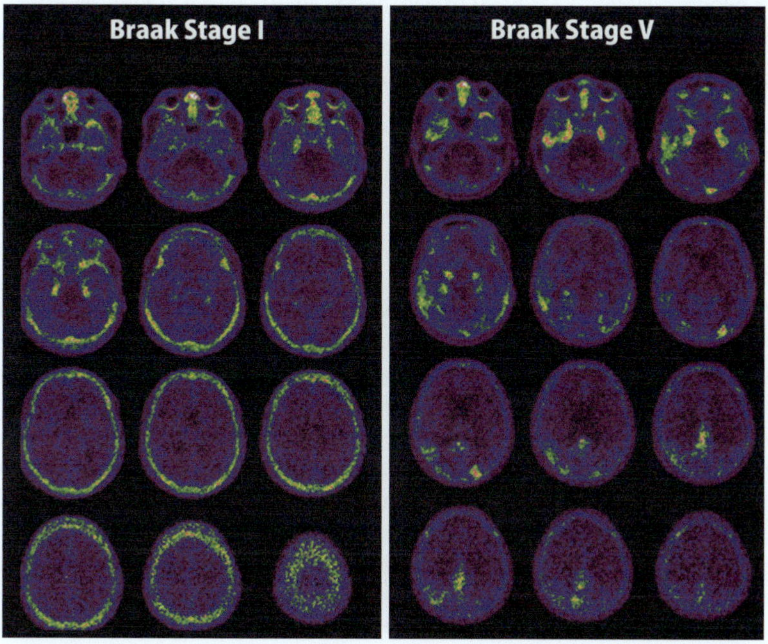


**Fig. 3.5** Tau PET images with $^{18}$F-MK6240. Tau PET with $^{18}$F-MK6240 shows progressive tau accumulation according to Braak stage: stage I—uptake restricted to the medial temporal lobe; stage V—extensive neocortical uptake involving the temporoparietal cortex

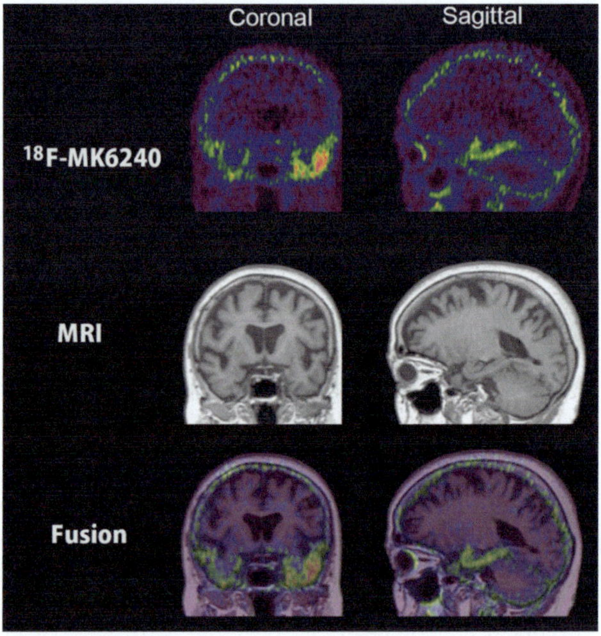


**Fig. 3.6** Hook-like tau uptake in the medial temporal lobe. A sagittal $^{18}$F-MK6240 PET image from a patient with AD demonstrates a characteristic *"hook-like"* pattern, with intense tau uptake extending from the amygdala and entorhinal cortex to the parahippocampal gyrus, and weaker uptake in the hippocampus

with neocortical uptake typical of AD. Nonbrain off-target signals such as meninges are not considered positive uptake.

This spatial classification helps monitor disease progression and stratify individuals in clinical or research settings.

Clinically, tau PET provides a direct window into neuronal injury and disease staging. Unlike amyloid deposition—which plateaus early in the disease course—tau accumulation continues to increase in parallel with cognitive decline and cortical atrophy. Longitudinal studies consistently show that changes in tau PET signals correlate more strongly with both cognitive trajectories and brain volume loss than amyloid measures. Consequently, tau imaging has emerged as the most sensitive biomarker of disease progression and therapeutic response, particularly in evaluating the efficacy of disease-modifying drugs targeting tau pathology.

The integration among tau PET into clinical trials has further refined the design of precision therapeutics. By enabling stratification based on molecular stage and regional tau burden, tau imaging supports individualized treatment monitoring and the assessment of drug target engagement. In this way, molecular PET—first through amyloid and now through tau—has completed the transition of AD diagnosis from a syndromic to a biological definition, transforming both clinical practice and the conceptual understanding of neurodegenerative disease.

## 3.4 Clinical Translation and Ethical Implications

The translation of molecular neuroimaging from the research domain to clinical practice is among the most significant transformations in modern neurology. Whereas early applications of PET focused primarily on elucidating disease mechanisms, this field now is central inpatient stratification, therapeutic eligibility, and longitudinal monitoring. This transition has elevated PET from a research tool to a clinical biomarker platform, shaping the landscape of precision medicine for AD and related disorders.

In Japan, the clinical translation of molecular neuroimaging has been closely intertwined with national health-insurance policies. Table 3.1 summarizes the list of neuroimaging modalities currently approved and reimbursed under the Japanese National Health Insurance system for the evaluation of dementia. This regulatory framework illustrates how Japan has progressively expanded coverage from morphological to molecular imaging, aligning insurance policy with the paradigm shift toward biomarker-based diagnosis.

### *3.4.1 Molecular Imaging as a Gatekeeper for Precision Therapeutics*

The clinical utility of molecular PET lies in its diagnostic accuracy but in its capacity to guide therapeutic decision-making. The advent of anti-amyloid monoclonal antibodies such as lecanemab and donanemab has established amyloid PET as an essential biomarker for confirming treatment eligibility [69, 70]. These agents specifically target amyloid-β aggregates, and their administration requires prior evidence of amyloid positivity—typically demonstrated by PET or CSF assays. In this context, PET functions as a gatekeeper for therapy, ensuring that disease-modifying drugs are administered to biologically appropriate candidates.

Similarly, tau PET is emerging as a pharmacodynamic biomarker for assessing downstream treatment effects. Early clinical trials increasingly incorporate serial

**Table 3.1** Neuroimaging modalities for dementia diagnosis currently covered by the Japanese National Health Insurance

| Imaging modality | Indicated disease |
|---|---|
| CT | Cerebrovascular disease, brain tumor |
| MRI | Neurodegenerative disorders, cerebrovascular disease, brain tumor |
| Brain perfusion SPECT | Neurodegenerative disorders, cerebrovascular disease |
| Dopamine transporter SPECT | Dementia with Lewy bodies |
| Metaiodobenzylguanidine | Dementia with Lewy bodies |
| Amyloid PET | Alzheimer's disease |

tau imaging to evaluate whether anti-amyloid interventions attenuate tau propagation or cortical neurodegeneration. This dynamic use of PET transforms it from a diagnostic modality into a quantitative endpoint for therapeutic efficacy, aligning imaging biomarkers with the regulatory models of the U.S. FDA and Japan's PMDA. As a result, molecular PET now serves as a translational bridge connecting molecular pathology, therapeutic development, and clinical outcome assessment.

### 3.4.2 Integration into Clinical Guidelines and Reimbursement Systems

In Japan, the inclusion of amyloid PET in national dementia care guidelines and its partial insurance reimbursement mark pivotal milestones in its clinical adoption. These developments were driven by both scientific validation and health policy initiatives that recognized the importance of biomarker-supported diagnosis in disease-modifying therapies. Hospitals certified as Advanced Dementia Imaging Centers are increasingly incorporating amyloid PET into standardized diagnostic algorithms, often in conjunction with MRI, SPECT, or CSF biomarker testing.

However, challenges persist. The high cost of PET imaging and tracer synthesis continues to limit accessibility, particularly outside major urban areas. Reimbursement remains restricted to specific indications—such as eligibility assessment for antiamyloid therapy. Broader implementation will require cost-effectiveness analyses demonstrating that biomarker-guided diagnosis improves patient outcomes and optimizes healthcare resource allocation. Ongoing health economic modeling efforts in Japan are evaluating how early and accurate diagnosis may reduce downstream costs associated with delayed or inappropriate treatment.

### 3.4.3 Clinical Workflow and Multidisciplinary Coordination

The integration among molecular imaging into routine clinical workflows necessitates close collaboration among neurologists, psychiatrists, radiologists, nuclear medicine physicians, and radiological technicians. Standardized acquisition protocols, reconstruction pipelines, and quantitative analysis tools are essential to ensure reproducibility across centers.

Interdisciplinary case conferences are increasingly being adopted to jointly review PET, CSF, and plasma biomarker data before establishing a final diagnosis. This integrated method exemplifies the emerging multimodal biomarker paradigm, in which molecular and structural imaging are interpreted in concert with fluid biomarkers to provide a holistic view of disease state and progression.

### 3.4.4 Ethical Challenges of Biomarker Disclosure

Despite these advances, molecular imaging introduces profound ethical and psychosocial challenges. The detection of amyloid or tau pathology in cognitively normal individuals raises complex questions regarding disclosure, counseling, and potential social or insurance discrimination. Unlike conventional diagnostic findings, biomarker results carry probabilistic meaning—they indicate elevated risk rather than definitive disease. This inherent uncertainty complicates communication between clinicians and patients and challenges the informed-consent process in both clinical and research settings.

Ethical models emphasize the necessity of pretest counseling, post-test interpretation, and psychological support for individuals receiving biomarker information. Disclosure should be accompanied by clear explanations of predictive limitations and the fact that biomarker positivity does not guarantee clinical progression.

### 3.4.5 Equity, Accessibility, and Global Health Considerations

The introduction of molecular PET has also magnified healthcare inequities at both national and global levels. Its high cost, reliance on radiochemistry infrastructure, and concentration in tertiary medical centers limit access primarily to affluent regions. In Japan, where PET scanners are predominantly located in metropolitan hospitals, rural populations often experience delayed or limited access to definitive molecular diagnosis. This geographic disparity mirrors global patterns, where molecular neuroimaging remains concentrated in high-income countries, leaving low- and middle-income regions underserved.

Addressing these inequities will require innovative policy and technological solutions. The development of low-cost, long-lived tracers, centralized radiopharmacies, and mobile PET units could expand access to underserved populations. Moreover, the integration among plasma biomarkers as preliminary screening tools can triage patients for confirmatory PET imaging [71], improving cost-efficiency and resource allocation. Collaborative models among public institutions, academic centers, and industry stakeholders will be essential to ensure equitable dissemination of molecular diagnostic technologies worldwide.

### 3.4.6 The Societal and Philosophical Impact of Molecular Diagnosis

Beyond its clinical applications, molecular neuroimaging has reshaped the philosophical boundaries of diagnosis. By revealing pathology decades before symptom onset, PET challenges traditional distinctions between health, disease, and normal aging. Individuals who are biologically positive but clinically asymptomatic occupy a new liminal state—neither healthy nor ill in the conventional sense. This ontological ambiguity raises profound questions about identity, stigma, and the social meaning of diagnosis.

Public perception of dementia is likewise evolving. Early detection is increasingly viewed as a form of empowerment, enabling individuals to engage proactively in lifestyle modification, clinical research, and preventive care. Nevertheless, this shift demands careful public education to prevent misunderstanding of biomarker results and undue anxiety. Communication strategies that emphasize risk mitigation, hope, and therapeutic progress are crucial for maintaining trust between clinicians, patients, and society.

## 3.5 Conclusions

Molecular neuroimaging has fundamentally redefined the diagnostic and conceptual model of Alzheimer's disease (AD) and related neurodegenerative disorders. The ability to visualize the pathological hallmarks—amyloid-β plaques and tau neurofibrillary tangles—in vivo has transformed AD research from a descriptive and clinical discipline into a quantitative and biological science.

This progress marks a technological innovation but a transition that reshapes how diseases are defined, detected, and treated. The transition from structural and functional imaging to molecular and computational imaging has opened a new era in neuroscience.

Today, molecular PET serves multiple pivotal roles:

As a diagnostic gatekeeper: it determines eligibility for disease-modifying therapies, including antiamyloid and anti-tau treatments.

As a quantitative marker of disease activity and therapeutic response: it provides biological indices for objectively tracking disease progression and treatment effects.

As a translational bridge between research, clinical practice, and society: through spatial visualization of neuropathology, it supports clinical decision-making, drug development, and ethical policy formation.

As a result of these achievements, AD is no longer regarded as a "clinical syndrome" but rather as a "measurable biological process." This new perspective forms the foundation of precision neurology, enabling individualized prediction, prevention, and therapeutic monitoring.

Looking ahead, the integration among molecular imaging, multimodal data fusion, AI, and computational modeling will enable systematic prediction of disease risk, staging, and treatment response at the individual level. In this emerging paradigm, molecular neuroimaging is expected to function as a technique for "seeing" lesions but as a scientific foundation for understanding and controlling neurodegenerative diseases.

## References


1. Matsuda H, Ito K, Ishii K, et al. Quantitative evaluation of $^{18}$F-Flutemetamol PET in patients with cognitive impairment and suspected Alzheimer's disease: a multicenter study. Front Neurol. 2021;11:578753.
2. Petersen RC. Mild cognitive impairment as a diagnostic entity. J Intern Med. 2004;256:183–94.
3. Gauthier S, Reisberg B, Zaudig M, et al. Mild cognitive impairment. Lancet. 2006;367:1262–70.
4. Albert MS, DeKosky ST, Dickson D, et al. The diagnosis of mild cognitive impairment due to Alzheimer's disease: recommendations from the National Institute on Aging-Alzheimer's Association workgroups on diagnostic guidelines for Alzheimer's disease. Alzheimers Dement. 2011;7:270–9.
5. Matsuda H, Okita K, Motoi Y, et al. Clinical impact of amyloid PET using $^{18}$F-florbetapir in patients with cognitive impairment and suspected Alzheimer's disease: a multicenter study. Ann Nucl Med. 2022;36:1039–49.
6. Jack CR, Bennett DA, Blennow K, et al. A/T/N: an unbiased descriptive classification scheme for Alzheimer disease biomarkers. Neurology. 2016;87:539–47.
7. Frisoni GB, Jack CR, Bocchetta M, et al. The EADC-ADNI harmonized protocol for manual hippocampal segmentation on magnetic resonance: evidence of validity. Alzheimers Dement. 2015;11:111–25.
8. Frisoni GB, Fox NC, Jack CR Jr, et al. The clinical use of structural MRI in Alzheimer disease. Nat Rev Neurol. 2010;6:67–77.
9. Jack CR, Barkhof F, Bernstein MA, et al. Steps to standardization and validation of hippocampal volumetry as a biomarker in clinical trials and diagnostic criterion for Alzheimer's disease. Alzheimers Dement. 2011;7:474–85.
10. Fujishima M, Kawaguchi A, Maikusa N, et al. Sample size estimation for Alzheimer's disease trials from Japanese ADNI serial magnetic resonance imaging. J Alzheimer's Dis. 2017;56:75–88.
11. Fischl B, Salat DH, Busa E, et al. Whole brain segmentation: automated labeling of neuroanatomical structures in the human brain. Neuron. 2003;33:341–55.
12. Fujishima M, Maikusa N, Nakamura K, et al. Mild cognitive impairment, poor episodic memory, and late-life depression are associated with cerebral cortical thinning and increased white matter hyperintensities. Front Aging Neurosci. 2014;6:306.
13. Yushkevich PA, Pluta JB, Wang H, et al. Automated volumetry and regional thickness analysis of hippocampal subfields and medial temporal cortical structures in mild cognitive impairment. Hum Brain Mapp. 2015;36:258–87.
14. Ashburner J, Friston KJ. Voxel-based morphometry--the methods. Neuroimage. 2000;11:805–21.
15. Matsuda H, Mizumura S, Nemoto K, et al. Automatic voxel-based morphometry of structural MRI by SPM8 plus diffeomorphic anatomic registration through exponentiated lie algebra improves the diagnosis of probable Alzheimer disease. AJNR Am J Neuroradiol. 2012;33:1109–14.
16. Matsuda H. MRI morphometry in Alzheimer's disease. Ageing Res Rev. 2016;30:17–24.
17. Whitwell JL, Dickson DW, Murray ME, et al. Neuroimaging correlates of pathologically defined subtypes of Alzheimer's disease: a case-control study. Lancet Neurol. 2012;11:868–77.
18. Ferreira D, Nordberg A, Westman E. Biological subtypes of Alzheimer disease: a systematic review and meta-analysis. Neurology. 2020;94:436–48.
19. Matsunari I, Samuraki M, Chen WP, et al. Comparison of $^{18}$F-FDG PET and optimized voxel-based morphometry for detection of Alzheimer's disease: aging effect on diagnostic performance. J Nucl Med. 2007;48:1961–70.
20. Frisoni GB, Pievani M, Testa C, et al. The topography of grey matter involvement in early and late onset Alzheimer's disease. Brain. 2007;130:720–30.

21. Silverman DH. Brain $^{18}$F-FDG PET in the diagnosis of neurodegenerative dementias: comparison with perfusion SPECT and with clinical evaluations lacking nuclear imaging. J Nucl Med. 2004;45:594–607.
22. Minoshima S, Frey KA, Koeppe RA, et al. A diagnostic approach in Alzheimer's disease using three-dimensional stereotactic surface projections of fluorine-18-FDG PET. J Nucl Med. 1995;36:1238–48.
23. Matsuda H, Mizumura S, Nagao T, et al. Automated discrimination between very early Alzheimer disease and controls using an easy Z-score imaging system for multicenter brain perfusion single-photon emission tomography. AJNR Am J Neuroradiol. 2007;28:731–6.
24. Minoshima S, Giordani B, Berent S, et al. Metabolic reduction in the posterior cingulate cortex in very early Alzheimer's disease. Ann Neurol. 1997;42:85–94.
25. Kogure D, Matsuda H, Ohnishi T, et al. Longitudinal evaluation of early Alzheimer's disease using brain perfusion SPECT. J Nucl Med. 2000;41:1155–62.
26. Imabayashi E, Matsuda H, Asada T, et al. Superiority of 3-dimensional stereotactic surface projection analysis over visual inspection in discrimination of patients with very early Alzheimer's disease from controls using brain perfusion SPECT. J Nucl Med. 2004;45:1450–7.
27. Matsuda H. Role of neuroimaging in Alzheimer's disease, with emphasis on brain perfusion SPECT. J Nucl Med. 2007;48:1289–300.
28. Mathis CA, Wang Y, Holt DP, et al. Synthesis and evaluation of $^{11}$C-labeled 6-substituted 2-arylbenzothiazoles as amyloid imaging agents. J Med Chem. 2003;46:2740–54.
29. Klunk WE, Engler H, Nordberg A, et al. Imaging brain amyloid in Alzheimer's disease with Pittsburgh compound-B. Ann Neurol. 2004;55:306–19.
30. Bacskai BJ, Frosch MP, Freeman SH, et al. Molecular imaging with Pittsburgh compound B confirmed at autopsy: a case report. Arch Neurol. 2007;64:431–4.
31. Ikonomovic MD, Klunk WE, Abrahamson EE, et al. Post-mortem correlates of in vivo PiB-PET amyloid imaging in a typical case of Alzheimer's disease. Brain. 2008;131:1630–45.
32. Nelissen N, Van Laere K, Thurfjell L, et al. Phase 1 study of the Pittsburgh compound B derivative $^{18}$F-flutemetamol in healthy volunteers and patients with probable Alzheimer disease. J Nucl Med. 2009;50:1251–9.
33. Wong DF, Rosenberg PB, Zhou Y, et al. In vivo imaging of amyloid deposition in Alzheimer disease using the radioligand $^{18}$F-AV-45 (florbetapir [corrected] F 18). J Nucl Med. 2010;51:913–20.
34. Barthel H, Gertz HJ, Dresel S, et al. Cerebral amyloid-β PET with florbetaben ($^{18}$F) in patients with Alzheimer's disease and healthy controls: a multicentre phase 2 diagnostic study. Lancet Neurol. 2011;10:424–35.
35. Klunk WE, Koeppe RA, Price JC, et al. The centiloid project: standardizing quantitative amyloid plaque estimation by PET. Alzheimers Dement. 2015;11:1–15.e154.
36. Jagust WJ, Mattay VS, Krainak DM, et al. Quantitative brain amyloid PET. J Nucl Med. 2024;65:670–8.
37. Salvadó G, Molinuevo JL, Brugulat-Serrat A, et al. Centiloid cut-off values for optimal agreement between PET and CSF core AD biomarkers. Alzheimers Res Ther. 2019;11:27.
38. Jack CR Jr, Wiste HJ, Weigand SD, et al. Defining imaging biomarker cut points for brain aging and Alzheimer's disease. Alzheimers Dement. 2017;13:205–16.
39. Amadoru S, Doré V, McLean CA, et al. Comparison of amyloid PET measured in Centiloid units with neuropathological findings in Alzheimer's disease. Alzheimers Res Ther. 2020;12:22.
40. La Joie R, Ayakta N, Seeley WW, et al. Multisite study of the relationships between antemortem [$^{11}$C]PIB-PET Centiloid values and postmortem measures of Alzheimer's disease neuropathology. Alzheimers Dement. 2019;15:205–16.
41. Pemberton HG, Collij LE, Heeman F, et al. Quantification of amyloid PET for future clinical use: a state-of-the-art review. Eur J Nucl Med Mol Imaging. 2022;49:3508–28.
42. Milà-Alomà M, Salvadó G, Shekari M, et al. Comparative analysis of different definitions of amyloid-β positivity to detect early downstream pathophysiological alterations in preclinical Alzheimer. J Prev Alzheimers Dis. 2021;8:68–77.

43. Jovalekic A, Roé-Vellvé N, Koglin N, et al. Validation of quantitative assessment of florbetaben PET scans as an adjunct to the visual assessment across 15 software methods. Eur J Nucl Med Mol Imaging. 2023;50:3276–89.
44. Pemberton HG, Buckley C, Battle M, et al. Software compatibility analysis for quantitative measures of [$^{18}$F]flutemetamol amyloid PET burden in mild cognitive impairment. EJNMMI Res. 2023;13:48.
45. Matsuda H, Yamao T. Software development for quantitative analysis of brain amyloid PET. Brain Behav. 2022;12:e2499.
46. Matsuda H, Soma T, Okita K, et al. Development of software for measuring brain amyloid accumulation using $^{18}$ F-florbetapir PET and calculating global Centiloid scale and regional Z-score values. Brain Behav. 2023;13:e3092.
47. Zhang K, Mizuma H, Zhang X, et al. PET imaging of neural activity, β-amyloid, and tau in normal brain aging. Eur J Nucl Med Mol Imaging. 2021;48:3859–71.
48. Marquié M, Normandin MD, Vanderburg CR, et al. Validating novel tau positron emission tomography tracer [F-18]-AV-1451 (T807) on postmortem brain tissue. Ann Neurol. 2015;78:787–800.
49. Mattay VS, Fotenos AF, Ganley CJ, et al. Brain tau imaging: Food and Drug Administration approval of $^{18}$F-Flortaucipir injection. J Nucl Med. 2020;61:1411–2.
50. Jie CVML, Treyer V, Schibli R, Mu L. Tauvid™: the first FDA-approved PET tracer for imaging tau pathology in Alzheimer's disease. Pharmaceuticals (Basel). 2021;14:110.
51. Braak H, Braak E. Staging of Alzheimer's disease-related neurofibrillary changes. Neurobiol Aging. 1995;16:271–8.
52. Walji AM, Hostetler ED, Selnick H, et al. Discovery of 6-(Fluoro-($^{18}$)F)-3-(1H-pyrrolo[2,3-c]pyridin-1-yl)isoquinolin-5-amine ([($^{18}$)F]-MK-6240): a Positron Emission Tomography (PET) imaging agent for quantification of neurofibrillary tangles (NFTs). J Med Chem. 2016;59:4778–89.
53. Leuzy A, Pascoal TA, Strandberg O, et al. A multicenter comparison of [$^{18}$F]flortaucipir, [$^{18}$F]RO948, and [$^{18}$F]MK6240 tau PET tracers to detect a common target ROI for differential diagnosis. Eur J Nucl Med Mol Imaging. 2021;48:2295–305.
54. Hostetler ED, Walji AM, Zeng Z, et al. Preclinical characterization of $^{18}$F-MK-6240, a promising PET tracer for in vivo quantification of human neurofibrillary tangles. J Nucl Med. 2016;57:1599–606.
55. Pascoal TA, Shin M, Kang MS, et al. In vivo quantification of neurofibrillary tangles with [$^{18}$F]MK-6240. Alzheimer's Res Ther. 2018;10:74.
56. Betthauser TJ, Cody KA, Zammit MD, et al. In vivo characterization and quantification of neurofibrillary tau PET radioligand $^{18}$F-MK-6240 in humans from Alzheimer disease dementia to young controls. J Nucl Med. 2019;60:93–9.
57. Lohith TG, Bennacef I, Vandenberghe R, et al. Brain imaging of Alzheimer dementia patients and elderly controls with $^{18}$F-MK-6240, a PET tracer targeting neurofibrillary tangles. J Nucl Med. 2019;60:107–14.
58. Pascoal TA, Therriault J, Benedet AL, et al. $^{18}$F-MK-6240 PET for early and late detection of neurofibrillary tangles. Brain. 2020;143:2818–30.
59. Aguero C, Dhaynaut M, Normandin MD, et al. Autoradiography validation of novel tau PET tracer [F-18]-MK-6240 on human postmortem brain tissue. Acta Neuropathol Commun. 2019;7:37.
60. Salinas C, Lohith TG, Purohit A, et al. Test-retest characteristic of [$^{18}$F]MK-6240 quantitative outcomes in cognitively normal adults and subjects with Alzheimer's disease. J Cereb Blood Flow Metab. 2020;40:2179–87.
61. Gogola A, Minhas DS, Villemagne VL, et al. Direct comparison of the Tau PET tracers $^{18}$F-Flortaucipir and $^{18}$F-MK-6240 in human subjects. J Nucl Med. 2022;63:108–16.
62. Braak H, Braak E. Neuropathological stageing of Alzheimer-related changes. Acta Neuropathol. 1991;82:239–59.

63. Braak H, Alafuzoff I, Arzberger T, et al. Staging of Alzheimer disease-associated neurofibrillary pathology using paraffin sections and immunocytochemistry. Acta Neuropathol. 2006;112:389–404.
64. Macedo AC, Tissot C, Therriault J, et al. The use of tau PET to stage Alzheimer disease according to the Braak staging framework. J Nucl Med. 2023;64:1171–8.
65. Shuping JL, Matthews DC, Adamczuk K, et al. Development, initial validation, and application of a visual read method for [$^{18}$F]MK-6240 tau PET. Alzheimers Dement (NY). 2023;9(1):e12372.
66. Crary JF, Trojanowski JQ, Schneider JA, et al. Primary age-related tauopathy (PART): a common pathology associated with human aging. Acta Neuropathol. 2014;128:755–66.
67. Krishnadas N, Doré V, Groot C, et al. Mesial temporal tau in amyloid-β-negative cognitively normal older persons. Alzheimer's Res Ther. 2022;14:51.
68. Krishnadas N, Huang K, Schultz SA, et al. Visually identified Tau $^{18}$F-MK6240 PET patterns in symptomatic Alzheimer's disease. J Alzheimer's Dis. 2022;88:1627–37.
69. van Dyck CH, Swanson CJ, Aisen P, et al. Lecanemab in early Alzheimer's disease. N Engl J Med. 2023;388:9–21.
70. Sims JR, Zimmer JA, Evans CD, et al. Donanemab in early symptomatic Alzheimer disease: the TRAILBLAZER-ALZ 2 randomized clinical trial. JAMA. 2023;330:512–27.
71. Schöll M, Vrillon A, Ikeuchi T, et al. Cutting through the noise: a narrative review of Alzheimer's disease plasma biomarkers for routine clinical use. J Prev Alzheimers Dis. 2025;12:100056.

# Chapter 4
# Neuropsychiatric Manifestations Along with Aging, Mild and Major Neurocognitive Disorders

**Linda Chiu Wa Lam, Allen Ting Chun Lee, and Wai Chi Chan**

**Abstract** Neuropsychiatric symptoms (NPS) are not uncommon in late life. NPS are important clinical manifestations of neurocognitive disorders (NCD). However, it is also important to recognize that NPS are present in people with normal cognition. Some NPS may be related to early-onset functional psychiatric conditions presenting with a chronic course across the lifespan. Other NPS may be associated with underlying NCDs that may carry early diagnostic implications. This chapter outlines the profiles and clinical implications of NPS across the cognitive spectrum.

**Keywords** Neuropsychiatric symptoms · Neurocognitive disorders · Dementia · Affective dysregulation · Impulse dyscontrol · Psychosis

With global population aging, early diagnosis and management of neurocognitive disorders (NCD) have become major health concerns. While cognitive decline is a core feature of NCD, behavioral and psychiatric symptoms (NPS) are also integral to the clinical presentations. NPS not only adversely affect quality of life and everyday function, but also pose additional risks, increase carer burden, and cause stress, especially in the early stage of impairment [1, 2]. Owing to the heterogeneity of NPS, management strategies have been symptom-oriented and not frequently derived from the hypothesis on pathological mechanisms.

NPS in NCD have been described using different terminologies. The two most frequently quoted terms include neuropsychiatric symptoms and behavioral and psychological symptoms of dementia (BPSD). The Neuropsychiatric Inventory (NPI) has been a standard assessment adopted to measure NPS, ranging from

---

L. C. W. Lam (✉) · A. T. C. Lee
Department of Psychiatry, Faculty of Medicine, The Chinese University of Hong Kong, Ma Liu Shui, Hong Kong
e-mail: cwlam@cuhk.edu.hk

W. C. Chan
Department of Psychiatry, School of Clinical Medicine, The University of Hong Kong, Pok Fu Lam, Hong Kong



Y.-H. Yang (ed.), *Management of Dementia from the Preclinical Stage*,
https://doi.org/10.1007/978-981-95-5222-1_4

psychosis to vegetative syndromes (sleep and appetite disturbances) [3]. BPSD was coined in 1999 and defined as "symptoms of disturbed perception, thought content, mood or behavior that frequently occur in patients with dementia" [4, 5]. The International Psychogeriatric Association has recently updated the management approach to BPSD and refined the definition of psychosis in NCD, reflecting attempts to standardize descriptions for better management of these distressing symptoms in people living with NCD [6].

## 4.1 NPS in Major Neurocognitive Disorders

NPS comprise of broad range of noncognitive and behavioral changes found in patients with NCD. Major groups of symptoms consist of psychosis, mood disturbances, behavioral changes, euphoria, and vegetative symptoms [7]. NPS are highly prevalent in NCD. Over 90% of people with major NCDs are reported to have one or more NPS at any time [8]. Most NPS fluctuate with time, while overall severity and intensity generally peak in the moderate phase of global decline.

Depression, apathy, and irritability are common in mild NCD. Among people with major NCD, the most frequently reported disturbances were apathy, depression, and agitation/aggression. Psychosis is of lower prevalence, but its presence, especially persistent symptoms, was linked to clinically significant cognitive decline. While there might be little differences in the overall prevalence of NPS between Alzheimer-type and other NCDs, the pattern differs [9, 10].

The pathophysiological mechanisms of NPS in major NCD are diverse, representing the consequence of progressive neuronal death. It has been suggested that frontal circuitry disruption with impulsivity and disinhibition may be implicated in the more outwardly presented disorganized behaviors. In a study that examined NPS clusters in different NCDs, psychosis was differently distributed, with Lewy body disease (LBD) patients showing higher scores for hallucinations. There was a negative correlation between NPI total score and tau levels. Frontal atrophy scores were associated with psychosis, apathy, and agitation/aggression [11].

Perceptual disturbances, typically represented by visual hallucinations and misinterpretation, are reported in NCD associated with α-synucleinopathy with significant degeneration of the cholinergic pathway. A study assessed the association between cholinergic denervation and visual hallucinations in Parkinson's disease using positron emission tomography (PET) imaging of the cholinergic system (38 patients with Parkinson's disease and 10 healthy subjects). Cholinergic system integrity was assessed with PET imaging using 18F-fluoroethoxybenzovesamicol as the tracer. The Parkinson's disease group showed an extensive pattern of decreased tracer uptake throughout the brain. The VH+ group ($n$ = 13) showed decreased tracer uptake which covered most of the left ventral visual stream and extended towards superior temporal areas. Visual hallucinations in Parkinson's disease are associated with a marked cholinergic deficiency in the left ventral visual stream and the left superior temporal lobe, in addition to an extensive global cholinergic denervation [12].

## 4.2 NPS in Mild Neurocognitive Disorders

In the past few decades, attention to NPS has mainly focused on secondary impairments and caregiver burden. In most pivotal randomized controlled trials targeting on disease modification in Alzheimer's disease (AD), people with NPS were frequently excluded. This has led to limited information on the impact of new therapies on NPS. On the other hand, it is increasingly recognized that many NPS are found in the early stages of cognitive impairment. Early identification of NPS may assist in clinical diagnosis.

The term "mild behavioral impairment" (MBI) has been quoted and operationalized in the International Society to Advance Alzheimer's Research and Treatment—Alzheimer's Association research diagnostic criteria [13]. It is a construct that describes neuropsychiatric symptoms in people aged 50 years and older before the onset of clinically significant cognitive decline and dementia, and the behavioral changes are not entirely attributable to functional psychiatric disorders. MBI encompasses symptoms including decreased drive and motivation (apathy), affective dysregulation (mood and anxiety symptoms), impulse dyscontrol (agitation, impulsivity, and abnormal reward salience), social inappropriateness (social cognition impairment), and abnormal perception and thought content (psychotic symptoms including delusions and hallucinations). NPS in mild NCD may present as distinct psychiatric symptoms or manifest as more subtle behavioral changes. A greater number and severity of MBI have been associated with faster cognitive decline. MBI has gained increased recognition as presenting pre-dementia risk factors [14].

In a study examining the longitudinal association of the MBI with plasma biomarkers, including pTau181, after 1 year, abnormal perception was associated with steeper increases in plasma pTau181. Abnormal perception, decreased motivation, and impulse dyscontrol were also associated with markers of metabolic dysregulation, including homocysteine or insulin [15].

## 4.3 Affective Dysregulation

### *4.3.1 Depression*

Depression is the most commonly reported affective symptom in old age. The bidirectional relationship between depression and NCD has been widely studied. It is one of the 14 potentially modifiable factors for dementia quoted by the 2024 Lancet

Commission report on dementia prevention [16]. Depression may be a prodromal symptom representing underlying neurodegeneration, or it may be a contributory risk factor. Early-onset depression (or depressive symptoms) in adult life has been associated with a more than twofold increase in dementia risk. Multiple biological mechanisms may link depression to dementia, including cardiovascular disease, alterations in glucocorticoid steroid levels, hippocampal atrophy, inflammatory changes, and nerve growth factors deficits [17].

The risk is higher when depression is not properly managed. On the other hand, people with a history of depression but achieved remission have lower risks compared to those who remain depressed in old age. In a 6-year prospective study on health risk factors for dementia, people with depression in adulthood only did not have a higher incidence of dementia [18]. Having depression in both adulthood and late life was associated with a higher dementia risk, and improvement in depression in late life was associated with a lower risk, suggesting that persistent or recurrent lifetime depression is a risk factor for dementia [18]. Older adults with chronic depression should be monitored for cognitive decline. Early optimal treatment of depression is potentially important for dementia prevention.

### *4.3.2 Apathy*

Apathy is another common NPS that spans from early to severe cognitive impairment. Depression and apathy frequently coexist in NCD, but apathy appears to be a distinct symptom construct requiring different detection and intervention strategies. Apathy causes caregiver distress and exaggerates functional impairment. In moderate to severe cognitive impairment, the prevalence of apathy is generally higher. However, apathy occurring in mild NCD may be a sign of faster decline. In studies observing the risk prediction of apathy in mild NCD, apathy appeared to be associated with a higher risk of progression to major NCD. In the context of neurodegeneration, apathy is closely related to frontal subcortical circuitry disruption due to different pathological processes.

A study examined the association between apathy and cognitive decline in 1057 non-dementia older adults from the Alzheimer's Disease Neuroimaging Initiative database with up to 13 years of follow-up. Apathy was associated with faster impairment of cognition and an elevation of the Abeta burden. The effects of apathy on cognitive function were mediated by Abeta pathology and Abeta deposition in the prefrontal regions. The findings suggested that apathy is an early manifestation of cognitive decline and there may be bidirectional roles between apathy syndrome and Abeta pathology. Prefrontal Abeta pathology influenced the pathway from apathy to cognitive decline [19, 20]. In subcortical small vessel disease, ischemic changes or lacunar infarcts in the basal ganglia are implicated in the development of apathy and frontal network alterations [21]. On the other hand, in patient with frontotemporal lobar degeneration (FTLD), frontal atrophy is associated with a mixed presentation of disinhibition, impulsivity and apathy.

Interventions for apathy are diverse. Pharmacological options include alterations in dopaminergic, noradrenergic, and cholinergic transmissions. Nonpharmacological approaches are also heterogeneous, including cognitive stimulation, behavioral activation, and activity training. A recent review suggested that repetitive Transcranial Magnetic Stimulation and cognitive interventions are more effective than conventional interventions in improving apathy in patients with neurological diseases. However, there is a need for more nonpharmacological intervention studies with high quality and larger sample sizes for further exploration [22].

### *4.3.3 Anxiety*

Anxiety symptoms in people without significant cognitive impairment have been described as the "worried well." Increasing evidence has shown that functionally independent, anxious older adults are more likely to present with subtle and specific cognitive impairments, such as complex attention and episodic memory decline [23]. Long-term prospective studies also suggested that anxiety symptoms in people with no or mild cognitive impairment may be associated with a trend for more rapid deterioration. The Australian imaging, biomarker and lifestyle (AIBL) study of ageing observed that older adults with amyloid positivity in positron emission tomography (PET) with anxiety exhibited faster cognitive deterioration compared to people with amyloid positive who were not anxious [24].

Different mechanisms have been proposed to link anxiety and cognitive decline. Persistent anxiety, depression, and stress-related disorders reflect exaggerated stress response and are associated with inflammatory profile changes [25]. It would be of interest to further explore the association between anxiety, cognitive decline, and systemic inflammation. Late-onset anxiety symptoms may represent early involvement of the locus ceruleus in AD, disturbing neurotransmitter pathways that regulate mood symptoms [26]. Anxiety symptoms may be managed with both pharmacological and nonpharmacological interventions such as mindfulness-based cognitive therapy or relaxation. It would be of great interest to study if satisfactory management of anxiety symptoms will modulate the trajectories of cognitive decline in NCD.

## 4.4 Impulse Dyscontrol

Agitation, impulsivity, and irritability are NPS describing episodic maladaptive temper outbursts in response to everyday environmental stimuli of intensity that are generally not severe. With increasing cognitive impairment, a person's ability to interpret and react appropriately to environmental stimuli would be compromised. In people with mild NCD, the emergence of subtle irritability and agitation may be interpreted as self-centeredness and mental rigidity in old age. As NPS related to impulse dyscontrol are mostly reactive, it is important to carefully consider environmental triggers of agitation and irritability individually. Training of carers who appreciate the triggers and antecedents is important, as they would be able to minimize the escalation of behavioral outbursts due to impulse dyscontrol [27]. In conditions of severe disturbances that pose significant mental health risks, psychotropic medication may be considered after the failure of non-pharmacological interventions [28]. Brexpiprazole, a dopamine receptor modulator, has recently been approved by the Food and Drug Administration (FDA) office of the United States for the management of agitation in major NCD [29]. However, it is essential to note that antipsychotic medication has a black box warning for the treatment of psychosis in NCD.

## 4.5 Psychosis Syndromes

Psychosis syndromes are of regular occurrence in major NCD [9]. The prevalence of delusions and hallucinations varies among different subtypes of NCD. The prevalence of psychosis generally increases from mild to moderate severity. Hallucinations may be of varying forms and have been reported to vary in people with different types of NCD.

Visual hallucinations and related perceptual disturbances are characteristic symptoms and core clinical diagnostic symptoms in NCD due to Lewy body disease (LBD). Structural brain analysis suggested that white matter connecting the cortical regions to the nucleus basalis of Meynert and the thalamus was more affected in patients with hallucinations [30]. On the other hand, the clinical profiles of frontotemporal lobar degeneration (FTLD) are dominated by attention to disinhibition and social cognitive deficits. However, it is important to note that a subtype of FTLD (especially associated with C9orf72 expansion) is associated with prominent auditory hallucinations and delusions that may be confused with symptoms of functional psychotic disorders [31]. Late-onset psychotic symptoms in the absence of neurodegeneration are uncommon, and an accurate diagnosis is important to avoid exposure to antipsychotic medication with undesirable side effects.

## 4.6 Sleep Disturbances

Complaints about poor sleep are common in late life, from community-living older adults with normal aging to those with mild or major NCD [32, 33]. Older adults with normal cognition or mild NCD who had increased sleep disturbances (increased sleep latency, intermittent sleep, disturbed slow-wave sleep) have been reported to have higher odds for cognitive decline and increased amyloid burden [34]. It has been hypothesized that non-rapid eye movement (REM) sleep and slow-wave sleep disturbances are implicated in amyloid and tau accumulation at different stages of Alzheimer's disease (AD) [35–37]. Degeneration of the suprachiasmatic nucleus in

NCD, a regulator of sleep, contributes to the pathological mechanisms relating to disrupted sleep and cognitive decline [38]. As sleep habits are enduring lifestyle patterns, it will be of great interest to evaluate if better sleep hygiene in midlife is a protective factor against cognitive decline in late life.

Another sleep-related symptom with a specific bearing on early diagnosis is Rapid Eye Movement Behavioral Disorder (RBD). The prevalence of RBD in a population-based prospective cohort was estimated in Korea. The adjusted prevalence of RBD was 1.4% (95% CI: 1.0–1.8%) [39]. Consumption of hypnotics including zolpidem and certain short-acting benzodiazepines has been associated with RBD. In NCD associated with alpha-synucleinopathy (LBD), symptoms of Rapid Eye Movement (REM) sleep behavior are reported a few years before the onset of other clinical symptoms of Parkinson's disease or cognitive impairment [40, 41]. RBD also appears to be a phenotype that runs in families in probands with LBD and may aid early detection of preclinical conditions [42]. In the consensus criteria for NCD with Lewy bodies, RBD is considered a core symptom in the diagnosis [43].

## 4.7 NPS in Normal Cognition

Late-onset NPS are mainly studied from the perspective of neurodegeneration and frequently considered as adjuvant manifestations of NCD. However, primary psychiatric disorders are common in adulthood, with most running a chronic and episodic course, and may persist into old age. The management of early-onset psychiatric symptoms may be complicated by the emergence of medical comorbidities and cognitive decline.

There have been ongoing discussions as to whether functional psychiatric conditions are risk factors for NCD. Major depressive disorder in midlife is a well-recognized risk factor, with anxiety showing emerging evidence for NCD. Schizophrenia is associated with an early decline in cognitive function after symptom onset in adult life. Prospective studies reported that adult-onset schizophrenia showed an increased risk of NCD in late life after controlling for medical morbidities of cerebrovascular risk factors [44]. Very late-onset schizophrenia is uncommon, and recent reports also suggested a higher risk of cognitive decline in people presenting with late-onset psychosis [45].

## 4.8 Implications of NPS on Clinical Care

NPS represent a wide spectrum of symptoms, from subtle behavioral change to severe perceptual disturbances. Optimal management of NPS should be integral in the care plan for people with NCD. Further understanding of the mechanisms of different NPS in relation to specific or general degenerative etiologies is important in the development of evidence-based management.

## References

1. Tsai CF, et al. Health-related quality of life and mild behavioral impairment in older adults without dementia. Int J Geriatr Psychiatry. 2023;38(9):e6003.
2. Delgado C, et al. Neuropsychiatric symptoms in Alzheimer's disease are the main determinants of functional impairment in advanced everyday activities. J Alzheimer's Dis. 2019;67(1):381–92.
3. Cummings JL. The neuropsychiatric inventory: assessing psychopathology in dementia patients. Neurology. 1997;48(5 Suppl 6):S10–6.
4. Finkel SI. Managing the behavioral and psychological signs and symptoms of dementia. Int Clin Psychopharmacol. 1997;12(Suppl 4):S25–8.
5. Finkel SI, et al. Behavioral and psychological signs and symptoms of dementia: a consensus statement on current knowledge and implications for research and treatment. Int Psychogeriatr. 1996;8(Suppl 3):497–500.
6. Sano M, et al. International psychogeriatric association (IPA) consensus for defining psychosis in major and mild neurocognitive disorders. Int Psychogeriatr. 2022;34(3):203–7.
7. Cheng ST, Kwok T, Lam LC. Neuropsychiatric symptom clusters of Alzheimer's disease in Hong Kong Chinese: prevalence and confirmatory factor analysis of the neuropsychiatric inventory. Int Psychogeriatr. 2012;24(9):1465–73.
8. Kwon KJ, et al. Future therapeutic strategies for Alzheimer's disease: focus on behavioral and psychological symptoms. Int J Mol Sci. 2024;25(21):11338.
9. Lyketsos CG, et al. Prevalence of neuropsychiatric symptoms in dementia and mild cognitive impairment: results from the cardiovascular health study. JAMA. 2002;288(12):1475–83.
10. Bayram E, Shan G, Cummings JL. Associations between comorbid TDP-43, lewy body pathology, and neuropsychiatric symptoms in Alzheimer's disease. J Alzheimer's Dis. 2019;69(4):953–61.
11. Cotta Ramusino M, et al. Correlation of frontal atrophy and CSF tau levels with neuropsychiatric symptoms in patients with cognitive impairment: a memory clinic experience. Front Aging Neurosci. 2021;13:595758.
12. d'Angremont E, et al. Cholinergic deficiency in Parkinson's disease patients with visual hallucinations. Brain. 2024;147(10):3370–8.
13. Ismail Z, et al. Neuropsychiatric symptoms as early manifestations of emergent dementia: provisional diagnostic criteria for mild behavioral impairment. Alzheimers Dement. 2016;12(2):195–202.
14. Ferraro PM, et al. Mild behavioral impairment as a potential marker of predementia risk states in motor neuron diseases. Eur J Neurol. 2023;30(1):47–56.
15. Gonzalez-Bautista E, et al. Mild behavioral impairment domains are longitudinally associated with pTAU and metabolic biomarkers in dementia-free older adults. Alzheimers Dement. 2024;20(7):4692–701.
16. Livingston G, et al. Dementia prevention, intervention, and care: 2024 report of the lancet standing commission. Lancet. 2024;404(10452):572–628.
17. Byers AL, Yaffe K. Depression and risk of developing dementia. Nat Rev Neurol. 2011;7(6):323–31.
18. Lee ATC, et al. Risk of incident dementia varies with different onset and courses of depression. J Affect Disord. 2021;282:915–20.
19. Sun L, et al. Prefrontal Abeta pathology influencing the pathway from apathy to cognitive decline in non-dementia elderly. Transl Psychiatry. 2021;11(1):534.
20. Johansson M, et al. Development of apathy, anxiety, and depression in cognitively unimpaired older adults: effects of Alzheimer's disease pathology and cognitive decline. Biol Psychiatry. 2022;92(1):34–43.

21. Altunkaya S, et al. Dissociable functional brain networks associated with apathy in subcortical ischemic vascular disease and Alzheimer's disease. Front Aging Neurosci. 2021;13:717037.
22. Tan S, et al. Non-pharmacological intervention effects on apathy caused by central nervous system organic diseases: a network meta-analysis. Medicine (Baltimore). 2022;101(35):e30467.
23. Fung AWT, et al. Anxiety symptoms predicted decline in episodic memory in cognitively healthy older adults: a 3-year prospective study. Int J Geriatr Psychiatry. 2018;33(5):748–54.
24. Pietrzak RH, et al. Anxiety symptoms, cerebral amyloid burden and memory decline in healthy older adults without dementia: 3-year prospective cohort study. Br J Psychiatry. 2014;204:400–1.
25. Kuring JK, et al. Inflammatory markers in persons with clinically-significant depression, anxiety or PTSD: a systematic review and meta-analysis. J Psychiatry Res. 2023;168:279–92.
26. Haglund M, Sjobeck M, Englund E. Locus ceruleus degeneration is ubiquitous in Alzheimer's disease: possible implications for diagnosis and treatment. Neuropathology. 2006;26(6):528–32.
27. James IA, et al. Management of Agitation in behaviours that challenge in dementia care: multidisciplinary perspectives on non-pharmacological strategies. Clin Interv Aging. 2023;18:219–30.
28. Marcinkowska M, et al. Management of dementia-related psychosis, agitation and aggression: a review of the pharmacology and clinical effects of potential drug candidates. CNS Drugs. 2020;34(3):243–68.
29. Zhong K, Cummings J. A critical review of brexpiprazole oral tablets as the first drug approved to treat agitation symptoms associated with dementia due to Alzheimer's disease. Expert Rev Neurother. 2024;25:1–9.
30. Mehraram R, et al. Functional and structural brain network correlates of visual hallucinations in Lewy body dementia. Brain. 2022;145(6):2190–205.
31. Devenney EM, et al. The neural correlates and clinical characteristics of psychosis in the frontotemporal dementia continuum and the C9orf72 expansion. Neuroimage Clin. 2017;13:439–45.
32. Gordon NP, et al. Prevalence of sleep-related problems and risks in a community-dwelling older adult population: a cross-sectional survey-based study. BMC Public Health. 2022;22(1):2045.
33. Koren T, et al. Prevalence of sleep disturbances in people with dementia living in the community: a systematic review and meta-analysis. Ageing Res Rev. 2023;83:101782.
34. Mudalige D, et al. Longitudinal associations between mild behavioral impairment, sleep disturbance, and progression to dementia. J Alzheimers Dis Rep. 2023;7(1):1323–34.
35. Borges CR, et al. Amyloid profile is associated with sleep quality in preclinical but not in prodromal Alzheimer's disease older adults. Sleep Med. 2024;121:359–64.
36. Stankeviciute L, et al. Amyloid beta-independent sleep markers associated with early regional tau burden and cortical thinning. Alzheimers Dement (Amst). 2024;16(3):e12616.
37. Yoon SH, et al. Association of sleep disturbances with brain amyloid and tau burden, cortical atrophy, and cognitive dysfunction across the AD continuum. Neurology. 2023;101(21):e2162–71.
38. Van Erum J, Van Dam D, De Deyn PP. Sleep and Alzheimer's disease: a pivotal role for the suprachiasmatic nucleus. Sleep Med Rev. 2018;40:17–27.
39. Lee WJ, et al. REM sleep behavior disorder and its possible prodromes in general population: prevalence, polysomnography findings, and associated factors. Neurology. 2023;101(23):e2364–75.
40. Fujishiro H, et al. Early diagnosis of prodromal dementia with Lewy bodies using clinical history of probable REM sleep behaviour disorder and cardiac (123) I-MIBG scintigraphy in memory clinics. Psychogeriatrics. 2021;21(3):288–95.
41. Malkani RG, Wenger NS. REM sleep behavior disorder as a pathway to dementia: if, when, how, what, and why should physicians disclose the diagnosis and risk for dementia. Curr Sleep Med Rep. 2021;7(3):57–64.

42. Wang J, et al. Familial alpha-synucleinopathy spectrum features in patients with psychiatric REM sleep behaviour disorder. J Neurol Neurosurg Psychiatry. 2023;94(11):893–903.
43. McKeith IG, et al. Diagnosis and management of dementia with Lewy bodies: fourth consensus report of the DLB Consortium. Neurology. 2017;89(1):88–100.
44. Ribe AR, et al. Long-term risk of dementia in persons with schizophrenia: a Danish population-based cohort study. JAMA Psychiatry. 2015;72(11):1095–101.
45. Kodesh A, et al. Risk of dementia and death in very-late-onset schizophrenia-like psychosis: a national cohort study. Schizophr Res. 2020;223:220–6.

# Chapter 5
# Vascular Contribution and Risks to Cognitive Disorder

Yong-Jae Kim

**Abstract** Vascular health plays a crucial role in maintaining cognitive function, and vascular contributions to cognitive impairment and dementia are increasingly recognized as significant factors in brain health. This chapter discusses in depth the effects of vascular contributions on cognitive impairment, key mechanisms, relevant risk factors, and prevention and management strategies.

**Keywords** Vascular cognitive impairment · Vascular dementia · Cerebral infarction · Leukoaraiosis

## 5.1 Introduction

Cognitive disorders including vascular dementia are significant public health issues that are increasing worldwide. Vascular diseases are especially one of the leading causes of these cognitive impairments, highlighting the close association between vascular health and cognitive function. This chapter discusses in depth the effects of vascular contributions on cognitive impairment, key mechanisms, relevant risk factors, and prevention and management strategies.

Y.-J. Kim (✉)
Eunpyeong St. Mary's Hospital, Affiliated with the College of Medicine at Catholic, University of Korea in Seoul, Seoul, South Korea



Y.-H. Yang (ed.), *Management of Dementia from the Preclinical Stage*,
https://doi.org/10.1007/978-981-95-5222-1_5

## 5.2 The Mechanism of Vascular Contribution

### 5.2.1 Cerebral Infarction and Cerebral Hemorrhage

Cerebral infarction occurs when blood flow to the brain is blocked, resulting in a lack of oxygen and nutrients. Brain cells are highly sensitive to hypoxia, an oxygen-deficient state, and within minutes of the blockage, brain cells begin to be damaged. If this blockage persists, brain cells either become necrotic or die through programmed apoptosis. This causes direct damage to the neural networks around the affected area [18].

After a cerebral infarction, an inflammatory response is triggered in the damaged brain tissue. Inflammation increases the permeability of the blood-brain barrier, promoting the penetration of immune cells, which can cause additional brain damage. The inflammatory response also increases the production of free radicals, leading to oxidative stress and further brain cell damage [28]. Therefore, a recent study suggests that anti-inflammatory interventions can improve cognitive function in cases of cognitive decline following cerebral injury, as observed in animal research [41].

The brain attempts to form new neural pathways through neuroplasticity to compensate for areas damaged by cerebral infarction, but this process is not always successful. Cognitive decline can persist if the damaged networks are not properly restored [1].

When blood vessels rupture due to hypertension or vascular dysmorphia in cerebral hemorrhage, blood leaks into the brain tissue. This increases cerebral pressure by forming brain edema and hematoma. The leaked blood compresses and physically damages the brain tissue, destroying the neural network in the area. Additionally, bleeding increases the permeability of the blood-brain barrier, promoting an inflammatory response and the penetration of immune cells, causing further damage to brain tissue [38].

After a cerebral hemorrhage, iron accumulates during the process of blood decomposition, causing oxidative stress that is toxic to brain cells. Hemoglobin and its degradation product, hemosiderin, are particularly neurotoxic [16]. As with cerebral infarction, the brain attempts to reorganize the neural network through neuroplasticity even after cerebral hemorrhage. However, this process is limited due to the extensive damage to the affected area and its surroundings [1].

Let us look at the specific effects of these cerebral infarction and cerebral hemorrhage that lead to cognitive impairment. Both conditions directly damage areas that manage memory, such as the hippocampus, negatively affecting short-term and long-term memory formation [40]. The frontal lobe, responsible for planning, judgment, and problem-solving abilities, can suffer from deteriorated executive function when damaged by cerebral infarction or hemorrhage. Damage to language centers, such as Broca's area or Wernicke's area, impairs language expression and comprehension. Simultaneous damage to the frontal and parietal lobes results in attention loss, significantly impacting daily life [10].

### *5.2.2 Microbleeds and Microinfarcts*

Microbleed is a phenomenon in which bleeding occurs in small blood vessels in the brain, primarily detected through MRI scans. It is caused by degenerative changes in blood vessel walls, hypertension, amyloid vasculopathy, and other factors. Microbleed involves blood leaking into brain tissue, causing direct damage to surrounding tissues. This can damage the blood-brain barrier and trigger an inflammatory response. When bleeding occurs, immune cells rush to the damaged area, exacerbating inflammation and causing additional brain tissue damage, which reduces cognitive function. This mild chronic inflammation increases the production of free radicals, leading to oxidative damage to brain cells, thus sustaining and accelerating cognitive impairment.

Microinfarcts occur when small blood vessels in the brain become blocked, causing brain tissue to become necrotic. It can result from hypertension, diabetes, hyperlipidemia, and other causes. When small blood vessels are blocked, the affected area experiences reduced blood flow, leading to hypoxia and cell death. If the hypoxic state persists, nerve cells become necrotic, losing their function. This particularly damages the white matter, contributing to cognitive decline. Although microscopic infarctions occur in small areas, they have cascading effects along the brain's neural network, reducing neural connectivity and resulting in decreased information processing speed and cognitive function.

### *5.2.3 Leukoaraiosis*

Leukoaraiosis refers to chronic ischemic injury that primarily occurs in the white matter of the brain. This condition is mainly observed as hyperintensity in MRI scans and is characterized by impaired nerve connectivity due to white matter damage. It is primarily caused by chronic diseases such as hypertension, diabetes, and hyperlipidemia, which weaken nerve connectivity in the brain and lead to cognitive decline. Leukoaraiosis specifically affects executive function, information processing speed, and attention span. The severity of leukoaraiosis identified in MRI scans is associated with the degree of depression and cognitive impairment in stroke patients [43]. It is known that leukoaraiosis can improve with the treatment of hypertension. Additionally, monitoring for leukoaraiosis in individuals with normal cognitive function can help prevent cognitive impairment [14].

### *5.2.4 Types of Vascular Dementia*

Vascular dementia is characterized by memory loss and cognitive decline caused by cerebrovascular diseases, including infarcts and leukoaraiosis. Vascular dementia can be classified into several types based on the location of the lesion causing the vascular pathology or dementia. These types include multi-infarct dementia, subcortical ischemic vascular dementia, strategic infarct dementia, hypoperfusion dementia, and hemorrhage-associated dementia. Among them, strategic infarct dementia occurs due to a single lesion in areas such as the caudate nucleus, medial frontal lobe, or genu of the internal capsule. Leukoaraiosis, which means white matter hypotonicity, caused by small vessel cerebral infarction or incomplete infarction from microvascular disease, primarily affects the prefrontal-subcortical circuit. As a result, subcortical dysfunctions such as bradyphrenia and apraxia may appear, rather than traditional dementia symptoms like memory loss [12, 25].

## 5.3 Vascular Risk Factors

The main vascular risk factors for cognitive disorders include old age, hypertension, diabetes, smoking, cardiovascular disease, and atrial fibrillation. Cardiovascular disease, mild cognitive impairment (MCI), and dementia often occur together. Most vascular risk factors for cognitive disorders are preventable, so it is essential to manage these risk factors adequately before cognitive impairment occurs [17].

### *5.3.1 Hypertension*

Hypertension is one of the major risk factors for cerebrovascular disease, especially stroke. In examining the factors contributing to the development of stroke and stroke-related death, hypertension showed the greatest contribution, surpassing diabetes and dyslipidemia. The global and regional effects of potentially modifiable risk factors associated with acute stroke in 32 countries (INTERSTROKE) study comprehensively analyzed and identified the risk factors for stroke, confirming that hypertension poses the highest risk for developing stroke among all stroke risk factors [32].

Endothelial cells in the vessels are responsible for the relaxation and contraction of blood vessels, blood flow control, and anti-inflammatory and anticoagulant functions. Hypertension damages these vascular endothelial cells, leading to endothelial dysfunction. As a result, blood vessels become rigid, and blood flow is impaired, reducing the supply of oxygen and nutrients to the brain. This causes brain cell damage and eventually leads to cognitive decline [29].

If hypertension patients with normal cognitive function do not maintain proper blood pressure, the continuous high blood pressure damages small blood vessels in the brain, causing microvascular lesions. This results in chronic ischemic damage to both white matter and gray matter in the brain, leading to leukoaraiosis and microbleeds, which ultimately cause cognitive impairment as mentioned above [44].

Hypertension can also induce an inflammatory response by damaging vascular endothelial cells. It promotes the secretion of inflammatory mediators such as cytokines, causing additional brain damage. If proper blood pressure is not maintained, cognitive decline is accelerated by continuous inflammatory reactions [4]. Increased oxidative stress is also associated with hypertension and promotes the production of reactive oxygen species. Brain damage caused by oxidative stress can lead to apoptosis, resulting in permanent cognitive impairment [9].

Hypertension is known to reduce the thickness of the cerebral cortex, particularly affecting the frontal and parietal lobes. Without proper blood pressure management, this can lead to cognitive declines such as impaired executive function, reduced attention span, and slower information processing speed [2].

Patients with hypertension and normal cognitive function should maintain proper blood pressure (≥ 140/90 mmHg) to prevent cognitive decline. Among antihypertensive drugs, calcium channel blockers and renin-angiotensin system blockers are known to be associated with the prevention of cognitive decline as well as dementia [35]. However, intensive blood pressure management in the elderly may cause hypotension or blood pressure variability, potentially leading to cognitive decline. Therefore, appropriate blood pressure management is essential in adult patients with hypertension to prevent cognitive decline, but careful monitoring is required in the elderly [50].

The systolic blood pressure intervention-trial memory and cognition in decreased hypertension (SPRINT-MIND) study compared the risk of developing dementia in patients with hypertension when the treatment goal for systolic blood pressure was set at 120 mmHg versus 140 mmHg. The risk of developing dementia in the group with systolic blood pressure targeted to 120 mmHg tended to decrease by 15% compared to the 140 mmHg control group, but this was not statistically significant. In contrast, the risk of developing mild cognitive impairment was significantly lower by 19% in the 120 mmHg group than in the 140 mmHg control group. The results of this study provide important evidence for identifying the association between antihypertensive treatment and cognitive decline in patients with hypertension [20]. In addition, the post hoc analysis of the SPRINT-MIND study revealed that high variability in systolic blood pressure was associated with an increased risk of dementia [8].

According to several randomized controlled studies, antihypertensive treatment in patients with hypertension reduces the risk of dementia by approximately 7–11%. In particular, in elderly patients with hypertension, antihypertensive treatment is associated with a lower risk of developing dementia. This trend was observed in very old and frail patients with hypertension. However, intensive antihypertensive treatment in elderly individuals with hypertension may increase the risk of orthostatic hypotension and related complications. The optimal target blood pressure and the best antihypertensive drugs for elderly patients with orthostatic hypotension still need to be studied. Additionally, research is needed to determine the optimal target blood pressure and antihypertensive drugs to prevent both cardiovascular disease and cognitive decline [5, 33].

### 5.3.2 Diabetes

Diabetes has a complex mechanism, with insulin resistance playing an important role. Diabetes is known as a modifiable risk factor for dementia, and individuals with diabetes have a higher risk of cognitive decline than those without diabetes. Therefore, it is essential to understand the effect of diabetes on cognitive decline [37].

Hyperglycemia in patients with diabetes increases metabolic stress in brain neurons and promotes oxidative stress and inflammatory reactions, causing brain cell damage. Diabetes can also cause mild chronic inflammatory conditions and is associated with increased oxidative stress [22].

Patients with diabetes have high insulin resistance, leading to a state where nerve cells do not receive insulin signals properly. This insulin resistance interferes with the proper signaling of nerve cells, promoting neuronal degeneration and increasing the risk of diseases such as Alzheimer's disease and vascular dementia. Animal studies have shown that diabetes affects glycogen metabolism in the brain, disrupting the metabolic balance and energy supply, damaging the homeostasis of energy and neurotransmitters [39].

Similarly to hypertension, diabetes increases the risk of macrovascular complications such as arteriosclerosis. As a result, cerebrovascular narrowing can increase the risk of cerebral infarction, cerebral hemorrhage, and other cerebrovascular diseases [46].

Elderly patients with diabetes are known to have a higher risk of cognitive decline, including vascular dementia, compared to elderly patients without diabetes. Therefore, the American Diabetes Association recommends that elderly patients with diabetes should take cognitive function screening tests at the first visit, annually, and as needed, for early diagnosis of mild cognitive impairment and dementia [13].

### 5.3.3 Dyslipidemia

Dyslipidemia refers to an abnormal balance of lipids (cholesterol and triglycerides) in the blood. Dyslipidemia can negatively affect cognitive function through various mechanisms. The primary mechanisms include arteriosclerosis, inflammatory reactions, oxidative stress, changes in brain structure, and beta-amyloid accumulation, all of which can lead to cognitive decline and impairment. Active management of hyperlipidemia is crucial for maintaining cognitive health.

Dyslipidemia typically involves increased levels of low-density lipoprotein (LDL) cholesterol and decreased levels of high-density lipoprotein (HDL) cholesterol, which promote arteriosclerosis. Arteriosclerosis refers to a condition in which lipid deposits build up on the walls of arteries, narrowing and stiffening the blood vessels. These vascular changes reduce blood flow to the brain, limiting the supply of oxygen and nutrients needed for brain cells [21].

Dyslipidemia is also associated with chronic inflammation. Plaque accumulation in the arteries due to dyslipidemia promotes an inflammatory response. Inflammatory mediators damage brain tissue and impair the function of brain neurons, causing cognitive impairment. The exacerbation of arteriosclerosis caused by dyslipidemia leads to the overproduction of reactive oxygen species, which can cause oxidative stress. This eventually promotes the death of brain neurons, resulting in decreased cognitive function [3].

Accumulation of amyloid beta in the brain is a major cause of Alzheimer's disease. Recently, studies have investigated the association between cholesterol and amyloid beta. The results vary across studies, indicating different outcomes for this association. Due to the complex role of cholesterol and the difficulty in researching amyloid beta accumulation in humans, a clear mechanism for the relationship between the two needs to be elucidated in the future [23, 36].

Several studies have shown that patients with dyslipidemia tend to score low on cognitive function evaluations. To manage dyslipidemia in preventing cognitive decline, the treatment with cholesterol-lowering agents such as statins, along with a low-carb, low-fat diet, and regular, appropriate exercise, is essential [15, 48].

According to the American Heart Association (AHA) guidelines published in 2023, among patients with atherosclerotic cardiovascular disease (ASCVD), such as those who have had a myocardial infarction within the prior year, peripheral artery disease, type 2 diabetes, and polyvascular disease, it is recommended to lower their LDL cholesterol levels below the reinforced target goal to reduce their risk of ASCVD-related complications. Regarding lowering LDL cholesterol levels, some past studies have reported a relationship between statin therapy and low LDL cholesterol levels with an increased risk of cognitive disorders, such as dementia, but the exact causal relationship is not yet certain. Therefore, it is recommended to set the lower LDL cholesterol target goal according to the individual's ASCVD risk and treat them accordingly, compared to past guidelines. There is no solid evidence that cholesterol-lowering medications such as statins, PCSK9 inhibitors, and ezetimibe increase the risk of bleeding, including hemorrhagic stroke, in the treatment of dyslipidemia. There is also little evidence that maintaining a very low LDL cholesterol level increases the risk of hemorrhagic stroke, unless patients with inherently low LDL-C levels are particularly susceptible to hemorrhagic stroke. Therefore, among individuals with a high risk of ASCVD, lowering the LDL cholesterol level according to the target goal of AHA guidelines should not be hindered by concerns about the risk of hemorrhagic stroke, which has not yet been proven [19].

### *5.3.4 Smoking and Alcohol Consumption*

Smoking, like chronic diseases, can cause cognitive decline through a number of mechanisms. Fortunately, the rate of tobacco use is decreasing worldwide, but in recent years, the rate of e-cigarettes use has been increasing. Therefore, smoking cessation education is required in clinical practices.

Smoking constricts blood vessels and reduces blood flow through harmful chemicals such as nicotine and carbon monoxide. This reduction in blood flow, particularly to the brain, limits the supply of oxygen and nutrients. As a result, decreased brain blood flow adversely affects brain cell metabolism, causing persistent hypoxia and resulting in brain cell damage [31]. Chronic inflammation and increased oxidative stress persist in smokers, which is associated with an increased risk of Alzheimer's disease and vascular dementia [6].

Smoking causes imbalances in neurotransmitters such as dopamine and serotonin. While nicotine temporarily increases dopamine secretion, it decreases the sensitivity of dopamine receptors over time. This imbalance of neurotransmitters can lead to various cognitive declines, such as mood disorders, attention deficits, and memory loss [45].

According to previous studies, nicotine is associated with amyloid beta accumulation in smokers. Additionally, heavy smokers are known to have higher levels of tau protein than non-smokers. This relationship suggests a high risk of Alzheimer's disease or cognitive impairment in smokers. However, further research is needed to elucidate the exact mechanism [24, 47].

When smokers quit smoking, the negative effects on the brain are largely reduced. Brain blood flow improves, oxidative stress and inflammation decrease, and neurotransmitter levels in the brain return to balance. Therefore, smoking cessation education is needed to prevent cognitive impairment, even in those who have not yet shown signs of cognitive decline [42].

Alcohol consumption affects cognitive function in both the short and long terms. It can interfere with the function of the hippocampus, leading to temporary forgetfulness (also called "memory blackout") by impairing short-term memory. Additionally, alcohol consumption inhibits the function of the prefrontal cortex, reducing attention and concentration and thereby impairing the ability to perform complex tasks. When consuming alcohol, the central nervous system is inhibited, slowing reaction times and reducing judgment and decision-making abilities [49].

Continuous long-term alcohol consumption causes brain atrophy, leading to chronic memory loss. In particular, long-term alcohol abuse can result in alcoholic dementia. Persistent alcohol consumption impairs not only memory but also learning ability, problem-solving skills, and logical thinking. In severe cases, alcohol can damage brain cells, leading to encephalopathy such as Wernicke-Korsakoff syndrome, which causes memory damage, confusion, and motor dysfunction [34].

From a neurophysiological perspective, alcohol consumption activates gamma-aminobutyric acid (GABA) receptors and inhibits glutamate receptors, thereby reducing the excitation of the central nervous system. This can cause excessive sedation and temporary cognitive decline [7].

The negative effects of excessive alcohol consumption may differ depending on genetic factors [11]. The elderly and women may be more sensitive to alcohol [26, 30] Previously, in the case of patients with mental disorders, the negative effects of alcohol may be further increased [27].

Avoiding alcohol or drinking less is necessary to prevent cognitive decline caused by alcohol consumption. Long-term alcohol abuse adversely affects cognitive function permanently, so it is crucial to detect signs of alcohol abuse early even in patients with normal cognitive function.

## 5.4 Conclusions

Cognitive decline, including vascular dementia, is closely associated with cerebrovascular disease. Vascular dementia can be prevented by properly treating and managing important risk factors such as hypertension, diabetes, dyslipidemia, smoking, and alcohol drinking to prevent atherosclerosis of the cerebrovascular system. In particular, it is crucial to effectively manage hypertension, diabetes, and dyslipidemia in elderly patients, as these are major risk factors for cerebrovascular diseases to help prevent vascular dementia.

## References

1. Alia C, Spalletti C, Lai S, Panarese A, Lamola G, Bertolucci F, Vallone F, Di Garbo A, Chisari C, Micera S, Caleo M. Neuroplastic changes following brain ischemia and their contribution to stroke recovery: novel approaches in neurorehabilitation. Front Cell Neurosci. 2017;11:76.
2. Alosco ML, Gunstad J, Xu X, Clark US, Labbe DR, Riskin-Jones HH, Terrero G, Schwarz NF, Walsh EG, Poppas A, Cohen RA, Sweet LH. The impact of hypertension on cerebral perfusion and cortical thickness in older adults. J Am Soc Hypertens. 2014;8:561–70.
3. Amiya E. Interaction of hyperlipidemia and reactive oxygen species: insights from the lipid-raft platform. World J Cardiol. 2016;8:689–94.
4. Baggeroer CE, Cambronero FE, Savan NA, Jefferson AL, Santisteban MM. Basic mechanisms of brain injury and cognitive decline in hypertension. Hypertension. 2024;81:34–44.
5. Canavan M, O'donnell MJ. Hypertension and cognitive impairment: A review of mechanisms and key concepts. Front Neurol. 2022;13:821135.
6. Choi D, Choi S, Park SM. Effect of smoking cessation on the risk of dementia: a longitudinal study. Ann Clin Transl Neurol. 2018;5:1192–9.
7. Davies M. The role of GABAA receptors in mediating the effects of alcohol in the central nervous system. J Psychiatry Neurosci. 2003;28:263–74.
8. De Havenon A, Anadani M, Prabhakaran S, Wong KH, Yaghi S, Rost N. Increased blood pressure variability and the risk of probable dementia or mild cognitive impairment: A post hoc analysis of the SPRINT MIND trial. J Am Heart Assoc. 2021;10:e022206.
9. Di Chiara T, Del Cuore A, Daidone M, Scaglione S, Norrito RL, Puleo MG, Scaglione R, Pinto A, Tuttolomondo A. Pathogenetic mechanisms of hypertension-brain-induced complications: focus on molecular mediators. Int J Mol Sci. 2022;23:2445.
10. Duncan KR. Neuropsychiatric symptoms after stroke. Curr Psychiatry. 2022;21:31.
11. Edenberg HJ, Foroud T. Genetics and alcoholism. Nat Rev Gastroenterol Hepatol. 2013;10:487–94.
12. Elahi FM, Miller BL. A clinicopathological approach to the diagnosis of dementia. Nat Rev Neurol. 2017;13:457–76.

13. Elsayed NA, Aleppo G, Aroda VR, Bannuru RR, Brown FM, Bruemmer D, Collins BS, Hilliard ME, Isaacs D, Johnson EL, Kahan S, Khunti K, Leon J, Lyons SK, Perry ML, Prahalad P, Pratley RE, Jeffrie Seley J, Stanton RC, Gabbay RA, Association OBOTAD. 13. Older adults: standards of care in diabetes—2023. Diabetes Care. 2022;46:S216–29.
14. Filley CM. Cognitive dysfunction in white matter disorders: new perspectives in treatment and recovery. J Neuropsychiatry Clin Neurosci. 2021;33:349–55.
15. Fu M, Bakulski KM, Higgins C, Ware EB. Mendelian randomization of dyslipidemia on cognitive impairment among older Americans. Front Neurol. 2021;12:660212.
16. Galea I, Durnford A, Glazier J, Mitchell S, Kohli S, Foulkes L, Norman J, Darekar A, Love S, Bulters DO, Nicoll JAR, Boche D. Iron deposition in the brain after aneurysmal subarachnoid hemorrhage. Stroke. 2022;53:1633–42.
17. Ganguli M, Fu B, Snitz BE, Unverzagt FW, Loewenstein DA, Hughes TF, Chang C-CH. Vascular risk factors and cognitive decline in a population sample. Alzheimer Dis Assoc Disord. 2014;28:9–15.
18. Girnar GA, Mahajan HS. Cerebral ischemic stroke and different approaches for treatment of stroke. Future J Pharm Sci. 2021;7:134.
19. Goldstein LB, Toth PP, Dearborn-Tomazos JL, Giugliano RP, Hirsh BJ, Pena JM, Selim MH, Woo D, American Heart Association Council On Arteriosclerosis T, Vascular B, Council On C, Stroke N, Council On Peripheral Vascular D, Stroke C. Aggressive LDL-C lowering and the brain: impact on risk for dementia and hemorrhagic stroke: A scientific statement from the American Heart Association. Arterioscler Thromb Vasc Biol. 2023;43:e404–42.
20. Group TSMIFTSR. Effect of intensive vs standard blood pressure control on probable dementia: A randomized clinical trial. JAMA. 2019;321:553–61.
21. Ha SH, Kim BJ. Dyslipidemia treatment and cerebrovascular disease: evidence regarding the mechanism of stroke. J Lipid Atheroscler. 2024;13:139–54.
22. Hoyos CM, Stephen C, Turner A, Ireland C, Naismith SL, Duffy SL. Brain oxidative stress and cognitive function in older adults with diabetes and pre-diabetes who are at risk for dementia. Diabetes Res Clin Pract. 2022;184:109178.
23. Hu N, Gao L, Jiang Y, Wei S, Shang S, Chen C, Dang L, Wang J, Huo K, Deng M, Wang J, Qu Q. The relationship between blood lipids and plasma amyloid beta is depend on blood pressure: a population-based cross-sectional study. Lipids Health Dis. 2020;19:8.
24. Hu H, Fu JT, Bi YL, Ma YH, Huang YY, Wang X, Tan L, Yu JT. Tau pathologies mediate the association of cigarette smoking with cognitive impairment in older adults without dementia: the CABLE study. J Alzheimer's Dis. 2022;86:1849–59.
25. Lee AY. Vascular dementia. Chonnam Med J. 2011;47:66–71.
26. Meier P, Seitz HK. Age, alcohol metabolism and liver disease. Curr Opin Clin Nutr Metab Care. 2008;11:21–6.
27. Milani RM, Perrino L. Chapter 4 - Alcohol and mental health: co-occurring alcohol use and mental health disorders. In: Frings D, Albery IP, editors. The handbook of alcohol use. Academic Press; 2021.
28. Milosevich E, Demeyere N, Pendlebury ST. Infection, inflammation, and poststroke cognitive impairment. J Am Heart Assoc. 2024;13:e9130.
29. Mone P, Gambardella J, Pansini A, De Donato A, Martinelli G, Boccalone E, Matarese A, Frullone S, Santulli G. Cognitive impairment in frail hypertensive elderly patients: role of hyperglycemia. Cells. 2021;10:2115.
30. Mumenthaler MS, Taylor JL, O'hara R, Yesavage JA. Gender differences in moderate drinking effects. Alcohol Res Health. 1999;23:55–64.
31. Nah S, Choi S, Lee SU, Kim GW, Lee YH, Han S. Effects of smoking on delayed neuropsychiatric sequelae in acute carbon monoxide poisoning: A prospective observational study. Medicine (Baltimore). 2021;100:e26032.
32. O'donnell MJ, Chin SL, Rangarajan S, Xavier D, Liu L, Zhang H, Rao-Melacini P, Zhang X, Pais P, Agapay S, Lopez-Jaramillo P, Damasceno A, Langhorne P, Mcqueen MJ, Rosengren A, Dehghan M, Hankey GJ, Dans AL, Elsayed A, Avezum A, Mondo C, Diener HC, Ryglewicz

D, Czlonkowska A, Pogosova N, Weimar C, Iqbal R, Diaz R, Yusoff K, Yusufali A, Oguz A, Wang X, Penaherrera E, Lanas F, Ogah OS, Ogunniyi A, Iversen HK, Malaga G, Rumboldt Z, Oveisgharan S, Al Hussain F, Magazi D, Nilanont Y, Ferguson J, Pare G, Yusuf S, Investigators I. Global and regional effects of potentially modifiable risk factors associated with acute stroke in 32 countries (INTERSTROKE): a case-control study. Lancet. 2016;388:761–75.

33. Rea F, Corrao G, Mancia G. Risk of dementia during antihypertensive drug therapy in the elderly. J Am Coll Cardiol. 2024;83:1194–203.
34. Ridley NJ, Draper B, Withall A. Alcohol-related dementia: an update of the evidence. Alzheimer's Res Ther. 2013;5:3.
35. Rouch L, Cestac P, Hanon O, Cool C, Helmer C, Bouhanick B, Chamontin B, Dartigues JF, Vellas B, Andrieu S. Antihypertensive drugs, prevention of cognitive decline and dementia: a systematic review of observational studies, randomized controlled trials and meta-analyses, with discussion of potential mechanisms. CNS Drugs. 2015;29:113–30.
36. Rudajev V, Novotny J. Cholesterol as a key player in amyloid beta-mediated toxicity in Alzheimer's disease. Front Mol Neurosci. 2022;15:937056.
37. Sebastian MJ, Khan SK, Pappachan JM, Jeeyavudeen MS. Diabetes and cognitive function: an evidence-based current perspective. World J Diabetes. 2023;14:92–109.
38. Shao Z, Tu S, Shao A. Pathophysiological mechanisms and potential therapeutic targets in intracerebral hemorrhage. Front Pharmacol. 2019;10:1079.
39. Sickmann HM, Waagepetersen HS. Effects of diabetes on brain metabolism--is brain glycogen a significant player? Metab Brain Dis. 2015;30:335–43.
40. Szabo K. Hippocampal stroke. *Front Neurol Neurosci.* 2014;34:150–6.
41. Tack RWP, Amboni C, Van Nuijs D, Pekna M, Vergouwen MDI, Rinkel GJE, Hol EM. Inflammation, anti-inflammatory interventions, and post-stroke cognitive impairment: a systematic review and meta-analysis of human and animal studies. Transl Stroke Res. 2023;16:535.
42. Tavee J. Smoking cessation for the neurologic patient. Neurol Clin Pract. 2012;2:112–21.
43. Tziaka E, Christidi F, Tsiptsios D, Sousanidou A, Karatzetzou S, Tsiakiri A, Doskas TK, Tsamakis K, Retzepis N, Konstantinidis C, Kokkotis C, Serdari A, Aggelousis N, Vadikolias K. Leukoaraiosis as a predictor of depression and cognitive impairment among stroke survivors: A systematic review. Neurol Int. 2023;15:238–72.
44. Ungvari Z, Toth P, Tarantini S, Prodan CI, Sorond F, Merkely B, Csiszar A. Hypertension-induced cognitive impairment: from pathophysiology to public health. Nat Rev Nephrol. 2021;17:639–54.
45. Valentine G, Sofuoglu M. Cognitive effects of nicotine: recent progress. Curr Neuropharmacol. 2018;16:403–14.
46. Viigimaa M, Sachinidis A, Toumpourleka M, Koutsampasopoulos K, Alliksoo S, Titma T. Macrovascular complications of type 2 diabetes mellitus. Curr Vasc Pharmacol. 2020;18:110–6.
47. Wallin C, Sholts SB, Österlund N, Luo J, Jarvet J, Roos PM, Ilag L, Gräslund A, Wärmländer S. Alzheimer's disease and cigarette smoke components: effects of nicotine, PAHs, and Cd(II), Cr(III), Pb(II), Pb(IV) ions on amyloid-β peptide aggregation. Sci Rep. 2017;7:14423.
48. Wee J, Sukudom S, Bhat S, Marklund M, Peiris NJ, Hoyos CM, Patel S, Naismith SL, Dwivedi G, Misra A. The relationship between midlife dyslipidemia and lifetime incidence of dementia: A systematic review and meta-analysis of cohort studies. Alzheimers Dement (Amst). 2023;15:e12395.
49. White AM. What happened? Alcohol, memory blackouts, and the brain. Alcohol Res Health. 2003;27:186–96.
50. Yang W, Luo H, Ma Y, Si S, Zhao H. Effects of antihypertensive drugs on cognitive function in elderly patients with hypertension: A review. Aging Dis. 2021;12:841–51.

# Chapter 6
# Neuropathological Diagnoses of Dementia

**Rajka M. Liscic**

**Abstract** Alzheimer's disease (AD) is a progressive neurodegenerative disease of the brain and the most common cause of dementia among elderly people worldwide, accounting for at least two-thirds of all dementia cases. Macroscopically, a general cerebral atrophy is a hallmark of AD. Microscopically, prone features include diffuse and neuritic extracellular plaques composed of amyloid beta (Aβ) peptides frequently surrounded by dystrophic neurites, and intraneuronal neurofibrillary tangles (NFT) composed of paired helical filaments of phosphorylated tau proteins. These hallmark pathologies are often accompanied by reactive microgliosis and synapse loss. The neuropathological staging of AD in research centers may be performed using the Braak and Braak (1991) staging, where NFT and neuritic plaques exhibit a distribution pattern used to classify the degree of pathology into six stages.

Frontotemporal dementia is a lesser known but equally devastating condition. Frontotemporal lobar degeneration (FTLD) represents a group of disorders that is considered to be clinically and pathologically distinct from AD. Macroscopically, there may be focal atrophy of the frontal and temporal lobes with variable involvement of the striatum. FTLD is genetically, neuropathologically, and clinically heterogeneous and may present as a dementia with three major clinical syndromes dominated by behavioral, language, and motor disorders, respectively. Most of these diseases are characterized by the pathological aggregation of misfolded proteins, either in neurons or glial cells, or both. About half of these cases have abnormal intracellular cytoplasmic accumulations of the microtubule-associated protein tau (MAPT). The characteristic aggregate-forming protein in non-tau FTLD is either TAR DNA-binding protein 43 (TDP-43), the most frequent protein or RNA-binding Fused in Sarcoma (FUS) protein or FUS. Additionally, inflammation mediated by activated microglia is an important component of AD pathophysiology, and neuritic plaques and neurofibrillary tangles are foci of a local inflammatory response.

R. M. Liscic (✉)
Department of Neurology, Median Klinik, Bad Wildungen, Germany

Josip Juraj Strossmayer University of Osijek, School of Medicine, Osijek, Croatia



Y.-H. Yang (ed.), *Management of Dementia from the Preclinical Stage*,
https://doi.org/10.1007/978-981-95-5222-1_6

The pathogenic mechanisms implicated in neurodegenerative disorders are not linked to individual clinical entities. Neuroinflammation is probably a common cause across the disease spectrum. In contrast, neurodegenerative pathogenesis shows a considerable overlap in protein misfolding and aggregation. The overlapping proteinopathies /comorbidities exist throughout the entire spectrum of most neurodegenerative disorders. Notably, these comorbidities may often influence the main pathology and affect both disease progression, cognitive decline and duration of the disease.

**Keywords** Alzheimer's disease · Frontotemporal dementia · Amyloid · Tau · Pathological diagnosis · AD staging

## 6.1 Introduction

Alzheimer's disease (AD) is a progressive neurodegenerative disease and the most frequent cause of dementia among elderly people worldwide, accounting for at least two-thirds of all dementia cases [1]. Macroscopically, AD is characterized by generalized cerebral atrophy, in particular, the medial temporal lobe being most affected (Fig. 6.1). Microscopically, AD is characterized by two lesions: the neurofibrillary tangles (tau aggregates forming neurofibrillary tangles) and the neuritic plaques (amyloid beta—Aβ) (Fig. 6.2) accompanied by synaptic loss and vascular amyloid deposits. Plaques contain a protein Aβ, which morphologically may present differently as either including diffuse plaques and compact or neuritic plaques. Aβ can, however, also be found in many superficial blood vessels referred to as cerebral amyloid angiopathy, which is frequently surrounded by dystrophic neurites and intraneuronal neurofibrillary tangles (NFT). These NFTs are composed of paired

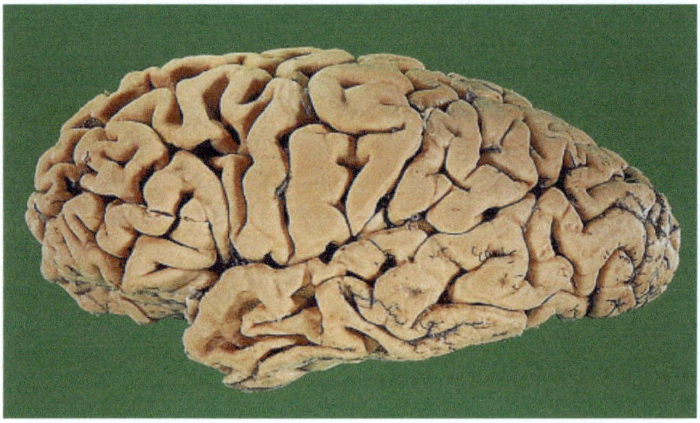

**Fig. 6.1** Lateral view showing severe atrophy of the temporal lobe with less severe atrophy of the parietal and frontal lobes. The occipital lobe is spared. The pattern of atrophy typically seen in AD is characteristic, but not specific for the disease. (Courtesy of Professor Nigel J. Cairns, PhD, FRCPath, University of Exeter, Exeter, UK)

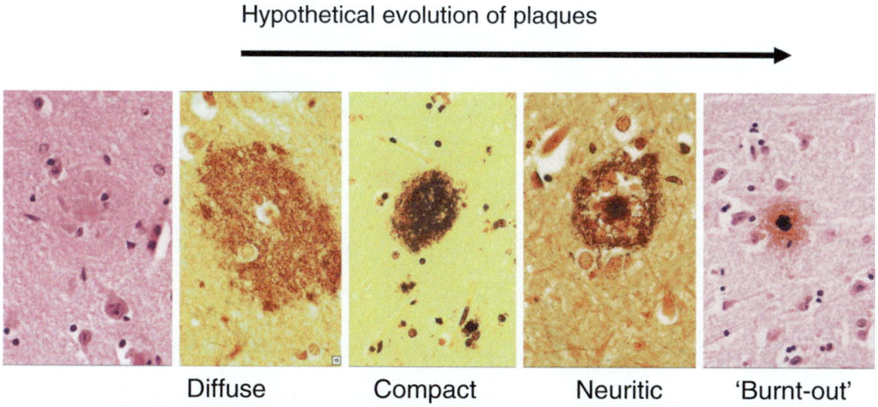


**Fig. 6.2** The evolution of plaques in the course of Alzheimer's disease. Diffuse plaques, are extracellular defined focal aggregates of amyloid and pre-amyloid material and are about 60–300 mm in diameter. They are, also called benign plaques, and occur much earlier than the neuritic plaques, thus supporting the idea of a therapeutic interventions in the early stage of the disease. Neuronal cell processes traversing the plaque appear normal and do not contain tau protein. Diffuse plaques may be detected by using silver stains sensitive for amyloid, but are best demonstrated by immunohistochemistry for Aβ peptide after formic acid pretreatment of sections. (Courtesy of Professor Nigel J. Cairns, PhD, MRCPath, University of Exeter, Exeter, UK)

helical filaments of phosphorylated tau proteins [2]. These lesions are typically accompanied by reactive astrocytosis, microgliosis, and loss of neurons and synapses. The neuropathological diagnosis of AD has been based on the criteria of Khachaturian [3], the Consortium to Establish a Registry for Alzheimer's Disease [2], and the National Institutes of Aging-Reagan Institute (NIA-Reagan Institute) criteria [4]. The latter criteria are most often used in the clinic today. The neuropathological staging of AD in research centers may be performed using the Braak & Braak staging [5], where NFT and neuritic plaques present a characteristic distribution pattern used to classify the degree of pathology into six stages.

The first two stages are characterized by either mild or severe alteration of the transentorhinal layer pre-alpha (stages I-II). The two forms of limbic stages (stages III-IV) are marked by a conspicuous involvement of layer pre-alpha neurons in both the transenthorinal region and the entorhinal cortex. In addition, there is mild involvement of the Ammon's horn sector 1. The predominant feature of the two isocortical stages (stages V-VI) is the destruction of virtually all isocortical association areas (Figs. 6.3 and 6.4).

Abnormal metabolism of Aβ is considered the major pathogenic mechanism in AD, initiating the "amyloid cascade hypothesis." Dysfunctional Aβ clearance has been hypothesized to be a reason for Aβ accumulation in patients with sporadic AD, which typically precedes spreading of tau, neuronal loss, and ultimately clinical manifestations by up to 20–30 years [6]. Therefore, an imbalance between the production and clearance of Aβ is generally recognized as an initiating factor in early-onset AD, and the common late-onset form of AD may be characterized by an

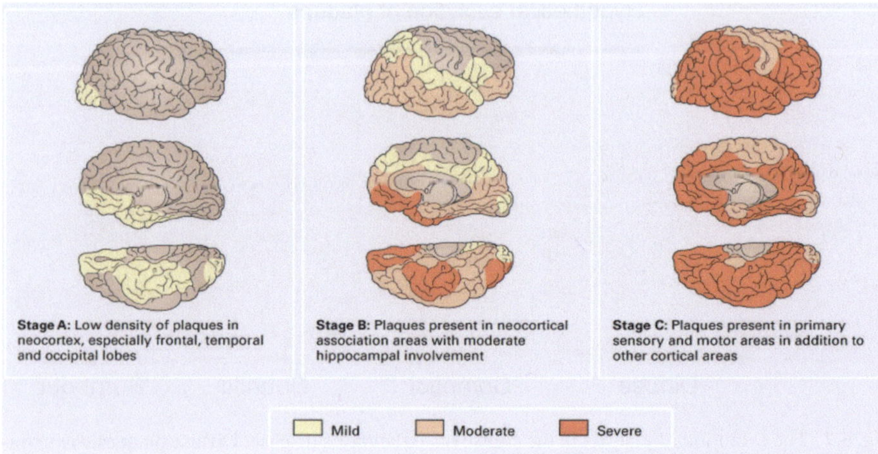


*(Braak H et al. Acta Neuropathologica 1991;82:239-259)*

**Fig. 6.3** Braak & Braak staging. Amyloid beta plaques show poor correlation with dementia severity. On contrary, NFT (neurofibrillary tangles) intraneuronal structure composed of paired helical filaments of phosphorylated tau protein show good correlation with dementia severity

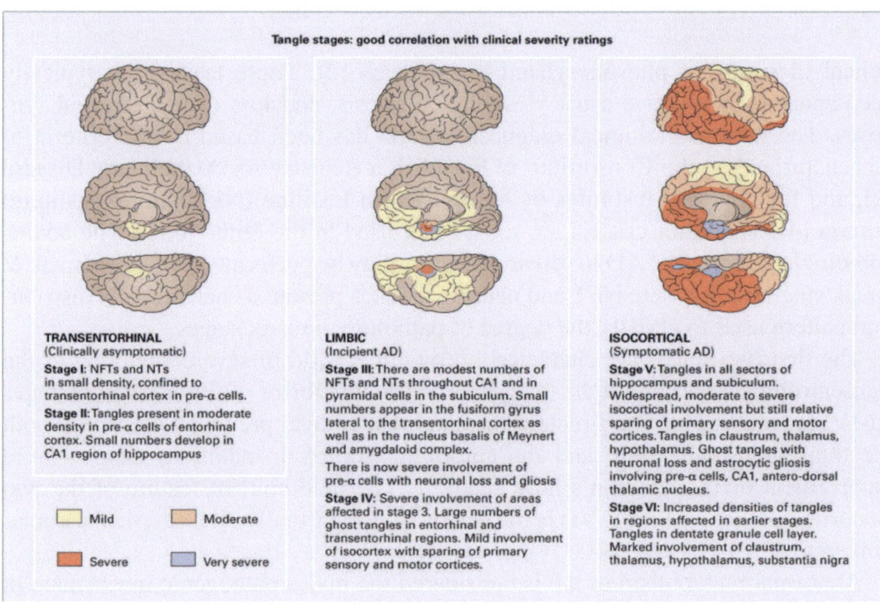


**Fig. 6.4** Braak & Braak staging: Neurofibrilary tangels (NFT) stages: good correlation with severity of dementia

overall impairment in Aβ clearance. Improving Aβ production/clearance is a promising therapeutic strategy for AD [7].

The etiological mechanisms underlying the neuropathological changes in AD still remain unclear. In recent years, however, neuroinflammatory factors and environmental and genetic factors, as well are becoming more important [8].

Out of all AD cases, up to 3% are familial, caused by an autosomal dominant mutation with three thus far identified genes: the amyloid precursor protein (*APP*), presenilin 1 (*PSEN 1*), and presenilin 2 (*PSEN 2*) [9]. The Aβ peptide is cleaved from the APP by the sequential activities of β-secretase and γ-secretase enzymes. Aβ occurs in multiple forms, including those ranging from 37 to 43 amino acids in length. Among these, Aβ42 seems to be essential for initiating Aβ aggregation and is considered central to the amyloid cascade hypothesis of AD [6, 10, 11]. The Apolipoprotein E (APOE) ε4 allele is the most important genetic risk factor for sporadic AD [12]. Sporadic AD (about 97% of cases), however, often results from a combination of genetic and environmental risk factors, with neuroinflammation, contributing to the neuron damage and death.

The microtubule-associated protein (MAP) tau is a major protein component of the intraneuronal NFT and is elevated in the Cerebrospinal Fluid (CSF) of most AD patients. Human tau is transcribed from the *MAPT* gene located on chromosome 17. Tau is produced intracellularly and is expressed predominantly in the axons of CNS neurons. Total-tau, as a biomarker of neuronal injury, can transiently increase after any acute brain injury, such as stroke or physical trauma [14]. The abnormal phosphorylated tau (p-tau), which is three to four-fold more hyperphosphorylated than tau in the normal adult brain, has increased specificity for discriminating AD from other dementias (e.g., FTLD or dementia with Lewy body (DLB) [15] and nondemented controls [16]).

The abnormally hyperphosphorylated tau in AD brain is distinguished from transiently hyperphosphorylated tau by its ability to sequester normal tau, MAP 1 and MAP 2 and disrupt microtubules. In its more hyperphosphorylated state, tau is polymerized into paired helical filaments (PHF) admixed with straight filaments (SF) forming NFT. The cytosolic abnormally hyperphosphorylated tau, because of oligomerization, unlike normal tau, may cause accumulation of tau and self-assembly into PHF/SF, which loses its ability to sequester normal MAPs [35].

Clinically, AD is presented either as an AD *single disease*: sporadic AD, familial AD or adult Down's Syndrome (Trisome 21), or as an AD *combined disease:* AD with coexisting Lewy body-related pathology [18], TDP-43 pathology [37, 39], or AD with Pick's disease or other tauopathies [34], or with cerebrovascular disease as a common comorbidity in patients with AD [38].

In inflammation, astrocytosis and activated microglia are important components of AD pathophysiology with neuritic plaques as the foci of the local inflammatory response [36, 37]. Aβ neuritic plaques are surrounded by activated microglia, cytokines, and complement components, which are called inflammatory foci. In contrast, diffuse plaques without reactive microglia are regarded as necessary features for AD but not sufficient to generate clinical features [13]. While Alzheimer's disease is the most common form of dementia, frontotemporal dementia is a lesser-known but equally devastating condition.

Frontotemporal lobar degeneration (FTLD) represents a group of heterogeneous disorders that is considered to be clinically and pathologically distinct from AD [17], although FTLD may be mistaken for AD in early clinical stages [18]. FTLD is the second most common form of dementia in people under the age of 65 years after AD [19].

Clinical FTLD may be associated with a variety of different neuropathological entities, which macroscopically typically show symmetric focal atrophy of the frontal and/or temporal lobes. In some patients, there is asymmetry of atrophy, typically reflected in perisylvian loss on one side of the brain. Macroscopic atrophy of the basal ganglia and loss of pigmentation from the substantia nigra may be seen in a proportion of cases. Additionally, FTLD individuals may have parkinsonian features. FTLD may be associated with motor neuron disease [22], progressive supranuclear palsy [23], and corticobasal degeneration [24].

Based on neuropathologic criteria [20, 21], and [44], the FTLDs are classified into three distinct neuropathologic categories, according to molecular pathology of the misfolded proteins within the inclusion: FTLD-tau, FTLD-TDP, and FTLD-FUS with additional rare entities. FTLD with microtubule-associated protein tau *(MAPT)* mutation has inclusions of 3R, 4R or 3R and 4R tau protein, while the characteristic aggregate-forming protein in non-tau FTLD is either TDP-43 or FUS. After tau and TDP-43, FUS/TLS immunohistochemistry defines a third, less frequent, group of FTLD entities collectively called FTLD-FUS [41, 43]. FTLD-TDP is the most frequent FTLD entity, which encompasses most cases of FTLD-U [39, 42].

Although the clinical features of FTLD appear to be distinct from AD [25–27], some studies show clinical overlap [28, 29]. Nonetheless, pathologically confirmed cases of FTLD alone or in combination with AD apparently meet AD criteria during life [28], suggesting that the clinical distinction between the two disorders may be challenging in some individuals. Also, a strong association between the APOE ε4 allele and AD has been established [30], although the evidence for an association in FTLD is equivocal.

The pathogenic mechanisms implicated in all neurodegenerative disorders are not linked to individual clinical entities. In contrast, these pathologies show a considerable overlap in protein misfolding and aggregation, defects in endosomal-lysosomal network and clearance of damaged proteins by autophagy or proteasomes. The overlapping proteinopathies/comorbidities exist throughout the entire spectrum of most neurodegenerative disorders. Notably, these comorbidities may often influence the main pathology and affect both disease progression, cognitive decline and duration of the disease [13, 40]. Besides the TDP-43 pathology found in AD [37], another type of comorbidity that may be found in AD is α-synuclein in brain inclusions of AD patients [30, 31].

Liscic et al. [31] found in the sample of 48 FTLD cases a predominant spectrum of FTLD-MND type neuropathological entity causing FTLD [20] with ubiquitin/p62-positive, tau- and α-synuclein inclusions (FTLD-U) now called FTLD-TDP, as it contains the TDP-43 protein. This protein now defines a novel class of neurodegenerative diseases collectively called TDP-43 proteinopathies [44].

Deposition of Aβ in FTLD patients is generally sparse or absent, and when present rarely exceeds a level expected for the age of the subject. Some authors, however, have highlighted the presence of Aβ within the brains of people with FTDP-17, which suggests a synergistic influence of tau mutation with amyloid metabolism [32, 33, 35, 36]. Comparison of these individuals showed them to have a later age at onset of disease, and a higher *APOE* ε4 allele frequency in the FTLD, indicating that the possession of an *APOE* ε4 allele, late age at onset, and survival time are likely to increase the probability of AD pathology in cases with FTLD compounding the overlap of FTLD and AD clinical phenotypes is neuropathologic AD in one-fourth of FTLD individuals [31, 32].

## 6.2 Conclusions

Alzheimer's disease (AD) is a progressive neurodegenerative disease of the brain and the most common cause of dementia among elderly people, accounting for at least two-thirds of all dementia cases. The neuropathological hallmarks of AD include neuritic plaques composed of dystrophic neurites containing abnormal tau and amyloid beta (Aβ) filaments and intraneuronal neurofibrillary tangles (NFT) composed of paired helical filaments (PHF) made of phosphorylated tau protein. These brain lesions are typically accompanied by astrocytosis and reactive microgliosis, synapse and neuron loss.

Frontotemporal lobar degeneration (FTLD) represents a group of disorders that is considered clinically and pathologically distinct from AD. FTLD is genetically, neuropathologically, and clinically heterogeneous and may present as a dementia with three major clinical syndromes dominated by behavioral, language, and motor disorders, respectively. Most of these diseases are characterized by the pathological aggregation of misfolded proteins, either in neurons or glial cells, or both. About half of these cases have abnormal intracellular cytoplasmic accumulations of the microtubule-associated protein tau (MAPT). The characteristic aggregate-forming protein in non-tau FTLD is either TDP-43 or FUS.

Neuroinflammation plays an important role in AD pathology, which is mediated by activated microglia, and neuritic plaques and neurofibrillary tangles are foci of a local inflammatory response.

The pathogenic mechanisms implicated in neurodegenerative disorders are not linked to individual clinical entities. In contrast, neurodegenerative pathogenesis shows a considerable overlap in protein misfolding and aggregation. Although in the early stages of disease pathogenesis there may be only one molecular pathology, e.g., Aβ, as the disease progresses, additional molecular pathologies are often also found, e.g., tauopathy, TDP-43 proteinopathy and synucleinopathy. The overlapping proteinopathies/comorbidities exist throughout the entire spectrum of most neurodegenerative disorders. Notably, these comorbidities may influence the main pathology and affect both disease progression, cognitive decline and duration of the disease, as well as the efficacy of disease-modifying therapies for this devastating disorder.

**Acknowledgments** The author thanks Nigel J. Cairns, PhD, FRCPath, Professor of Pathology and Immunology for his invaluable help.

## References

1. Jonsson T, Atwal JK, Steinberg S, et al. A mutation in APP protects against Alzheimer's disease and age-related cognitive decline. Nature. 2012;488:96–9.
2. Mirra SS, Heyman A, McKeel D, et al. The consortium to establish a registry for Alzheimer's disease (CERAD). Part II. Standardization of the neuropathologic assessment of Alzheimer's disease. Neurology. 1991;41:479–86.
3. Khachaturian ZS. Diagnosis of Alzheimer's disease. Arch Neurol. 1985;42:1097–105.
4. The National Institute on Aging and Reagan Institute Working Group. Consensus recommendations for the postmortem diagnosis of Alzheimer's disease. The National Institute on Aging, and Regan Institute Working Group on Diagnostic Criteria for the Neuropathological Assessment of Alzheimer's Disease. Neurobiol Aging. 1997;18:S1–2.
5. Braak H, Braak E. Neuropathological staging of Alzheimer-related changes. Acta Neuropathol (Berl). 1991;82:239–59.
6. Duboi B, Feldman HH, Jacova C, et al. Advancing research diagnostic criteria for Alzheimer's disease: the IWG-2 criteria. Lancet Neurol. 2014;13:614–29.
7. Sperling RA, Aisen PS, Beckett LA, et al. Toward defining the preclinical stages of Alzheimer's disease: recommendations from the National Institute on Aging-Alzheimer's Association work groups on diagnostic guidelines for Alzheimer's disease. Alzheimers Dement. 2011;7:280–92.
8. Reitz C, Brayne C, Mayeux R. Epidemiology of Alzheimer disease. Nat Rev Neurol. 2011;7:137–52.
9. Schellenberg GD, Montine TJ. The genetics and neuropathology of Alzheimer's disease. Acta Neuropathol. 2012;124:305–23.
10. Hardy J, Selkoe DJ. The amyloid hypothesis of Alzheimer's disease: progress and problems on the road to therapeutics. Science. 2002;297:352–6.
11. Hampel H, Hardy J, Blennow K, et al. The amyloid-β pathway in Alzheimer's disease. Mol Psychiatry. 2021;26(10):5481–503.
12. Strittmatter WJ, Roses AD. Apolipoprotein E and Alzheimer disease. Annu Rev Neurosci. 1996;19:53–77.
13. De Marchi F, Munitic I, Vidatic L, et al. Overlapping neuroimmune mechanisms and therapeutic targets in neurodegenerative disorders. Biomedicine. 2023;11(10):2793.
14. Fagan AM, Mintun MA, Shah AR, et al. Cerebrospinal fluid tau and ptau(181) increase with cortical amyloid deposition in cognitively normal individuals: implications for future clinical trials of Alzheimer's disease. EMBO Mol Med. 2009;1(8–9):371–80.
15. Hampel H, Buerger K, Zinkowski R, et al. Measurement of phosphorylated tau epitopes in the differential diagnosis of Alzheimer disease: a comparative cerebrospinal fluid study. Arch Gen Psychiatry. 2004;61(1):95–102.
16. Bateman R, Munsell L, Morris J, et al. Human amyloid-β synthesis and clearance rates as measured in cerebrospinal fluid in vivo. Nat Med. 2006;12:856–61.
17. Foster NL, Wilhelmsen K, Sima AA, et al. Frontotemporal dementia and parkinsonism linked to chromosome 17: a consensus conference. Ann Neurol. 1997;41:706–15.
18. Klatka LA, Schiffer RB, Powers JM, et al. Incorrect diagnosis of Alzheimer's disease: a clinicopathological study. Arch Neurol. 1996;53:35–42.

19. Ratnavalli E, Brayne C, Dawson K, et al. The prevalence of frontotemporal dementia. Neurology. 2002;58:2615–21.
20. McKhann GM, Albert MS, Grossman M, et al. Clinical and pathological diagnosis of frontotemporal dementia: report of the work Group on Frontotemporal Dementia and Pick's Disease. Arch Neurol. 2001;58(18):1803–9.
21. Cairns NJ, Bigio EH, Mackenzie IR, et al. Neuropathologic diagnosis and nosologic criteria for frontotemporal lobar degeneration: consensus of the Consortium for Frontotemporal Lobar Degeneration. Acta Neuropathol (Berl). 2007;114:5–22.
22. Neary D, Snowden JS, Mann DMA, et al. Frontal lobe dementia and motor neuron disease. J Neurol Neurosurg Psychiatry. 1990;53:23–32.
23. Hauw JJ, Daniel SE, Dickson D, et al. Preliminary NINDS neuropathologic criteria for Steele-Richardson-Olszewski syndrome (progressive supranuclear palsy). Neurology. 1994;44:2015–9.
24. Dickson DW, Bergeron C, Chin SS, Duyckaerts C, Horoupian D, Ikeda K, Jellinger K, Lantos PL, Lippa CF, Mirra SS, Tabaton M, Vonsattel JP, Wakabayashi K, Litvan I. Office of rare diseases neuropathologic criteria for corticobasal degeneration. J Neuropathol Exp Neurol. 2002;61(11):935–46.
25. Rosen HJ, Hartikainen KM, Jagust W, et al. Utility of clinical criteria in differentiating frontotemporal lobar degeneration (FTLD) from AD. Neurology. 2002;58:1608–15.
26. Rascovsky K, Salmon DP, Ho GJ, et al. Cognitive profiles differ in autopsy-confirmed frontotemporal dementia and AD. Neurology. 2002;58:1801–8.
27. Knopman DS, Boeve BF, Parisi JE, et al. Antemortem diagnosis of frontotemporal lobar degeneration. Ann Neurol. 2005;57:480–8.
28. Varma AR, Snowden JS, Lloyd JJ, et al. Evaluation of the NINCDS-ADRDA criteria in the differentiation of Alzheimer's disease and frontotemporal dementia. J Neurol Neurosurg Psychiatry. 1999;66:184–8.
29. Johnson JK, Head E, Kim R, et al. Clinical and pathological evidence for a frontal variant of Alzheimer disease. Arch Neurol. 1999;56:1233–9.
30. Twohig D, Nielsen HM. Alfa-Synuclein in the pathophysiology of Alzheimer's disease. Mol Neurodegener. 2019;14:1–19.
31. Liscic RM, Storandt M, Cairns NJ, et al. Clinical and psychometric distinction of frontotemporal and Alzheimer dementias. Arch Neurol. 2007;64:535–40.
32. Mann D, McDonagh A, Pickering-Brown S, et al. Amyloid b protein deposition in patients with frontotemporal lobar degeneration: relationship to age and Apolipoprotein E genotype. Neurosci Lett. 2001;304:161–4.
33. McLean CA, Maher F, Dark F, et al. Tau pathology in frontotemporal dementia with parkinsonism (FTDP-17)—an Australian pedigree. Brain Pathol. 2000;10:529.
34. Morris JC, Cole M, Banker BQ, et al. Hereditary dysphasic dementia and the pick-Alzheimer spectrum. Ann Neurol. 1984;16:455–66.
35. Iqbal K, Liu F, Gong CX, Grundke-Iqbal I. Tau in Alzheimer disease and related tauopathies. Curr Alzheimer Res. 2010;7(8):656–64.
36. Heneka MT, Carson MJ, El Khoury J, Landreth GE, Brosseron F, Feinstein DL, Jacobs AH, Wyss-Coray T, Vitorica J, Ransohoff RM, Herrup K, Frautschy SA, Finsen B, Brown GC, Verkhratsky A, Yamanaka K, Koistinaho J, Latz E, Halle A, Petzold GC, Town T, Morgan D, Shinohara ML, Perry VH, Holmes C, Bazan NG, Brooks DJ, Hunot S, Joseph B, Deigendesch N, Garaschuk O, Boddeke E, Dinarello CA, Breitner JC, Cole GM, Golenbock DT, Kummer MP. Neuroinflammation in Alzheimer's disease. Lancet Neurol. 2015;14(4):388–405.
37. Amador-Ortiz C, Lin WL, Ahmed Z, Personett D, Davies P, Duara R, Graff-Radford NR, Hutton ML, Dickson DW. TDP-43 immunoreactivity in hippocampal sclerosis and Alzheimer's disease. Ann Neurol. 2007;61(5):435–45.
38. Klohs J. An integrated view on vascular dysfunction in Alzheimer's disease. Neurodegener Dis. 2019;19(3–4):109–27.

39. Arai T, Hasegawa M, Akiyama H, Ikeda K, Nonaka T, Mori H, Mann D, Tsuchiya K, Yoshida M, Hashizume Y, Oda T. TDP-43 is a component of ubiquitin-positive tau-negative inclusions in frontotemporal lobar degeneration and amyotrophic lateral sclerosis. Biochem Biophys Res Commun. 2006;351(3):602–11.
40. Boon, Baayla DC, Peng Z, Kouri N, Hinkle KM, Lachner C, et al. Retrospective evaluation of neuropathologic proxies of the minimal atrophy subtype compared with corticolimbic Alzheimer disease subtypes. Neurology. 2023;101(14):1412–23.
41. Mackenzie IR, Neumann M, Bigio EH, et al. Nomenclature and nosology for neuropathologic subtypes of frontotemporal lobar degeneration: an update. Acta Neuropathol. 2010;119:1–4.
42. Neumann M, Sampathu DM, Kwong LK, et al. Ubiquitinated TDP-43 in frontotemporal lobar degeneration and amyotrophic lateral sclerosis. Science. 2006;314:130–3.
43. Neumann M. Frontotemporal lobar degeneration and amyotrophic lateral sclerosis: molecular similarities and differences. Rev Neurol (Paris). 2013;169:793–8.
44. Hortobagyi T, Cairns NJ. Amyotrophic lateral sclerosis and non-tau frontotemporal lobar degeneration. In: Kovacs GG, Alafuzoff I, editors. Handbook of clinical neurology, neuropathology, vol. 145. Elsevier; 2018. p. 369–81.

# Chapter 7
# Systemic Amyloid-β Metabolism in Alzheimer's Disease

**Dong-Yu Fan, Jun Wang, Ben J. Gu, Colin L. Masters, and Yan-Jiang Wang**

**Abstract** Alzheimer's disease (AD) is increasingly acknowledged not only as a neurological disorder but also as a condition modulated by systemic factors. While amyloid-β (Aβ) peptides are classically associated with brain pathology, compelling evidence suggests that significant Aβ production and metabolism also occur in peripheral organs and tissues. This review synthesizes the current understanding of systemic Aβ metabolic processes and their critical role in the pathogenesis of AD. We detail the biogenesis of Aβ in both the central nervous system (CNS) and periphery, establishing the existence of interconnected central and peripheral Aβ pools. Crucially, we examine the multiple pathways mediating Aβ clearance from the brain into the periphery, including transport across the blood-brain barrier (BBB) and the blood-cerebrospinal fluid barrier (BCSFB), clearance via the glymphatic and meningeal lymphatic systems, and drainage along intramural periarterial pathways and arachnoid granule pathways. Once in the periphery, brain-derived Aβ is cleared by various mechanisms involving blood components (monocytes, enzymes, erythrocytes), the liver (primary site of degradation), kidneys (filtration and excretion), spleen (phagocytosis by macrophages), and potentially other organs

D.-Y. Fan · J. Wang
Department of Neurology, Daping Hospital, Third Military Medical University, Chongqing, China

Chongqing Key Laboratory of Ageing and Brain Diseases, Chongqing, China

B. J. Gu · C. L. Masters
The Florey Institute, The University of Melbourne, Parkville, VIC, Australia
e-mail: ben.gu@innatephagolab.com.au; c.masters@florey.edu.au

Y.-J. Wang (✉)
Department of Neurology, Daping Hospital, Third Military Medical University, Chongqing, China

Chongqing Key Laboratory of Ageing and Brain Diseases, Chongqing, China

State Key Laboratory of Trauma, Burn and Combined Injury, Institute of Surgery Research, Daping Hospital, Third Military Medical University, Chongqing, China



Y.-H. Yang (ed.), *Management of Dementia from the Preclinical Stage*,
https://doi.org/10.1007/978-981-95-5222-1_7

like the skin and gut. Importantly, a range of systemic diseases – including metabolic disorders (diabetes and dyslipidemia), immune dysfunction, cardiovascular disease, hepatic/renal dysfunction, sleep/respiratory disorders, gut microbiome disturbances, blood abnormalities, infections, systemic inflammation, and bone diseases – are linked to impaired peripheral Aβ clearance and an increased risk of AD. These systemic abnormalities often form bidirectional feedback loops with AD brain pathology. The emerging understanding of the intricate cross-talk between central and peripheral Aβ pools suggests that peripheral Aβ clearance dysfunction is a major contributor to Aβ accumulation in sporadic AD. Consequently, targeting systemic Aβ metabolism and improving peripheral clearance represent promising therapeutic strategies for AD, complementing current brain-centric approaches like anti-Aβ antibodies. Future research should prioritize comprehensive therapeutic approaches and the control of comorbid systemic conditions to enhance prevention and treatment approaches for AD.

**Keywords** Alzheimer's disease · Amyloid-β · Systemic comorbidities · Systemic metabolism · Peripheral clearance

## 7.1 Introduction

The increasing occurrence of Alzheimer's disease (AD) and associated socioeconomic burdens have increased with increasing age worldwide. The extracellular senile plaques formed by the deposition of peptides are the specific hallmark of AD. Abnormal metabolism of amyloid-β (Aβ) has been proposed as a significant pathomechanism in AD, supported by compelling evidence and the results of recent clinical trials using anti-Aβ antibodies [1–3]. This disorder is primarily attributed to the overproduction of Aβ resulting from mutations in the amyloid precursor protein (APP) and PS1/2 genes in individuals with familial AD, a subtype that constitutes approximately 1% of all AD cases, whereas impaired Aβ clearance is hypothesized to be the primary mechanism underlying Aβ accumulation in individuals with sporadic AD, a form that represents approximately 99% of all AD cases [4]. Therefore, an imbalance between the production and clearance of Aβ is generally recognized as the initiating factor of AD, and the common late-onset form of AD is characterized by an overall impairment in Aβ clearance [5].

Enhancing the clearance of Aβ has emerged as a well-recognized and promising therapeutic approach for AD [6]. Currently, approved pharmacological treatments for AD are broadly categorized into symptomatic therapies and disease-modifying therapies (DMTs). Symptomatic medications, such as memantine, provide only temporary improvement or stabilization of neuropsychiatric symptoms and are unable to reverse or halt the progression of AD. Thus, DMT interventions that directly modify AD-specific pathobiological changes in the brain are urgently needed. To date, numerous therapeutic strategies have been developed to slow the clinical progression of AD by reducing cerebral Aβ levels [7, 8], most recently through the administration of monoclonal anti-Aβ antibodies [9, 10]. Recently, three DMT interventions, aducanumab [2], lecanemab [3], and donanemab [11], have achieved some clinical success and have been approved by the FDA for the treatment of mild cognitive impairment or mild dementia due to AD. Nonetheless, the current Aβ-targeting approaches can only slow the progression of AD but cannot reverse or even halt the disease process; thus, their cognitive benefits are limited. Increasing our understanding of the molecular pathogenesis of AD is still necessary to develop effective treatments for AD.

AD is traditionally classified as a neurodegenerative disorder of the brain. However, accumulating evidence in recent years has demonstrated that systemic abnormalities in peripheral organs and tissues contribute to the development of AD-related neuropathology and cognitive decline [12–18]. Large-scale epidemiological studies have consistently demonstrated associations between systemic comorbidities and the risks of AD and dementia [19–21]. Systemic factors originating from the peripheral nervous system can access the brain and contribute to brain aging, neurodegeneration, and the pathogenesis of AD [22–25]. Therefore, systemic organs and tissues play a role in the pathogenesis and progression of AD. Elucidating the mechanisms by which the peripheral system influences the onset and progression of AD could provide valuable insights for developing novel intervention strategies [26]. Given that Aβ is a major pathological hallmark of AD and a central focus of research in this condition, this section focuses on systemic disturbances in Aβ metabolism in AD. We discuss the cross-talk between peripheral and central Aβ pools and describe how systemic abnormalities interact with the pathogenesis of AD in the brain. Based on these findings, we suggest that interactions between the brain and the periphery might play critical roles in the development and progression of AD.

## 7.2 Aβ Biogenesis and Catabolism

Normal Aβ metabolism and the maintenance of homeostatic balance between Aβ production and clearance are essential for preserving cerebral health. The physiological metabolism of Aβ occurs not only in the brain but also in the peripheral tissues, and bidirectional communication between these compartments is feasible (Fig. 7.1).

### *7.2.1 Central and Peripheral Production of Aβ*

The Aβ that accumulates in the brain is traditionally thought to be derived from the cleavage of amyloid-β precursor protein (APP) in brain cells, including neurons, microglia, and astrocytes. However, studies have demonstrated that Aβ is widely

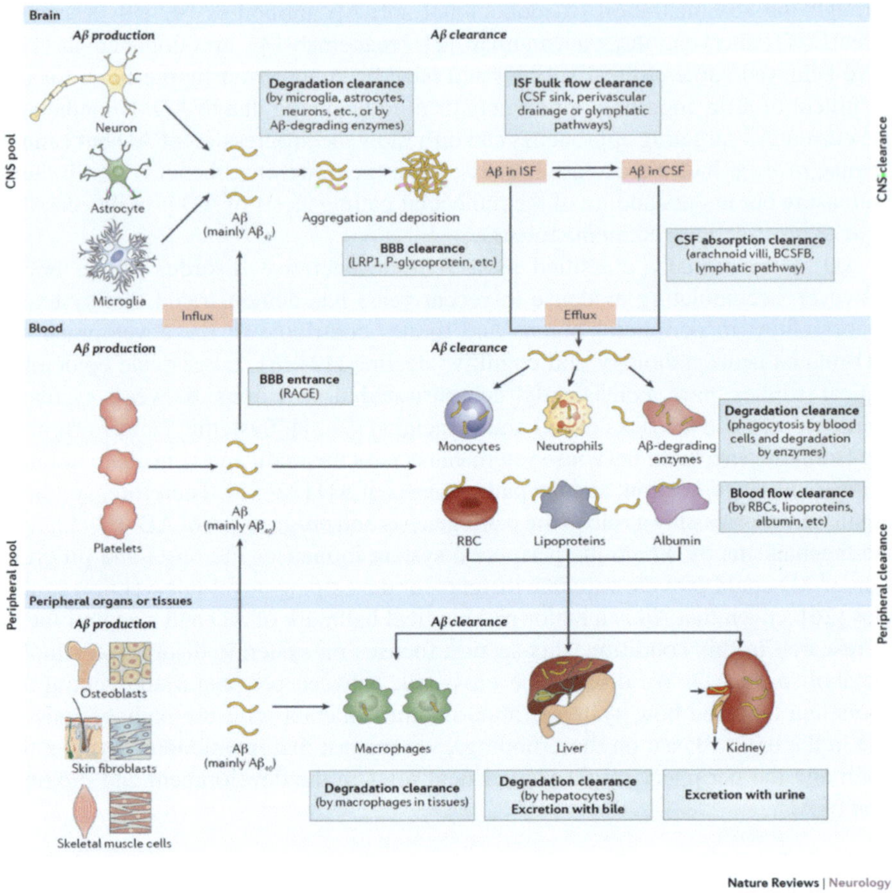


**Fig. 7.1** Physiological metabolism of Aβ in the brain and periphery. Amyloid-β (Aβ) is generated by neurons, microglia and astrocytes in the brain and by platelets, skin fibroblasts, osteoblasts, and skeletal muscle cells in the periphery. The CNS and peripheral pools of Aβ can interact; some Aβ peptides in the CNS are cleared via phagocytosis or proteolytic degradation, whereas others are released into the blood via the blood-brain barrier (BBB), interstitial fluid (ISF) bulk flow, or cerebrospinal fluid (CSF) egress pathways. Some Aβ peptides in the blood are phagocytosed by cells, such as monocytes or neutrophils, whereas other Aβ molecules are transported by carriers (such as erythrocytes, albumin, and lipoproteins) to peripheral organs or tissues, where they are eventually degraded by macrophages or hepatocytes or excreted from the body via the liver or kidney. BCSFB blood-CSF barrier; RBC red blood cell. (Material from: Wang et al. [109], Macmillan Publishers Limited, part of Springer Nature)

expressed in peripheral organs and tissues, including the adrenal gland, kidney, heart, liver, spleen, pancreas, and skeletal muscle [27, 28], as well as in peripheral cell types such as platelets, skin fibroblasts, skeletal muscle cells, and osteoblasts [29–31]. Aβ production, in both the brain and peripheral tissues, is lower in cognitively normal older adults compared to individuals with AD (Table 7.1). Given that skeletal muscle accounts for approximately one-quarter of human body weight and represents only one of numerous peripheral sources of Aβ, peripherally derived Aβ is likely to constitute a significant proportion of the total. However, the accumulation of Aβ aggregates in older adults, both with and without AD, is a significant factor influencing the $A\beta_{42}$ to $A\beta_{40}$ ratio in the brain and peripheral tissues. The levels and profiles of the predominant Aβ species in the brain and peripheral tissues should be assessed in young individuals without evidence of Aβ deposition in future studies.

Significant differences have been observed between the central and peripheral pools of Aβ. First, $A\beta_{42}$, the most aggregation-prone and neurotoxic isoform of Aβ, is the predominant molecular species in the brain, whereas $A\beta_{40}$ predominates in peripheral tissues. However, the mechanism underlying this difference remains unclear. A possible explanation is the differential expression of APP isoforms in the brain and periphery. APP695 is the predominant isoform expressed in neurons, whereas APP751 and APP770 are the predominant isoforms expressed in peripheral cells, including platelets and leukocytes [32]. Another possible explanation is that the tissue microenvironment of the CNS and periphery is different, which may influence the differential processing of APP by γ-secretase and lead to the generation of distinct Aβ species [27, 28]. Second, Aβ levels in the central compartment are higher than those in the peripheral compartment. The concentrations of Aβ are 5–15 times higher than those in plasma [33, 34]. One possible explanation is that the processing of APP in peripheral cells, unlike in neurons, likely occurs through α-cleavage rather than β-cleavage [35, 36], leading to reduced Aβ production. Another interpretation for the lower Aβ levels in peripheral tissues is that the

**Table 7.1** Amounts of Aβ generated in the CNS and periphery

| Source of Aβ | Cognitively normal elderly individuals | Patients with AD | References |
|---|---|---|---|
| *Brain gray matter* | | | |
| Total Aβ[a] | 3.2 μg/g | 13.1 μg/g | [5, 315] |
| $A\beta_{1-42}$ | 0.78 μg/g | 6.1 μg/g | [5] |
| $A\beta_{1-40}$ | 0.2 μg/g | 0.6 μg/g | [5] |
| *Packed quiescent platelets*[b] | | | |
| $A\beta_{1-40}$ | 84 ng/ml | Not available | [28] |
| $A\beta_{1-42}$ | 1.7 ng/ml | Not available | [28] |
| *Packed-activated platelets* | | | |
| $A\beta_{1-40}$ | 56.8 ng/ml | Not available | [28] |
| $A\beta_{1-42}$ | 1.6 ng/ml | Not available | [28] |
| *Skeletal muscle*[c] | | | |
| $A\beta_{1-40}$ | 29.8 ng/g | 37.8 ng/g | [28] |
| $A\beta_{1-42}$ | 10.2 ng/g | 15.7 ng/g | [28] |

[a]Includes $A\beta_{1-40}$, $A\beta_{1-42}$, $A\beta_{n-40}$, and $A\beta_{n-42}$

[b]Suggested to be the primary source of soluble Aβ (which is mainly $A\beta_{1-40}$) in the circulation [316, 317]

[c]Aβ might also be generated by skin fibroblasts and osteoblasts [28, 29, 31, 318], although these findings have not yet been confirmed

periphery contains high levels of Aβ-binding proteins, such as lipoproteins and albumin [37], as well as Aβ-binding cells, including erythrocytes [38], all of which facilitate Aβ transport and clearance. Additionally, the large volume of the circulatory system and the dilution effect of blood contribute efficiently to reducing Aβ concentrations.

The above factors may also contribute to explaining why Aβ aggregates are predominantly deposited in the brain and cerebral vessel walls, and rarely in peripheral organs, despite reports of Aβ aggregate detection in the skin, subcutaneous tissue, intestinal tissues, and heart [39–41]. The aggregation of Aβ peptides, including oligomerization and fibrillogenesis, is influenced by the relative proportions of Aβ species, their concentrations, solution pH, temperature, ionic strength, and incubation time [42]. Therefore, in the periphery, a higher proportion of $A\beta_{40}$ may promote the sequestration of $A\beta_{42}$ into stable complexes, thereby inhibiting its oligomerization and aggregation [43], whereas an elevated level of $A\beta_{42}$ in the brain may increase its susceptibility to aggregation.

### 7.2.2 Central Clearance and Peripheral Efflux of Aβ

Several potential pathways contribute to Aβ clearance from the brain, including phagocytosis and endocytosis mediated by various cell types—such as microglia, perivascular macrophages, and astrocytes—and proteolytic degradation by enzymes such as neprilysin (NEP), insulin-degrading enzyme (IDE), and matrix metalloproteinases (MMPs). Several pathways, including the blood-brain barrier, the blood-CSF barrier, the lymphatic-related pathway, intramural periarterial drainage (IPAD), also known as perivascular drainage, and arachnoid granules, have been demonstrated to mediate substantial Aβ efflux from the brain to the periphery [44] (Table 7.2). Moreover, certain endogenous inhibitors of Aβ aggregation, such as the secreted ectodomain of the neurotrophin p75 [45] and the N-terminal domain of myelin basic protein [46], can prevent Aβ deposition in the brain and promote its efflux into the systemic circulation.

1. Blood-Brain Barrier (BBB) Pathway

The blood-brain barrier (BBB) is composed of capillary endothelial cells joined by tight junctions, adherent junctions, and gap junctions. Due to its tight junctions, the BBB exhibits lower permeability to solutes compared to the peripheral vasculature [47]. The cellular components of the BBB are in contact with the basement membrane, which originates from endothelial cells and pericytes and undergoes age-related changes, including microvascular fibrosis and alterations in the relative proportions of type IV collagen, proteoglycans, and laminin [48]. Numerous studies have indicated that pathological alterations within the neurovascular unit—comprising neurons, glial cells, and pericytes—play a critical role in the initiation and progression of AD, reinforcing the association between BBB dysfunction and

**Table 7.2** Mechanisms of Aβ efflux from the brain to the periphery

| Clearance mechanism | Structure/location | Direction of Aβ transports | Alteration in AD | Comments |
|---|---|---|---|---|
| Blood–brain barrier (BBB) | Capillary endothelial cells separated by tight junctions, adherens junctions, and gap junctions | Bidirectional | Aβ clearance decreased by 30% | LRP1 and ABCB1 are key transcytosis-related transporters of Aβ across the BBB; paracellular transport of Aβ also occurs |
| Blood-cerebrospinal fluid barrier (BCSFB) | Choroid epithelial cells separated by tight junctions, adherens junctions, and desmosomes | Bidirectional | Impaired Aβ clearance may precede Aβ deposition in individuals with LOAD | Choroid plexus epithelial cells enclose stroma containing peripheral blood capillaries; LRP1 and ABCB1 are BCSFB efflux transporters |
| Lymphatic-related drainage | Meningeal lymphatics; paravascular space surrounding cerebral arteries and veins; perineural pathways | Unidirectional | Reduced in transgenic mouse models of AD | Decreased AQP4 expression adjacent to cerebral vessels in patients with AD suggests decreased glymphatic drainage |
| Intramural periarterial drainage (IPAD) | Perivascular space within the basement membrane of cerebral artery smooth muscle cells | Unidirectional | The frequent presence of CAA in AD patients suggests reduced IPAD-mediated clearance of Aβ | The pattern of Aβ deposition in CAA patients is similar to pattern of Aβ drainage by IPAD |
| Arachnoid granule–venous sinus pathway | Arachnoid villi and granulations in the walls of major venous sinuses | Unidirectional | Unclear if impaired arachnoid granule drainage contributes to an increased Aβ burden | Major pathway of CSF efflux in humans, the drainage of Aβ needs to be studied |

*ABCB1* ATP-binding cassette subfamily B member 1; *AD* Alzheimer's disease; *AQP4* aquaporin-4; *BBB* blood–brain barrier; *BCSFB* blood–cerebrospinal fluid barrier; *CAA* cerebral amyloid angiopathy; *IPAD* intramural periarterial drainage; *LOAD* late-onset Alzheimer's disease; *LRP1* low-density lipoprotein receptor-related protein 1

neurodegeneration processes [49]. Some studies have shown that the percentage of Aβ cleared by the BBB is estimated to be 62–85%, although Roberts et al. suggested that the direct transport of Aβ across the human BBB may contribute to only 25% of its clearance from the brain [50–52]. In patients with AD, BBB-mediated clearance of Aβ is reduced by approximately 30% [5]. Impaired elimination of Aβ across the BBB is widely considered to contribute to the pathogenesis of both cerebral amyloid angiopathy (CAA) and AD [53].

Aβ efflux is primarily mediated through its specific receptors expressed on the brain endothelial cells. Low-density lipoprotein receptor-related protein 1 (LRP1) and ATP-binding cassette subfamily B member 1 (ABCB1, commonly referred to as P-glycoprotein 1) are critical mediators of Aβ clearance across the BBB [54–56]. Several LRP1 ligands, including apolipoprotein E (ApoE), α2-microglobulin (α2M), and tissue-type plasminogen activator, are co-deposited with Aβ in senile plaques and participate in its clearance from the brain [57]. The affinity of Aβ40 for LRP1 is higher than that of Aβ peptides containing greater β-sheet contents, such as Aβ42, resulting in less efficient clearance of Aβ42 from the brain [58]. In addition, LRP2, the largest member of the low-density lipoprotein receptor (LDLR) family, mediates the endocytosis of Aβ and its subsequent clearance across the BBB following binding to apolipoprotein J (ApoJ, also known as clusterin) [58].

LRP1 and ABCB1 have been proposed to functionally interact through the phosphatidylinositol-binding clathrin assembly protein (PICALM) [59]; therefore, in patients with AD, Aβ-induced downregulation of PICALM may contribute to impaired Aβ clearance across the BBB [60]. In addition to these mechanisms, several other receptors mediate Aβ efflux, including insulin-sensitive and ANP-sensitive transporters [61]; however, their relative contributions remain poorly understood, and further research is required to clarify their roles in the pathogenesis of AD.

In contrast, circulating Aβ enters the brain primarily via the receptors for advanced glycation end products (RAGE), a multiligand influx receptor belonging to the immunoglobulin family and expressed on the luminal surface of cerebral blood vessels [62]. The expression levels of LRP1, ABCB1, and RAGE at the BBB are altered in AD models prior to Aβ deposition, which may contribute to Aβ accumulation in the brain [63].

2. Blood-CSF Barrier (BCSFB) Pathway.

The blood-CSF barrier (BCSFB) is the barrier constituted by the tight junctions between the epithelial cells of the choroid plexus that regulates the passage of solutes between the CSF and blood, which is the main source of CSF. Its functions include the transport of glucose and other nutrients from the blood to the CSF, the reabsorption and clearance of metabolic waste products from the CSF, and the maintenance of CNS homeostasis through the modulation of solute exchange between the CSF and brain parenchyma [64]. Choroid plexus blood flow has been estimated to be 5–10 times higher than that in the cerebral vasculature [65, 66]. Active solute transport occurs bidirectionally across the choroid plexus, although for Aβ, clearance from the CSF into the peripheral blood predominates. The permeability of Aβ across the choroid plexus is approximately 10 times greater than that across the BBB in either direction [67, 68].

The choroid plexus exhibits a substantial capacity for Aβ uptake from the CSF. The Aβ transporters LRP1, ABCB1, LRP2, and RAGE are expressed on the epithelium of the BCSFB [69]. LRP1 and ABCB1 are believed to function at the BCSFB as Aβ efflux transporters, whereas LRP2 mediates bidirectional Aβ transport from both the CSF and the bloodstream into the choroid plexus [70]. The choroid plexus is also capable of both producing and degrading Aβ, as IDE, NEP, and endothelin-converting enzyme-1 are expressed in choroidal epithelial cells [68, 71]. $A\beta_{42}$ oligomers can increase the permeability of the BCSFB by activating MMPs [72]. Impaired choroid plexus function has been proposed as an early pathogenic event in late-onset Alzheimer's disease (LOAD), potentially preceding cerebral Aβ deposition [73]; however, some studies have reported that changes in BCSFB permeability are not associated with AD severity [74]. The relationship between BCSFB dysfunction and AD progression remains unclear and requires further elucidation.

3. Lymphatic-Related Drainage Pathways

In 2012, Iliff et al. described a pathway for the cerebral clearance of other solutes through the paravascular space, which they termed the "glymphatic system" due to its functional resemblance to lymphatic drainage [75]. In this system, cerebrospinal fluid (CSF) enters the brain via para-arterial spaces, mixes with interstitial fluid (ISF), and subsequently exits the brain through paravenous spaces [76, 77]. Currently, it is widely believed that Aβ is cleared from the brain through glymphatic and other related pathways.

The first lymphatic pathway involves the meningeal lymphatics, which are specialized in draining CSF to deep cervical lymph nodes, enabling the removal of metabolic waste and macromolecules from the brain, not only in rodents but also in humans [78, 79]. This discovery was made possible by newly developed magnetic resonance imaging (MRI) protocols capable of distinguishing lymphatic flow from blood flow at the meninges, allowing visualization of continuous and substantial meningeal lymphatic outflow [80, 81]. In young adult AD transgenic mice, prolonged induction of aging-like meningeal lymphatic dysfunction demonstrated that impaired meningeal lymphatic drainage leads to increased Aβ deposition in both the meninges and the brain [80]. This effect is believed to result from compromised glymphatic clearance of Aβ due to diminished meningeal lymphatic function, inadequate drainage of Aβ from the CSF into deep cervical lymph nodes (LNs), and the development of detrimental inflammatory responses in the meninges and brain [82–84]. Recently, altered activation of brain border-associated macrophages (BAMs) has been directly linked to disruptions in vascular integrity and glymphatic function [85]. Future studies should aim to elucidate the specific mechanisms underlying the reduced perivascular lymphatic inflow and outflow observed following impaired meningeal lymphatic drainage.

The second lymphatic pathway is the paravascular space, a narrow compartment situated between the irregular surface of the leptomeningeal membrane and the outer basement membrane of vessel walls, as well as the glial endfeet [86, 87]. This space has been proposed to be part of the glymphatic pathway [75]. Also known as the Virchow–Robin space (VRS), the paravascular space surrounds the cerebral vasculature, including both arteries and veins. Notably, it differs from the perivascular space, which is located within the middle layers of the basement membrane of arterial smooth muscle cells [88], as described in the next section, paravascular drainage of solutes from the CSF depends on the expression of aquaporin-4 (AQP4) and efficient arterial pulsations, suggesting that rhythmic vessel wall movements may provide the driving force for solute clearance from the brain [89, 90]. Vasomotion—defined as low-frequency contractions and dilations of vascular smooth muscle cells—has also been implicated in regulating glymphatic flow [91]. Notably, sleep enhances glymphatic fluid transport by expanding the interstitial space through reduced noradrenergic tone, thereby decreasing resistance to fluid movement [92].

The third lymphatic pathway is the perineural outflow pathway, through which CSF drains into deep cervical lymph nodes. Emerging evidence indicates that CSF exists along cranial nerves, particularly in the nasal and optic regions [93, 94]. More specifically, perineural drainage via the olfactory nerve—the first cranial nerve (CN I), which traverses the cribriform plate to reach the nasal mucosa—is considered the most significant route for CSF lymphatic outflow across multiple species [94–97]. In addition, the optic nerve (CN II) and trigeminal nerve (CN V) also exhibit perineural drainage patterns [94]. These pathways collectively represent potential routes for the clearance of neurotoxic proteins, such as amyloid-β (Aβ), from the brain.

4. Intramural Periarterial Drainage (IPAD)-Mediated Clearance of Aβ

Intramural periarterial drainage (IPAD), also known as perivascular drainage, facilitates the clearance of ISF from the brain to cervical lymph nodes via basement membranes in capillary walls, the tunica media of arteries, and the wall of the internal carotid artery in the neck [98]. In contrast to conventional lymphatic drainage, the flow pattern observed in these studies occurs in the opposite direction to cerebral blood flow [99]. IPAD was initially proposed to be driven by arterial pulsations, specifically by the reflected (or "rebound") wave that follows each primary pulse wave [100]. However, this hypothesis has been challenged by subsequent studies suggesting that vasomotion—generated by spontaneous contractions and relaxations of vascular smooth muscle cells—may serve as the primary driving force behind IPAD [101, 102].

Aβ deposition in the basement membranes of capillaries and arterial walls in individuals with cerebral amyloid angiopathy (CAA) almost certainly obstructs perivascular drainage pathways, resulting in increased impedance to solute clearance from the brain. CAA is present in up to 90% of AD patients and is associated with more rapid disease progression [103]. With advancing age, arterial walls lose elasticity, and vessel stiffening may impair the perivascular drainage of ISF and solutes in older adults [104].

5. Arachnoid Granule–Venous Sinus Pathway

CSF is directly drained into the peripheral blood through arachnoid villi and granulations located in the walls of major venous sinuses [99]. Some researchers have proposed that this drainage occurs via gaps between endothelial cells and/or through hydrostatic pressure-dependent pinocytosis [100, 105]. In humans, the majority of CSF appears to be cleared through this pathway; however, in newborn lambs, the nasal route serves as the primary drainage pathway because arachnoid villi do not fully develop until later stages of maturation [106, 107]. Furthermore, considerable species differences in the size and structure of arachnoid villi and granulations have been documented—for instance, those in experimental animals are markedly smaller and structurally simpler than human arachnoid granulations—indicating that findings from animal models may not accurately reflect human physiological conditions. Therefore, the role of the arachnoid granule–venous sinus pathway in transporting Aβ and other metabolic waste products from the brain to the periphery in humans requires further investigation.

The drainage pathways for CSF and ISF appear to differ, and the proportion of ISF that drains into the CSF remains poorly understood. A previous study indicated that 10–15% of ISF drains into the CSF in rats [108], and a similar extent of drainage may occur in humans [99]. In addition, another study demonstrated that direct transport of Aβ across the BBB accounts for approximately 25% of Aβ clearance, while Aβ absorption in the CSF contributes to approximately 25% of total CNS Aβ clearance in humans [52]. However, the primary mechanism by which Aβ is eliminated from the brain, as well as the precise contributions of each of these pathways to overall Aβ clearance, remains unclear. Nevertheless, these pathways function synergistically to remove pathological proteins such as Aβ from the brain to the periphery, indicating a physiological connection between peripheral tissues and organs and the metabolism of brain-derived waste products [109].

## 7.3 Clearance of Brain-Derived Aβ in the Periphery

CNS clearance of Aβ is estimated to be reduced by approximately 30% in AD patients [5], yet the extent and mechanisms underlying peripheral Aβ clearance remain poorly understood. Studies have indicated that approximately 40–60% of brain-derived Aβ is cleared in the periphery [50, 110, 111]. Several peripheral tissues and organs have been shown to participate in Aβ catabolism.

A recent study revealed that ligation of deep cervical lymph nodes exacerbates AD-like pathology in APP/PS1 mice [83], suggesting that obstruction or dysfunction of brain drainage pathways is a contributing factor to AD progression. Targeting meningeal lymphatics with vascular endothelial growth factor C (VEGF-C) enhances the clearance of CSF macromolecules via meningeal lymphatic vessels and improves learning and memory performance in animal models [80, 112]. These findings indicate that physiological mechanisms actively transport pathological molecules from the brain to the periphery for degradation. The central and peripheral clearance pathways likely interact and function synergistically to eliminate Aβ from the brain, underscoring the critical role of peripheral clearance in the removal of brain-derived Aβ.

### 7.3.1 Blood Component-Mediated Aβ Clearance

Multiple components in the blood have been shown to participate in the clearance of circulating amyloid-β (Aβ). Studies have demonstrated that bone marrow transplantation (BMT) reverses age-related impairments in cognitive function and synaptic plasticity in aged mice [113]. A recent study revealed that amelioration of cerebral amyloidosis is associated with enhanced Aβ clearance by peripheral monocytes [114].

1. Monocytes

Monocytes are a key component of the innate immune system. Circulating monocytes give rise to various tissue-resident macrophages throughout the body and specialized cell populations, such as microglia in the brain. Peripheral monocytes can take up Aβ from the bloodstream, and Aβ phagocytosis by these cells is impaired in AD patients [115, 116].

Multiple lines of evidence highlight the crucial role of monocytes in AD. A reduced capacity of peripheral monocytes to capture Aβ leads to elevated Aβ levels [117]. Aβ uptake by blood monocytes declines with aging and is further diminished in AD patients; reduced expression of Toll-like receptor 2 (TLR2) has been observed in monocytes from individuals with AD [118]. A specific subset of circulating monocytes can adhere to Aβ-rich cerebral vasculature and effectively clear Aβ microaggregates by internalizing them and transporting them from the brain's vascular compartment into the bloodstream [119].

A recent study observed monocytes infiltrating from the blood into the CSF and migrating from the central nervous system (CNS) to peripheral lymph nodes and back into the bloodstream, revealing that Aβ-binding monocytes may contribute to CNS Aβ clearance [120]. Moreover, impaired Aβ phagocytosis in monocytes has been associated with reduced metabolic activity toward Aβ, cellular senescence, and dysregulated phagocytic function in AD mouse models, highlighting the importance of restoring monocyte energy metabolism as a potential therapeutic strategy for AD [17].

Several potential therapeutic strategies targeting monocytes in patients with AD have been developed in recent years. Early modulation of monocytes by the nonerythropoietic peptide ARA 290 has been shown to slow the progression of AD-like pathology in mouse models, suggesting a promising therapeutic approach for AD [121]. Bone marrow transplantation (BMT) from young donors significantly reduced cerebral Aβ plaque burden in aged APP/PS1 mice, and this improvement was associated with enhanced Aβ clearance by peripheral monocytes [114]. These findings indicate that monocytes play a critical role in clearing Aβ from the circulation and that impaired phagocytic function of monocytes contributes to AD pathogenesis.

2. Enzymes

Secreted enzymes that exhibit affinity for specific domains within the Aβ amino acid sequence and possess the ability to cleave these peptides into shorter, less pathogenic forms are essential for the catabolism of circulating Aβ. These include insulin-degrading enzyme (IDE), neprilysin (NEP) and its homologues endothelin-converting enzyme (ECE), angiotensin-converting enzyme (ACE), matrix metalloproteinase-9 (MMP-9), and plasmin—the central proteolytic component of the plasminogen system.

IDE is a well-validated Aβ-degrading enzyme that was originally identified as a regulator of plasma insulin levels. It is primarily a soluble cytoplasmic enzyme, although a secreted form also exists [122]. IDE activity levels are inversely correlated with brain Aβ burden [123], and IDE knockout animals exhibit a significant increase in cerebral Aβ levels, indicating that loss of this enzyme's activity may contribute to the pathogenesis of AD [124].

NEP is a ubiquitous circulating protease that is highly abundant in the kidney and lung. NEP is widely regarded as the most potent amyloid-β (Aβ)-degrading enzyme [125, 126]. NEP dysfunction leads to increased endogenous Aβ levels in the mouse brain in a gene dose-dependent manner [127]. These findings indicate that NEP may exert significant effects on AD pathogenesis by promoting Aβ clearance.

ACE is highly expressed by endothelial cells throughout the body and is well known for its role in regulating salt and fluid balance. This enzyme has been shown to degrade Aβ and, more importantly, to cleave Aβ42 into the less toxic Aβ40 isoform [128, 129]. Genetic studies have demonstrated an association between reduced plasma ACE levels and increased risk of AD [130, 131]. Furthermore, ACE overexpression in myelomonocytes results in decreased brain Aβ levels [132], supporting a potential role for ACE in Aβ clearance. In addition, endothelin-converting enzyme-1 (ECE-1), plasmin, and matrix metalloproteinase-9 (MMP-9) are also involved in Aβ degradation [133, 134], and compelling evidence indicates a major role for MMP-9 in degrading compact Aβ plaques [135, 136], underscoring its significant contribution to Aβ clearance.

3. Erythrocytes

Recent evidence indicates that Aβ undergoes erythrocyte-mediated immune adherence throughout its clearance pathway: Aβ activates the complement system in serum, and complement-opsonized Aβ peptides are captured by erythrocytes via complement receptor 1 (CR1) and transported to the liver and spleen for elimination [137, 138]. CR1 expression is reduced in the erythrocytes of patients with AD, and single-nucleotide polymorphisms (SNPs) associated with lower erythrocyte CR1 levels are linked to increased AD risk, whereas a CR1 SNP associated with higher CR1 expression correlates with reduced AD risk [139]. These findings help establish a mechanistic link between CR1 polymorphisms and the risk of AD [140]. Furthermore, Aβ-specific antibodies can markedly enhance complement activation and Aβ opsonization, thereby promoting Aβ capture by human erythrocytes and macrophages [141]. These results indicate that the peripheral mechanism of Aβ clearance mediated by immunotherapies cannot be overlooked and highlight a potential role for interactions among autoantibodies, Aβ, and erythrocytes in AD pathogenesis. Additionally, erythrocyte counts are lower in AD patients compared to cognitively normal controls [142]. Collectively, these studies suggest that erythrocyte-mediated clearance—a major pathway for eliminating circulating pathogens—represents a significant mechanism for the removal of circulating amyloid-β (Aβ).

### 7.3.2 Liver-Mediated Aβ Clearance

The liver is a vital metabolic organ responsible for protein synthesis, metabolic regulation, and detoxification of harmful substances in the body. Circulating Aβ is primarily cleared through degradation by hepatocytes—which accounts for over 60% of total clearance—or via biliary excretion and catabolism [143]. Upon entering the peripheral circulation, Aβ typically binds to plasma proteins such as albumin, ApoE, apolipoprotein J (ApoJ), transthyretin (TTR), and α-2-macroglobulin (α-2M), all of which have been shown to interact with Aβ [37, 144–147]. However, in human plasma, soluble low-density lipoprotein receptor-related protein 1 (sLRP1), which sequesters 70% to 90% of circulating Aβ, is the predominant Aβ-binding protein [148].

Although various receptors, such as scavenger receptor A (SR-A) and the receptor for advanced glycation end products (RAGE), are expressed in the liver, low-density lipoprotein receptor-related protein 1 (LRP1) has been identified as the primary receptor mediating hepatic Aβ uptake [149]. Recent studies have demonstrated that approximately 13.9% of Aβ42 and 8.9% of Aβ40 are cleared from the bloodstream during a single pass through the liver, and that enhancing hepatic Aβ clearance via LRP1 overexpression attenuates cerebral Aβ deposition and cognitive deficits in APP/PS1 mice [18, 149, 150]. These findings underscore the critical role of the liver in Aβ clearance and in the pathophysiology of AD, suggesting that targeting hepatic Aβ clearance may represent a novel therapeutic strategy for AD.

### 7.3.3 Kidney-Mediated Aβ Clearance

The kidney is the primary excretory organ responsible for maintaining metabolite homeostasis by filtering and regulating minerals from the blood. Previous studies have shown that protein uptake in renal tubules is primarily mediated by two receptors—megalin and cubilin—expressed on renal tubular epithelial cells [151]. Following intracranial or intravenous injection of I125-labeled Aβ, radioactivity is subsequently detected in the kidneys and urine [111]. Moreover, soluble Aβ has been detected in human urine [152]. These findings suggest that the kidney may contribute to the physiological clearance of Aβ by filtering it from the bloodstream into the urine. A recent study demonstrated that Aβ levels in renal arterial blood are higher than those in renal venous blood, indicating net renal extraction of Aβ, and that unilateral nephrectomy leads to increased brain Aβ deposition. In contrast, long-term furosemide treatment attenuates AD pathology and cognitive deficits in APP/PS1 mice [15]. These findings suggest that kidney-mediated Aβ excretion significantly impacts the removal of Aβ from the brain.

### 7.3.4 Spleen-Mediated Aβ Clearance

The spleen is an organ that functions as a blood filter and performs essential immune functions, housing a diverse population of immune cells, including monocytes and macrophages, which play critical roles in the innate immune system [153]. Like their counterparts in other tissues, splenic monocytes and macrophages contribute to the clearance of peripheral Aβ [16, 154]. A recent study by Yu et al. demonstrated that the spleen plays a significant role in the peripheral clearance of Aβ, with splenic monocytes and macrophages being key mediators in this process. In contrast, splenectomy leads to increased accumulation of Aβ and may accelerate the onset of AD [16, 155].

### 7.3.5 Aβ Clearance Mediated by Other Peripheral Organs

Several studies have reported the detection of Aβ deposits in non-neural tissues, including the skin, subcutaneous tissue, and intestines in humans, as well as the gastrointestinal tract in animal models [39, 156, 157]. The presence of Aβ deposits in the intestine and skin is likely attributable to circulating Aβ in the bloodstream, suggesting that these peripheral tissues may actively participate in systemic Aβ metabolism.

The skin has long been recognized as an immune organ. Both the skin and the brain, which originate from the embryonic ectoderm, are physiologically and pathologically interconnected. Aβ34, a specific Aβ peptide variant, has been identified in human skin and may serve as a potential biomarker of Aβ degradation [158]. Aβ deposition has also been observed in the skin of patients with AD [39]. Although amyloid precursor protein (APP) expression has been detected in situ in the mammalian epidermis, predominantly in basal keratinocytes [159, 160], the origin of these Aβ deposits—whether from circulating blood or local cutaneous cells—remains unclear. Our previous studies demonstrated that radiolabeled Aβ accumulates primarily in the skin following intravenous injection [111]. These findings suggest that the skin may participate in peripheral Aβ metabolism. Sweat secretion represents another potential pathway for Aβ excretion; however, the extent to which the skin contributes to systemic Aβ clearance remains to be determined. Further research is required to address this question.

The gastrointestinal tract is a lymphoid organ densely populated with macrophages and other immune cells, giving it the potential capacity to clear amyloid-β (Aβ). Accumulating evidence indicates that the gut microbiota is altered in patients with AD [161, 162], suggesting involvement of the brain–gut–microbiota axis in AD pathogenesis. A recent study found that Aβ aggregates are detectable in human feces and that their concentrations are elevated in AD patients compared to healthy controls. However, the origin of digestion-resistant Aβ aggregates in feces—whether they are secreted via the liver and bile or directly from the enteric nervous system—remains to be elucidated [163]. Therefore, investigating the role of the gastrointestinal system in peripheral amyloid-β metabolism is essential.

### 7.3.6 *Therapeutic Strategies for Aβ Clearance in the Periphery*

Peripheral interventions have garnered increasing attention in recent years, demonstrating positive outcomes in reducing brain Aβ levels and the incidence of dementia. These peripheral approaches include plasma exchange programs [164, 165], dialysis (peritoneal dialysis and hemodialysis) [166], young bone marrow transplantation (BMT) [113, 114], management of cardiovascular risk factors [167], treatment of sleep-disordered breathing with continuous positive airway pressure (CPAP) [168, 169], reduction of peripheral blood cholesterol levels using statins [170], enhancement of phagocytic activity and function of peripheral blood monocytes via proteolytic degradation [154, 171], targeting enzymatic processes such as neprilysin (NEP) and angiotensin-converting enzyme (ACE) [172], development of nanozymes [173], and various therapeutic agents designed to promote peripheral Aβ clearance, including inorganic nanoparticles, polymer nanoparticles, and liposomes [174, 175]. Collectively, these findings suggest that "systemic therapeutic strategies" may help reduce cerebral Aβ burden and attenuate disease pathology, warranting further investigation.

## 7.4 Systemic Diseases Increase the AD Risk Via Peripheral Aβ Clearance

An increasing number of studies indicate that systemic abnormalities can exacerbate the progression of AD. Conversely, downstream effects originating from pathological processes in the AD brain can also contribute to these systemic disorders, thereby establishing bidirectional feedback loops. Below, we discuss the interactions between central and peripheral Aβ metabolism within a systemic framework.

### 7.4.1 Metabolic Disorders

1. Diabetes Mellitus

Numerous epidemiological studies, informed by preclinical, clinical, and postmortem evidence, have established a significant association between diabetes mellitus (DM) and AD [176, 177]. Individuals with diabetes are estimated to have a 1.5- to 2.0-fold higher risk of developing AD compared to healthy controls [178, 179]. The precise mechanisms by which diabetes influences Aβ catabolism and increases AD risk remain unclear. However, extensive research has revealed multiple key molecular interactions underlying these two conditions, including impaired insulin signaling, hypercholesterolemia, compromised clearance capacity, oxidative stress, protein misfolding, BBB disruption, and reduced cellular energy metabolism—all of which can impact Aβ peptide metabolism [177, 180]. These interactions are discussed in greater detail below.

In patients with diabetes mellitus (DM), accompanied by hyperinsulinemia and hyperglycemia [181], excess insulin can competitively inhibit insulin-degrading enzyme (IDE)-mediated Aβ degradation, leading to impaired clearance of Aβ peptides [182, 183]. However, studies have reported beneficial effects of insulin on both cognitive function and hepatic clearance of circulating Aβ peptides [184]. Furthermore, amylin—a misfolded protein deposited in the pancreas of patients with type 2 diabetes mellitus—can enter the brain, where it accelerates and exacerbates Aβ misfolding and aggregation [177]. Conversely, Aβ peptides have also been detected in the pancreas of DM patients [177]. This cross-seeding potential between islet amyloid polypeptide (IAPP) and Aβ peptides suggests a significant molecular link between DM and AD [185]. Additionally, DM-associated hyperglycemia may contribute to BBB disruption, which impairs Aβ peptide clearance and may promote Aβ deposition, as observed in the brains of aged rats [186, 187].

In summary, multiple significant molecular interactions exist between diabetes mellitus (DM) and AD that influence Aβ peptide metabolism. Further research is required to elucidate the precise mechanisms underlying these interactions.

2. Lipid and Lipoprotein Risk Factors

Abnormalities in lipid metabolism influence Aβ peptide metabolism and are associated with an increased risk of AD pathogenesis [188, 189]. Genome-wide association studies (GWAS) have identified several AD risk genes that are closely linked to lipid metabolism, including APOE, BIN1, CLU, SORL1, PICALM, and PLD3 [190]. The impact of apolipoprotein E (ApoE) on Aβ peptide metabolism varies depending on its specific isoform and lipidation status [191–193].

Cholesterol, the primary structural component of cell membranes, has been extensively studied in the context of neurodegenerative diseases. Brain cholesterol levels can influence Aβ synthesis, clearance, and neurotoxicity. Elevated serum cholesterol levels are associated with increased cerebral Aβ burden [194, 195]. In contrast, reduced membrane cholesterol levels decrease the activity of BACE1 and γ-secretase, leading to diminished Aβ peptide production both in vitro and in vivo

[196, 197]. Abnormal cholesterol levels may reflect unmeasured genetic factors or dietary patterns that could contribute to AD pathogenesis [194, 195]. For instance, cell membrane fluidity is highly dependent on lipid composition. Membrane fluidity plays a critical role in APP processing, cellular phagocytosis, and membrane-dependent biological processes—including endocytosis, phagocytosis, micropinocytosis, and autophagy—all of which impact Aβ peptide metabolism. Increased membrane fluidity in platelets and leukocytes has been reported in patients with AD or Down syndrome [198–201].

In contrast to cholesterol, fatty acids such as polyunsaturated fatty acids (PUFAs) and monounsaturated fatty acids (MUFAs) suppress Aβ peptide production. In addition, high dietary intake of docosahexaenoic acid (DHA), a polyunsaturated fatty acid that helps maintain membrane fluidity, inhibits Aβ peptide deposition and is associated with improved cognitive performance in both experimental animals and patients [202, 203].

### 7.4.2 Disorders of Systemic Immunity

Immune system abnormalities are now considered major pathological factors in AD. Approximately half of the AD risk genes (*BIN1*, *TREM2*, *CD33*, etc.) are involved in immune processes [204, 205]. Variants in these genes, particularly *TREM2* and *CD33*, are associated with impaired phagocytic function of peripheral monocytes or macrophages and altered Aβ accumulation in the brains of individuals with AD [171, 206], providing compelling evidence for a link between immune function and AD pathogenesis. In recent years, numerous studies have highlighted the critical role of immune cell dysfunction in the development of AD [207]. Reduced expression of Aβ phagocytic receptors and Aβ-degrading enzymes, along with diminished phagocytic activity of mononuclear phagocytes and neutrophils, may hinder Aβ degradation and clearance [208–210]. Lymphocytes—including B cells, T cells, and natural killer cells—also contribute to Aβ clearance through immunoglobulin-mediated adaptive phagocytosis [211, 212].

With respect to adaptive immunity, autoreactive antibodies associated with AD pathogenesis have been investigated. Specifically, elevated levels of pathogenic autoreactive antibodies and reduced levels of protective antibodies may influence Aβ clearance and deposition. Notably, the aging immune system exhibits a decline in immune cell production, reduced diversity of the immune repertoire, and an accumulation of dysfunctional immune cells. These alterations are collectively termed immunosenescence, which not only contributes to systemic aging—including brain aging [213]—but also increases susceptibility to age-related disorders such as AD [214]. Rejuvenation of aged immune cells has been identified as a potential therapeutic strategy for AD [113, 114]. Future research should focus on exploring novel approaches to restore immune cell function, thereby enhancing the potential for clinical translation.

### *7.4.3 Cardiovascular Disease*

For decades, researchers have recognized a link between various cardiovascular abnormalities and AD. Emerging evidence indicates that cardiovascular disease (CVD) is a major comorbidity in individuals with sporadic AD. Hypertension, a low cardiac index, and heart failure (HF) are associated with dementia and may also contribute to AD risk [215–217]. However, because both CVD and AD are complex, multifactorial, age-related conditions, their association may be partially explained by shared risk factors, including diabetes, hypertension, hypercholesterolemia, and stroke [218, 219].

Hypertension has been independently identified as a risk factor for AD, and multiple hypotheses have been proposed to explain the mechanisms by which hypertension contributes to AD: (1) vascular alterations leading to cerebral infarcts, (2) adverse effects on neuronal health promoting Aβ deposition in the brain, and (3) the development of cardiovascular disease that may increase susceptibility to AD [220]. Hypertension has also been suggested to promote AD through ischemia, oxidative stress, inflammation, and small-vessel disease [221, 222]. More recently, hypertension has been widely recognized as the most detrimental vascular risk factor for AD progression [223].

The severity of HF has been shown to be positively correlated with the degree of cognitive decline [224, 225]. Individuals with HF often exhibit regional brain atrophy and demyelination, as well as impaired axonal circuit functionality [226]. Moreover, genetic studies have revealed similar genetic profiles between patients with HF and patients with AD. In their familial forms, these two conditions involve variations in the *PSEN1* or *PSEN2* genes [227].

Similarly, atrial fibrillation (AF) shares epidemiological features with AD, and chronic AF may lead to inadequate cerebral perfusion, thereby accelerating Aβ plaque formation [228]. Cardiac systolic dysfunction can impair Aβ generation and clearance in the brain due to reduced cerebral blood flow [225, 229–231]. Regional cerebral blood flow and glucose uptake or metabolism are consistently reduced in Aβ-positive individuals with AD [232] and are inversely correlated with disease severity [233]. Indeed, some degree of cerebral small-vessel disease is nearly always present in conjunction with AD. Increased stiffness of small vessel walls may attenuate Aβ clearance through the BBB, interstitial fluid bulk flow, and glymphatic pathways, thus contributing to AD progression [234, 235]. In addition, impaired myocardial function and intramyocardial Aβ deposition observed in AD patients suggest that peripheral Aβ accumulation may adversely affect cardiac function in these individuals [41, 236].

However, a clear understanding of the interaction between comorbid cardiovascular disease (CVD) and AD remains incomplete. The majority of evidence indicates that CVD is an independent risk factor for cognitive impairment and exerts an additive rather than synergistic effect on the neurodegenerative processes underlying AD.

### 7.4.4 Hepatic Dysfunction

Circulating Aβ in the blood is primarily cleared through degradation by hepatocytes or direct excretion into bile [111, 237, 238]. Several clinical studies have documented a close association between hepatic dysfunction and AD. Plasma Aβ levels are inversely correlated with liver function, suggesting that impaired hepatic function reduces peripheral Aβ clearance [239]. Liver tissue from patients with AD contains lower levels of Aβ compared to that of cognitively normal individuals, indicating compromised hepatic Aβ clearance capacity in AD [28].

Recent studies have revealed that elevated Aspartate Aminotransferase (AST)/Alanine Aminotransferase (ALT) ratios and reduced ALT levels are associated with AD brain biomarkers and poorer cognitive performance, and that nonalcoholic fatty liver disease (NAFLD) is independently associated with lower cognitive function, linking hepatic dysfunction to AD pathogenesis [240, 241]. ApoE, a liver-synthesized protein critically involved in AD risk, regulates Aβ clearance through BBB transport, enzymatic degradation, and multiple other pathways [242]. Furthermore, central circadian rhythms may specifically influence Aβ pathogenesis [243]. Given that the liver is the primary peripheral organ communicating with the brain via the liver–brain axis, it may modulate Aβ clearance by regulating circadian rhythmicity [244].

Whether liver dysfunction also increases Aβ load in the brain remains unclear; however, enhancing LRP1-mediated hepatic Aβ uptake has been shown to alleviate both cerebral Aβ burden and cognitive impairment [149, 245]. These findings suggest that improving the liver's capacity for Aβ clearance represents a promising systemic therapeutic strategy for AD.

### 7.4.5 Renal Dysfunction

Studies have shown that renal disorders are risk factors for both cognitive impairment and dementia [246]. Serum Aβ levels are inversely correlated with measures of renal function—specifically, estimated glomerular filtration rate (eGFR) and serum creatinine levels—in patients with chronic kidney disease (CKD), defined as a gradual loss of renal function [247, 248]. Serum Aβ levels and brain Aβ deposition are significantly elevated in individuals with CKD [248, 249], and an association between CKD and increased risk of cognitive impairment has been established [250–252]. Aβ deposition is observed in the brains of CKD patients [249]. Moreover, human kidney donors exhibit reduced eGFRs and elevated circulating Aβ levels [253], suggesting that diminished renal functional reserve associated with living with a single kidney may impair peripheral Aβ clearance. Similar to other peripheral organs, the kidney contributes to systemic Aβ peptide clearance, thereby helping to reduce Aβ accumulation in the brain [15, 248]. Collectively, these findings indicate that impaired renal function may compromise peripheral Aβ clearance and could contribute to the development of cognitive decline in CKD patients. These data provide evidence that renal function plays a role in the pathogenesis of AD in humans.

A previous clinical study reported that the use of diuretics is associated with a reduced risk of AD [254]. Kidney transplantation has been shown to reduce plasma Aβ levels [253], and hemodialysis can alleviate Aβ deposition in the brains of patients with chronic kidney disease (CKD) [249]. These findings suggest that improving renal function may represent a promising therapeutic strategy for the prevention and treatment of AD.

### 7.4.6 Sleep and Respiratory Disorders

1. Sleep Disorders

Recent animal and human studies on Aβ metabolism support the associations among sleep quality, circadian cycles of Aβ clearance, and AD pathogenesis [255, 256]. Prospective studies have demonstrated that disturbances in sleep and circadian rhythms are correlated with early markers of neurodegeneration [257]. Poorer sleep quality, as well as shorter or longer sleep durations, are associated with increased Aβ burden in cortical and precuneal regions and greater cortical thinning, supporting a link between preclinical AD and sleep disorders [258, 259]. The risk of AD is elevated in older adults with chronic sleep deprivation (defined as less than 6 hours of sleep per day) [260]. Sleep disruption has been proposed to increase Aβ production and aggregation, impair glymphatic clearance of AD-related pathogenic proteins such as tau and Aβ, and exacerbate oxidative stress, inflammation, and synaptic damage [261, 262]. Memory-related neuroplasticity depends on stable sleep continuity for effective memory consolidation. Electroencephalographic (EEG) abnormalities, particularly reduced fast-frequency sleep spindles, are more pronounced in individuals with mild cognitive impairment (MCI) and AD [263]. Collectively, these findings underscore the role of sleep disturbances in the pathogenesis of AD.

2. Respiratory Disorders

Patients with AD have an increased incidence of respiratory disorders, including bronchopneumonia, obstructive sleep apnea (OSA), and sleep-disordered breathing [264, 265]. Certain preclinical neurodegenerative conditions, such as nonamnestic mild cognitive impairment, are more prevalent among individuals with chronic obstructive pulmonary disease (COPD) than in the general population [266]. Chronic impairment of lung function in younger individuals, as seen in COPD or asthma, is associated with a higher risk of developing mild cognitive impairment or dementia later in life [267]. Moreover, compared with healthy controls, patients with OSA or COPD exhibit elevated blood levels of Aβ, which negatively correlate with pulmonary function [268, 269]. OSA is also associated with alterations in CSF biomarkers of AD, including increased levels of phosphorylated tau and reduced levels of Aβ42 [270].

### 7.4.7 Gut Microbiome Disturbances

The establishment of the gut–brain axis has revealed a clear association between the gastrointestinal microbiota and cognitive function [264, 265]. Accumulating evidence indicates that the gut–brain axis plays a crucial role in the pathogenesis of various neurological disorders, including AD [266]. Gram-negative bacterial species, such as *Escherichia coli* K99, are the primary sources of bacteria-derived factors in the normal human brain, and these microbial components are elevated in AD brains, along with the bacterial cell wall component lipopolysaccharide (LPS) [267]. Lipopolysaccharide colocalizes with Aβ in amyloid plaques in AD brains, suggesting an involvement of gram-negative bacteria in AD pathogenesis [267]. Probiotic supplementation has been associated with improved cognitive performance in patients with AD [268], further supporting the role of the gut microbiota in AD development.

Recent studies have suggested that antibiotic treatment reduces cerebral Aβ peptide pathology in APP/PS1 mouse models. However, this effect was partially reversed by fecal microbiota transplantation from non-antibiotic-treated transgenic donors, indicating a strong link between the gut microbiota and cerebral proteinopathies [269]. Dietary interventions, such as soluble fiber intake, have been shown to modulate the gut microbiota and improve cognitive function in Alzheimer's disease mouse models [270]. Additionally, administration of dominant gut microbial strains has shown promise in restoring the abundance and composition of the intestinal microbiota, reducing neuroinflammation, and decreasing amyloid plaque deposition in the brain, offering a potential alternative to fecal microbiota transplantation for the treatment of Alzheimer's disease [271]. Further research is needed to elucidate the mechanisms underlying the interaction between the gut microbiota and Alzheimer's disease progression.

### 7.4.8 Blood Abnormalities

Recent studies have established a connection between peripheral blood dysfunction and AD [272, 273]. Beyond the monocytes and leukocytes previously discussed, other blood components also contribute to Aβ metabolism. Platelets from AD patients exhibit increased APP expression, altered APP isoform ratios, modified APP processing patterns, and elevated β-secretase activity [274–276], all of which significantly influence peripheral Aβ peptide production. Serum levels of albumin, a known Aβ carrier, are reduced in individuals with AD [277]. Additionally, both the quantity and function of erythrocytes—another major Aβ carrier—are impaired in these patients, with their red blood cells showing diminished capacity to bind Aβ [137, 142]. Moreover, the activity of Aβ-degrading enzymes is reported to be decreased in the serum of AD patients [278]. These changes impede Aβ transportation and clearance in the periphery.

In summary, understanding these changes or blood abnormalities, including alterations in platelet AβPP (increased expression, altered isoform ratio, differential processing pattern), Aβ peptide carriers (erythrocytes or albumin), and Aβ peptide-catabolizing proteases in blood serum, would help understand the pathogenesis of AD.

### *7.4.9 Pathogen Infection*

Infectious pathogens can activate the immune system, triggering elevated expression of proinflammatory molecules that may directly or indirectly contribute to AD pathology. In this context, evidence from epidemiological, molecular biological, neuropathological, and genetic studies supports a significant association between pathogen-induced inflammation and AD [279, 280]. For example, individuals exposed to infectious pathogens exhibit increased serum levels of Aβ peptides (i.e., Aβ40, Aβ42, and total Aβ) and inflammatory cytokines (i.e., IFN-γ, TNF-α, IL-1β, and IL-1β-6), supporting the role of pathogen-induced inflammation/infection in AD pathogenesis [279].

Recently, AD has been increasingly linked to infectious diseases following the detection of various microbes—including bacteria, fungi, and viruses—in the brain tissue of AD patients [281]. Several studies have proposed the "infection hypothesis," which posits that microbial infection may serve as an underlying etiological trigger for AD pathologies [282]. Cytomegalovirus (CMV), HSV-1, *Burkholderia* sp., *Chlamydia pneumoniae*, and *Helicobacter pylori* are considered the five main infectious agents affecting AD, and cognitive decline is more pronounced in patients infected with a greater number of pathogen species [279, 283]. Studies have demonstrated an association between herpes simplex virus types 1 and 2 (HHV-1/2), cytomegalovirus (CMV), and dementia [284]. Following primary infection, HHV establishes latency in the trigeminal ganglion and undergoes periodic reactivation. Under conditions of immunocompromise—such as aging, stress, immunosuppression, or peripheral infections—the virus can reactivate and contribute to cerebral neurodegeneration, thereby increasing the risk of AD [285–287]. In a long-term study of older adults, the presence of anti-HHV-1 antibodies was significantly associated with AD [288]. However, the precise mechanisms by which pathogens influence AD pathogenesis remain unclear. It is still uncertain whether microbial agents actively contribute to AD development or whether increased susceptibility to infections is a consequence of preclinical or early-stage AD.

### 7.4.10 Systemic Inflammation

Numerous studies have reported a significant association between inflammation and AD. Extensive crosstalk between systemic inflammation and central neuroinflammation represents a key neuropathological feature of AD [289, 290]. In the brain, microgliosis and chronic reactive gliosis contribute to sustained neuroinflammatory responses and the progression of AD pathology. Peripheral inflammation may influence the inflammatory state of the CNS [291, 292].

Several studies have demonstrated that conditions characterized by chronic systemic inflammation are associated with an increased risk of developing AD. For instance, chronic periodontitis—a common peripheral infection recognized as a "low-grade systemic inflammatory condition"—leads to the release of proinflammatory cytokines into the systemic circulation, contributing to both localized and systemic inflammation, thereby promoting AD pathogenesis [293, 294]. Similarly, a significant association has been reported between chronic systemic inflammation in patients with arthritis or rheumatoid arthritis (RA) and the development of dementia or AD. Notably, the presence of RA in midlife is linked to persistent systemic inflammation and poorer cognitive performance in later life [295]. These conditions are also associated with elevated levels of C-reactive protein and proinflammatory cytokines, such as tumor necrosis factor, IL-6, and IL-1β [293, 295]. These proinflammatory molecules could participate in AD pathogenesis either directly by affecting brain Aβ metabolism (via entry into the CNS through the BBB or neural afferent pathways such as the vagus nerve) [296, 297] or indirectly by affecting Aβ metabolism in the periphery. From a treatment perspective, substantial evidence from observational, epidemiologic, and laboratory studies has suggested that the use of anti-inflammatory medications, such as Nonsteroidal Antiinflammatory Drugs (NSAIDs), reduces the risk of AD [298]. Collectively, these findings indicate that chronic systemic inflammation may play a critical role in the development and progression of AD. In contrast, acute systemic inflammatory responses appear to exert protective effects against AD—at least in animal models—by recruiting monocyte-derived macrophages into the brain, where they facilitate Aβ clearance [299]. However, most findings in this area lack replication. Future research should include large-scale prospective studies and innovative methodologies to clarify the precise relationship between inflammation and Aβ metabolism.

### 7.4.11 Bone Diseases

Osteoporosis is a common skeletal disorder characterized by reduced bone density and bone mass resulting from multiple etiological factors. A 2005 cohort study found that women with low femoral neck bone mineral density (BMD) had approximately twice the risk of developing AD and dementia compared to those with higher BMD, whereas no significant association was observed in men [300]. Subsequent research and meta-analyses have consistently demonstrated a higher incidence of cognitive decline among individuals with osteoporosis [301–305]. Therefore, certain pathophysiological alterations in bone tissue may influence brain function. Conversely, AD also constitutes a risk factor for osteoporosis. Clinical evidence suggests that individuals with dementia exhibit poorer bone health and are at increased risk of fractures [306]. BMD was lower in the early AD group and was related to brain volume and memory ability, and a higher BMD was associated with better memory performance in AD patients [307, 308]. These findings suggest that neurological alterations in individuals with AD may have downstream effects on bone function. Recently, a Mendelian randomization analysis of large-scale bone mineral density (BMD) and AD genetic datasets demonstrated that low BMD is a causal risk factor for AD [309]. Systematic reviews and meta-analyses have shown associations among osteoarthritis, bone loss, and AD [310–312]. A longitudinal study demonstrated that osteoarthritis is associated with earlier Aβ deposition and increased Aβ-dependent tau accumulation over the follow-up period [313]. Changes in hippocampal functional connectivity and reduced levels of brain-derived neurotrophic factor (BDNF) are linked to subsequent cognitive decline in individuals with osteoarthritis [314]. Collectively, substantial clinical evidence supports an association between bone disorders and AD as well as dementia.

## 7.5 Conclusions

A growing number of findings suggest that AD may be more than just a brain disorder in the sense that systemic factors may interact with the brain to alter the AD process. First, although Aβ peptides are generated in the brain, a considerable amount of Aβ is also generated in peripheral systems. Second, Aβ can be cleared from peripheral organs and tissues, as well as the brain, by professional phagocytes that can transmigrate through the BBB. Third, Aβ deposits have been detected in both the brain and periphery. Finally, a series of systemic abnormalities is both driven by and contributes to AD progression. As discussed above, the central and peripheral Aβ pools interact and influence each other. For example, the rate of peripheral catabolism of Aβ appears to influence the rate of Aβ efflux from the brain, and peripherally derived Aβ can enter the brain, potentially accelerating cerebral AD pathology. Therefore, we hypothesize that the peripheral pool of Aβ is not simply associated with AD but is causally linked to this disease.

Several clinical trials attempting to treat AD have been launched in recent years, and three antibody-based DMT treatments targeting Aβ have achieved limited success by slowing early-stage AD progression. However, merely slowing cognitive decline is not enough to meet the clinical goal of AD treatment, which is to preserve patients' cognitive function. In fact, the close interaction between the brain and the periphery in Aβ metabolism may play a vital role in AD's natural history and offer new insights into its pathogenesis. This process is also affected by various systemic diseases. Future research should focus specifically on "systemic therapeutic strategies for AD prevention." Managing systemic diseases, including systemic aging, should be a key aspect of developing effective AD treatments.

## References


1. Bateman RJ, et al. Clinical and biomarker changes in dominantly inherited Alzheimer's disease. N Engl J Med. 2012;367:795–804. https://doi.org/10.1056/NEJMoa1202753.
2. Sevigny J, et al. The antibody aducanumab reduces Aβ plaques in Alzheimer's disease. Nature. 2016;537:50–6. https://doi.org/10.1038/nature19323.
3. van Dyck CH, et al. Lecanemab in early Alzheimer's disease. N Engl J Med. 2023;388:9–21. https://doi.org/10.1056/NEJMoa2212948.
4. Selkoe DJ, Hardy J. The amyloid hypothesis of Alzheimer's disease at 25 years. EMBO Mol Med. 2016;8:595–608. https://doi.org/10.15252/emmm.201606210.
5. Mawuenyega KG, et al. Decreased clearance of CNS beta-amyloid in Alzheimer's disease. Science. 2010;330:1774. https://doi.org/10.1126/science.1197623.
6. Sun BL, et al. Clinical research on Alzheimer's disease: Progress and perspectives. Neurosci Bull. 2018;34:1111–8. https://doi.org/10.1007/s12264-018-0249-z.
7. Moussa-Pacha NM, Abdin SM, Omar HA, Alniss H, Al-Tel TH. BACE1 inhibitors: Current status and future directions in treating Alzheimer's disease. Med Res Rev. 2020;40:339–84. https://doi.org/10.1002/med.21622.
8. Imbimbo BP, et al. Therapeutic intervention for Alzheimer's disease with γ-secretase inhibitors: still a viable option? Expert Opin Investig Drugs. 2011;20:325–41. https://doi.org/10.1517/13543784.2011.550572.
9. Doody RS, et al. Phase 3 trials of solanezumab for mild-to-moderate Alzheimer's disease. N Engl J Med. 2014;370:311–21. https://doi.org/10.1056/NEJMoa1312889.
10. Salloway S, et al. Two phase 3 trials of bapineuzumab in mild-to-moderate Alzheimer's disease. N Engl J Med. 2014;370:322–33. https://doi.org/10.1056/NEJMoa1304839.
11. Dyer O. Donanemab: FDA experts recommend approval of Alzheimer's drug. BMJ. 2024;385:q1327. https://doi.org/10.1136/bmj.q1327.
12. Kang HG, Park HY, Ryu HU, Suk SH. Bone mineral loss and cognitive impairment: The PRESENT project. Medicine (Baltimore). 2018;97:e12755. https://doi.org/10.1097/md.0000000000012755.
13. Sun HL, et al. Blood cell-produced amyloid-β induces cerebral Alzheimer-type pathologies and behavioral deficits. Mol Psychiatry. 2021;26:5568–77. https://doi.org/10.1038/s41380-020-0842-1.
14. Chen C, et al. Gut inflammation triggers C/EBPβ/δ-secretase-dependent gut-to-brain propagation of Aβ and Tau fibrils in Alzheimer's disease. EMBO J. 2021;40:e106320. https://doi.org/10.15252/embj.2020106320.
15. Tian DY, et al. Physiological clearance of amyloid-beta by the kidney and its therapeutic potential for Alzheimer's disease. Mol Psychiatry. 2021;26:6074–82. https://doi.org/10.1038/s41380-021-01073-6.
16. Yu ZY, et al. Physiological clearance of Aβ by spleen and splenectomy aggravates Alzheimer-type pathogenesis. Aging Cell. 2022;21:e13533. https://doi.org/10.1111/acel.13533.
17. Liu ZH, et al. Improving blood monocyte energy metabolism enhances its ability to phagocytose amyloid-β and prevents Alzheimer's disease-type pathology and cognitive deficits. Neurosci Bull. 2023;39:1775–88. https://doi.org/10.1007/s12264-023-01077-y.
18. Cheng Y, et al. Physiological β-amyloid clearance by the liver and its therapeutic potential for Alzheimer's disease. Acta Neuropathol. 2023;145:717–31. https://doi.org/10.1007/s00401-023-02559-z.

19. Grande G, et al. Multimorbidity burden and dementia risk in older adults: The role of inflammation and genetics. Alzheimers Dement. 2021;17:768–76. https://doi.org/10.1002/alz.12237.
20. Ben Hassen C, et al. Association between age at onset of multimorbidity and incidence of dementia: 30 year follow-up in Whitehall II prospective cohort study. BMJ. 2022;376:e068005. https://doi.org/10.1136/bmj-2021-068005.
21. Hu HY, et al. Association between multimorbidity status and incident dementia: a prospective cohort study of 245,483 participants. Transl Psychiatry. 2022;12:505. https://doi.org/10.1038/s41398-022-02268-3.
22. Pluvinage JV, Wyss-Coray T. Systemic factors as mediators of brain homeostasis, ageing and neurodegeneration (vol 21, pg 93, 2020). Nat Rev Neurosci. 2020;21:298. https://doi.org/10.1038/s41583-020-0293-3.
23. Liu CC, et al. Peripheral apoE4 enhances Alzheimer's pathology and impairs cognition by compromising cerebrovascular function. Nat Neurosci. 2022;25:1020-+. https://doi.org/10.1038/s41593-022-01127-0.
24. Giannisis A, et al. Brain integrity is altered by hepatic ε4 in humanized-liver mice. Mol Psychiatry. 2022;27:3533–43. https://doi.org/10.1038/s41380-022-01548-0.
25. Schroer AB, et al. Platelet factors attenuate inflammation and rescue cognition in ageing. Nature. 2023; https://doi.org/10.1038/s41586-023-06436-3.
26. Liu ZH, Wang YJ, Bu XL. Alzheimer's disease: targeting the peripheral circulation. Mol Neurodegener. 2023;18:3. https://doi.org/10.1186/s13024-023-00594-8.
27. Yankner BA, Mesulam MM. Seminars in medicine of the Beth Israel Hospital, Boston. beta-Amyloid and the pathogenesis of Alzheimer's disease. N Engl J Med. 1991;325:1849–57. https://doi.org/10.1056/NEJM199112263252605.
28. Roher AE, et al. Amyloid beta peptides in human plasma and tissues and their significance for Alzheimer's disease. Alzheimers Dement. 2009;5:18–29. https://doi.org/10.1016/j.jalz.2008.10.004S1552-5260(08)02896-3[pii].
29. Kuo YM, et al. Elevated abeta42 in skeletal muscle of Alzheimer disease patients suggests peripheral alterations of AbetaPP metabolism. Am J Pathol. 2000;156:797–805.
30. Davies TA, et al. Beta amyloid fragments derived from activated platelets deposit in cerebrovascular endothelium: usage of a novel blood brain barrier endothelial cell model system. Amyloid. 2000;7:153–65. https://doi.org/10.3109/13506120009146830.
31. Li S, Liu B, Zhang L, Rong L. Amyloid beta peptide is elevated in osteoporotic bone tissues and enhances osteoclast function. Bone. 2014;61:164–75. https://doi.org/10.1016/j.bone.2014.01.010.
32. Li QX, Fuller SJ, Beyreuther K, Masters CL. The amyloid precursor protein of Alzheimer disease in human brain and blood. J Leukoc Biol. 1999;66:567–74.
33. Toledo J, et al. Factors affecting Aβ plasma levels and their utility as biomarkers in ADNI. Acta Neuropathol. 2011;122:401–13.
34. Mehta PD, Pirttila T, Patrick BA, Barshatzky M, Mehta SP. Amyloid beta protein 1-40 and 1-42 levels in matched cerebrospinal fluid and plasma from patients with Alzheimer disease. Neurosci Lett. 2001;304:102–6.
35. Delvaux E, Bentley K, Stubbs V, Sabbagh M, Coleman P. Differential processing of amyloid precursor protein in brain and in peripheral blood leukocytes. Neurobiol Aging. 2013;34:1680–6.
36. Evin G, Zhu A, Holsinger RMD, Masters C, Li Q-X. Proteolytic processing of the Alzheimer's disease amyloid precursor protein in brain and platelets. J Neurosci Res. 2003;74:386–92.
37. Biere AL, et al. Amyloid beta-peptide is transported on lipoproteins and albumin in human plasma. J Biol Chem. 1996;271:32916–22. https://doi.org/10.1074/jbc.271.51.32916.
38. Kuo YM, et al. Amyloid-beta peptides interact with plasma proteins and erythrocytes: implications for their quantitation in plasma. Biochem Biophys Res Commun. 2000;268:750–6. https://doi.org/10.1006/bbrc.2000.2222.

39. Joachim CL, Mori H, Selkoe DJ. Amyloid beta-protein deposition in tissues other than brain in Alzheimer's disease. Nature. 1989;341:226–30. https://doi.org/10.1038/341226a0.
40. Koronyo Y, Salumbides B, Black K, Koronyo Hamaoui M. Alzheimer's disease in the retina: imaging retinal aβ plaques for early diagnosis and therapy assessment. Neurodegener Dis. 2012;10:285–93.
41. Troncone L, et al. Aβ amyloid pathology affects the hearts of patients with Alzheimer's disease: Mind the Heart. J Am Coll Cardiol. 2016;68:2395–407. https://doi.org/10.1016/j.jacc.2016.08.073.
42. Stine WB, Dahlgren K, Krafft G, LaDu M. In vitro characterization of conditions for amyloid-beta peptide oligomerization and fibrillogenesis. J Biol Chem. 2003;278:11612–22.
43. Murray M, et al. Amyloid beta protein: Abeta40 inhibits Abeta42 oligomerization. J Am Chem Soc. 2009;131:6316–7.
44. Tarasoff-Conway JM, et al. Clearance systems in the brain-implications for Alzheimer disease. Nat Rev Neurol. 2015;11:457–70. https://doi.org/10.1038/nrneurol.2015.119.
45. Yao XQ, et al. p75NTR ectodomain is a physiological neuroprotective molecule against amyloid-beta toxicity in the brain of Alzheimer's disease. Mol Psychiatry. 2015;20:1301–10. https://doi.org/10.1038/mp.2015.49.
46. Liao MC, et al. N-terminal domain of myelin basic protein inhibits amyloid beta-protein fibril assembly. J Biol Chem. 2010;285:35590–8. https://doi.org/10.1074/jbc.M110.169599.
47. Daneman R, Prat A. The blood-brain barrier. Cold Spring Harb Perspect Biol. 2015;7:a020412. https://doi.org/10.1101/cshperspect.a020412.
48. Candiello J, Cole GJ, Halfter W. Age-dependent changes in the structure, composition and biophysical properties of a human basement membrane. Matrix Biol. 2010;29:402–10. https://doi.org/10.1016/j.matbio.2010.03.004.
49. Bell RD, Zlokovic BV. Neurovascular mechanisms and blood-brain barrier disorder in Alzheimer's disease. Acta Neuropathol. 2009;118:103–13. https://doi.org/10.1007/s00401-009-0522-3.
50. Qosa H, et al. Differences in amyloid-β clearance across mouse and human blood-brain barrier models: kinetic analysis and mechanistic modeling. Neuropharmacology. 2014;79:668–78. https://doi.org/10.1016/j.neuropharm.2014.01.023.
51. Goulay R, Mena Romo L, Hol EM, Dijkhuizen RM. From stroke to dementia: a comprehensive review exposing tight interactions between stroke and Amyloid-β formation. Transl Stroke Res. 2020;11:601–14. https://doi.org/10.1007/s12975-019-00755-2.
52. Roberts KF, et al. Amyloid-β efflux from the central nervous system into the plasma. Ann Neurol. 2014;76:837–44. https://doi.org/10.1002/ana.24270.
53. Gireud-Goss M, Mack AF, McCullough LD, Urayama A. Cerebral amyloid angiopathy and blood-brain barrier dysfunction. Neuroscientist. 2021;27:668–84. https://doi.org/10.1177/1073858420954811.
54. Shibata M, et al. Clearance of Alzheimer's amyloid-ss(1-40) peptide from brain by LDL receptor-related protein-1 at the blood-brain barrier. J Clin Invest. 2000;106:1489–99. https://doi.org/10.1172/JCI10498.
55. Erickson MA, et al. Lipopolysaccharide impairs amyloid beta efflux from brain: altered vascular sequestration, cerebrospinal fluid reabsorption, peripheral clearance and transporter function at the blood-brain barrier. J Neuroinflammation. 2012;9:150. https://doi.org/10.1186/1742-2094-9-150.
56. Hartz AM, Miller DS, Bauer B. Restoring blood-brain barrier P-glycoprotein reduces brain amyloid-beta in a mouse model of Alzheimer's disease. Mol Pharmacol. 2010;77:715–23. https://doi.org/10.1124/mol.109.061754.
57. Rebeck GW, Harr SD, Strickland DK, Hyman BT. Multiple, diverse senile plaque-associated proteins are ligands of an apolipoprotein E receptor, the alpha 2-macroglobulin receptor/low-density-lipoprotein receptor-related protein. Ann Neurol. 1995;37:211–7. https://doi.org/10.1002/ana.410370212.

58. Deane R, et al. LRP/amyloid beta-peptide interaction mediates differential brain efflux of Abeta isoforms. Neuron. 2004;43:333–44.
59. Storck SE, et al. The concerted amyloid-beta clearance of LRP1 and ABCB1/P-gp across the blood-brain barrier is linked by PICALM. Brain Behav Immun. 2018;73:21–33. https://doi.org/10.1016/j.bbi.2018.07.017.
60. Zhao Z, et al. Central role for PICALM in amyloid-β blood-brain barrier transcytosis and clearance. Nat Neurosci. 2015;18:978–87. https://doi.org/10.1038/nn.4025.
61. Ito S, et al. Involvement of insulin-degrading enzyme in insulin- and atrial natriuretic peptide-sensitive internalization of amyloid-beta peptide in mouse brain capillary endothelial cells. J Alzheimer's Dis. 2014;38:185–200. https://doi.org/10.3233/JAD-122077.
62. Deane R, et al. RAGE mediates amyloid-beta peptide transport across the blood-brain barrier and accumulation in brain. Nat Med. 2003;9:907–13. https://doi.org/10.1038/nm890.
63. Montagne A, Zhao Z, Zlokovic BV. Alzheimer's disease: A matter of blood-brain barrier dysfunction? J Exp Med. 2017;214:3151–69. https://doi.org/10.1084/jem.20171406.
64. Damkier HH, Brown PD, Praetorius J. Cerebrospinal fluid secretion by the choroid plexus. Physiol Rev. 2013;93:1847–92. https://doi.org/10.1152/physrev.00004.2013.
65. Keep RF, Jones HC. A morphometric study on the development of the lateral ventricle choroid plexus, choroid plexus capillaries and ventricular ependyma in the rat. Brain Res Dev Brain Res. 1990;56:47–53. https://doi.org/10.1016/0165-3806(90)90163-s.
66. Hubert V, et al. Clinical imaging of choroid pexus in health and in brain disorders: A mini-review. Front Mol Neurosci. 2019;12:34. https://doi.org/10.3389/fnmol.2019.00034.
67. Crossgrove JS, Li GJ, Zheng W. The choroid plexus removes beta-amyloid from brain cerebrospinal fluid. Exp Biol Med (Maywood). 2005;230:771–6. https://doi.org/10.1177/153537020523001011.
68. Crossgrove JS, Smith EL, Zheng W. Macromolecules involved in production and metabolism of beta-amyloid at the brain barriers. Brain Res. 2007;1138:187–95. https://doi.org/10.1016/j.brainres.2006.12.022.
69. Kaur C, Rathnasamy G, Ling EA. The choroid plexus in healthy and diseased brain. J Neuropathol Exp Neurol. 2016;75:198–213. https://doi.org/10.1093/jnen/nlv030.
70. Pascale CL, et al. Amyloid-beta transporter expression at the blood-CSF barrier is age-dependent. Fluids Barriers CNS. 2011;8:21. https://doi.org/10.1186/2045-8118-8-21.
71. Behl M, Zhang Y, Zheng W. Involvement of insulin-degrading enzyme in the clearance of beta-amyloid at the blood-CSF barrier: Consequences of lead exposure. Cerebrospinal Fluid Res. 2009;6:11. https://doi.org/10.1186/1743-8454-6-11.
72. Brkic M, et al. Amyloid β Oligomers disrupt blood-CSF barrier integrity by activating matrix metalloproteinases. J Neurosci. 2015;35:12766–78. https://doi.org/10.1523/jneurosci.0006-15.2015.
73. Krzyzanowska A, Carro E. Pathological alteration in the choroid plexus of Alzheimer's disease: implication for new therapy approaches. Front Pharmacol. 2012;3:75. https://doi.org/10.3389/fphar.2012.00075.
74. Frölich L, et al. Integrity of the blood-CSF barrier in dementia of Alzheimer type: CSF/serum ratios of albumin and IgG. Eur Arch Psychiatry Clin Neurosci. 1991;240:363–6. https://doi.org/10.1007/bf02279767.
75. Iliff JJ, et al. A paravascular pathway facilitates CSF flow through the brain parenchyma and the clearance of interstitial solutes, including amyloid β. Sci Transl Med. 2012;4:147ra111. https://doi.org/10.1126/scitranslmed.3003748.
76. Plog BA, Nedergaard M. The glymphatic system in central nervous system health and disease: past, present, and future. Annu Rev Pathol. 2018;13:379–94. https://doi.org/10.1146/annurev-pathol-051217-111018.
77. Jessen NA, Munk AS, Lundgaard I, Nedergaard M. The glymphatic system: A beginner's guide. Neurochem Res. 2015;40:2583–99. https://doi.org/10.1007/s11064-015-1581-6.
78. Jacob L, et al. Conserved meningeal lymphatic drainage circuits in mice and humans. J Exp Med. 2022;219 https://doi.org/10.1084/jem.20220035.

79. Ahn JH, et al. Meningeal lymphatic vessels at the skull base drain cerebrospinal fluid. Nature. 2019;572:62–6. https://doi.org/10.1038/s41586-019-1419-5.
80. Da Mesquita S, et al. Functional aspects of meningeal lymphatics in ageing and Alzheimer's disease. Nature. 2018;560:185–91. https://doi.org/10.1038/s41586-018-0368-8.
81. Louveau A, et al. CNS lymphatic drainage and neuroinflammation are regulated by meningeal lymphatic vasculature. Nat Neurosci. 2018;21:1380–91. https://doi.org/10.1038/s41593-018-0227-9.
82. Da Mesquita S, et al. Aging-associated deficit in CCR7 is linked to worsened glymphatic function, cognition, neuroinflammation, and β-amyloid pathology. Sci Adv. 2021;7 https://doi.org/10.1126/sciadv.abe4601.
83. Wang L, et al. Deep cervical lymph node ligation aggravates AD-like pathology of APP/PS1 mice. Brain Pathol. 2019;29:176–92. https://doi.org/10.1111/bpa.12656.
84. Cao X, Xu H, Feng W, Su D, Xiao M. Deletion of aquaporin-4 aggravates brain pathology after blocking of the meningeal lymphatic drainage. Brain Res Bull. 2018;143:83–96. https://doi.org/10.1016/j.brainresbull.2018.10.007.
85. Drieu A, et al. Parenchymal border macrophages regulate the flow dynamics of the cerebrospinal fluid. Nature. 2022;611:585–93. https://doi.org/10.1038/s41586-022-05397-3.
86. Bakker EN, et al. Lymphatic clearance of the brain: Perivascular, paravascular and significance for neurodegenerative diseases. Cell Mol Neurobiol. 2016;36:181–94. https://doi.org/10.1007/s10571-015-0273-8.
87. Zhang ET, Inman CB, Weller RO. Interrelationships of the pia mater and the perivascular (Virchow-Robin) spaces in the human cerebrum. J Anat. 1990;170:111–23.
88. Bacyinski A, Xu M, Wang W, Hu J. The paravascular pathway for brain waste clearance: current understanding, significance and controversy. Front Neuroanat. 2017;11:101. https://doi.org/10.3389/fnana.2017.00101.
89. Schley D, Carare-Nnadi R, Please CP, Perry VH, Weller RO. Mechanisms to explain the reverse perivascular transport of solutes out of the brain. J Theor Biol. 2006;238:962–74. https://doi.org/10.1016/j.jtbi.2005.07.005.
90. Carare RO, et al. Solutes, but not cells, drain from the brain parenchyma along basement membranes of capillaries and arteries: significance for cerebral amyloid angiopathy and neuroimmunology. Neuropathol Appl Neurobiol. 2008;34:131–44. https://doi.org/10.1111/j.1365-2990.2007.00926.x.
91. Greenberg SM, et al. Cerebral amyloid angiopathy and Alzheimer disease - one peptide, two pathways. Nat Rev Neurol. 2020;16:30–42. https://doi.org/10.1038/s41582-019-0281-2.
92. Xie L, et al. Sleep drives metabolite clearance from the adult brain. Science. 2013;342:373–7. https://doi.org/10.1126/science.1241224.
93. Ma Q, et al. Rapid lymphatic efflux limits cerebrospinal fluid flow to the brain. Acta Neuropathol. 2019;137:151–65. https://doi.org/10.1007/s00401-018-1916-x.
94. Ma Q, Ineichen BV, Detmar M, Proulx ST. Outflow of cerebrospinal fluid is predominantly through lymphatic vessels and is reduced in aged mice. Nat Commun. 2017;8:1434. https://doi.org/10.1038/s41467-017-01484-6.
95. Norwood JN et al. Anatomical basis and physiological role of cerebrospinal fluid transport through the murine cribriform plate. eLife. 2019;8. https://doi.org/10.7554/eLife.44278.
96. Liu H, et al. Olfactory route for cerebrospinal fluid drainage into the cervical lymphatic system in a rabbit experimental model. Neural Regen Res. 2012;7:766–71. https://doi.org/10.3969/j.issn.1673-5374.2012.10.009.
97. Bradbury MW, Cserr HF, Westrop RJ. Drainage of cerebral interstitial fluid into deep cervical lymph of the rabbit. Am J Phys. 1981;240:F329–36. https://doi.org/10.1152/ajprenal.1981.240.4.F329.
98. Weller RO, Sharp MM, Christodoulides M, Carare RO, Møllgård K. The meninges as barriers and facilitators for the movement of fluid, cells and pathogens related to the rodent and human CNS. Acta Neuropathol. 2018;135:363–85. https://doi.org/10.1007/s00401-018-1809-z.

99. Weller RO, Djuanda E, Yow HY, Carare RO. Lymphatic drainage of the brain and the pathophysiology of neurological disease. Acta Neuropathol. 2009;117:1–14. https://doi.org/10.1007/s00401-008-0457-0.
100. Bothwell SW, Janigro D, Patabendige A. Cerebrospinal fluid dynamics and intracranial pressure elevation in neurological diseases. Fluids Barriers CNS. 2019;16:9. https://doi.org/10.1186/s12987-019-0129-6.
101. Aldea R, Weller RO, Wilcock DM, Carare RO, Richardson G. Cerebrovascular smooth muscle cells as the drivers of intramural periarterial drainage of the brain. Front Aging Neurosci. 2019;11:1. https://doi.org/10.3389/fnagi.2019.00001.
102. Di Marco LY, Farkas E, Martin C, Venneri A, Frangi AF. Is vasomotion in cerebral arteries impaired in Alzheimer's disease? J Alzheimer's Dis. 2015;46:35–53. https://doi.org/10.3233/jad-142976.
103. Boyle PA, et al. Cerebral amyloid angiopathy and cognitive outcomes in community-based older persons. Neurology. 2015;85:1930–6. https://doi.org/10.1212/wnl.0000000000002175.
104. Weller RO, Boche D, Nicoll JA. Microvasculature changes and cerebral amyloid angiopathy in Alzheimer's disease and their potential impact on therapy. Acta Neuropathol. 2009;118:87–102. https://doi.org/10.1007/s00401-009-0498-z.
105. Tripathi BJ, Tripathi RC. Vacuolar transcellular channels as a drainage pathway for cerebrospinal fluid. J Physiol. 1974;239:195–206. https://doi.org/10.1113/jphysiol.1974.sp010563.
106. Papaiconomou C, Bozanovic-Sosic R, Zakharov A, Johnston M. Does neonatal cerebrospinal fluid absorption occur via arachnoid projections or extracranial lymphatics? Am J Physiol. 2002;283:R869–76. https://doi.org/10.1152/ajpregu.00173.2002.
107. Zakharov A, et al. Integrating the roles of extracranial lymphatics and intracranial veins in cerebrospinal fluid absorption in sheep. Microvasc Res. 2004;67:96–104.
108. Szentistvanyi I, Patlak CS, Ellis RA, Cserr HF. Drainage of interstitial fluid from different regions of rat brain. Am J Phys. 1984;246:F835–44. https://doi.org/10.1152/ajprenal.1984.246.6.F835.
109. Wang J, Gu BJ, Masters CL, Wang YJ. A systemic view of Alzheimer disease - insights from amyloid-β metabolism beyond the brain. Nat Rev Neurol. 2017;13:612–23. https://doi.org/10.1038/nrneurol.2017.111.
110. Yuede CM, et al. Rapid in vivo measurement of beta-amyloid reveals biphasic clearance kinetics in an Alzheimer's mouse model. J Exp Med. 2016;213:677–85. https://doi.org/10.1084/jem.20151428.
111. Xiang Y, et al. Physiological amyloid-beta clearance in the periphery and its therapeutic potential for Alzheimer's disease. Acta Neuropathol. 2015;130:487–99. https://doi.org/10.1007/s00401-015-1477-1.
112. Wen YR, Yang JH, Wang X, Yao ZB. Induced dural lymphangiogenesis facilities soluble amyloid-beta clearance from brain in a transgenic mouse model of Alzheimer's disease. Neural Regen Res. 2018;13:709–16. https://doi.org/10.4103/1673-5374.230299.
113. Das MM, et al. Young bone marrow transplantation preserves learning and memory in old mice. Commun Biol. 2019;2:73. https://doi.org/10.1038/s42003-019-0298-5.
114. Sun PY, et al. Rejuvenation of peripheral immune cells attenuates Alzheimer's disease-like pathologies and behavioral deficits in a mouse model. Sci Adv. 2024;10:eadl1123. https://doi.org/10.1126/sciadv.adl1123.
115. Theriault P, ElAli A, Rivest S. The dynamics of monocytes and microglia in Alzheimer's disease. Alzheimer's Res Ther. 2015;7:41. https://doi.org/10.1186/s13195-015-0125-2.
116. Fiala M, et al. Ineffective phagocytosis of amyloid-beta by macrophages of Alzheimer's disease patients. J Alzheimer's Dis. 2005;7:221–32.; discussion 255-262,. https://doi.org/10.3233/jad-2005-7304.
117. Halle M, et al. Methods to monitor monocytes-mediated amyloid-beta uptake and phagocytosis in the context of adjuvanted immunotherapies. J Immunol Methods. 2015;424:64–79. https://doi.org/10.1016/j.jim.2015.05.002.

118. Chen SH, et al. Amyloid-beta uptake by blood monocytes is reduced with ageing and Alzheimer's disease. Transl Psychiatry. 2020;10:423. https://doi.org/10.1038/s41398-020-01113-9.
119. Michaud JP, Bellavance MA, Prefontaine P, Rivest S. Real-time in vivo imaging reveals the ability of monocytes to clear vascular amyloid beta. Cell Rep. 2013;5:646–53. https://doi.org/10.1016/j.celrep.2013.10.010.
120. Huang X, et al. Clearance and transport of amyloid β by peripheral monocytes correlate with Alzheimer's disease progression. Nat Commun. 2024;15:7998. https://doi.org/10.1038/s41467-024-52396-1.
121. Al-Onaizi MA, et al. Early monocyte modulation by the non-erythropoietic peptide ARA 290 decelerates AD-like pathology progression. Brain Behav Immun. 2022;99:363–82. https://doi.org/10.1016/j.bbi.2021.07.016.
122. Zhao J, Li L, Leissring MA. Insulin-degrading enzyme is exported via an unconventional protein secretion pathway. Mol Neurodegener. 2009;4:4. https://doi.org/10.1186/1750-1326-4-4.
123. Miller BC, et al. Amyloid-beta peptide levels in brain are inversely correlated with insulysin activity levels in vivo. Proc Natl Acad Sci USA. 2003;100:6221–6. https://doi.org/10.1073/pnas.1031520100.
124. Farris W, et al. Insulin-degrading enzyme regulates the levels of insulin, amyloid beta-protein, and the beta-amyloid precursor protein intracellular domain in vivo. Proc Natl Acad Sci USA. 2003;100:4162–7. https://doi.org/10.1073/pnas.0230450100.
125. Lim CS, Han JS. The antioxidant xanthorrhizol prevents amyloid-beta-induced oxidative modification and inactivation of neprilysin. Biosci Rep. 2018;38 https://doi.org/10.1042/BSR20171611.
126. Yasojima K, Akiyama H, McGeer EG, McGeer PL. Reduced neprilysin in high plaque areas of Alzheimer brain: a possible relationship to deficient degradation of beta-amyloid peptide. Neurosci Lett. 2001;297:97–100. https://doi.org/10.1016/s0304-3940(00)01675-x.
127. Huang SM, et al. Neprilysin-sensitive synapse-associated amyloid-beta peptide oligomers impair neuronal plasticity and cognitive function. J Biol Chem. 2006;281:17941–51. https://doi.org/10.1074/jbc.M601372200.
128. Hemming ML, Selkoe DJ. Amyloid beta-protein is degraded by cellular angiotensin-converting enzyme (ACE) and elevated by an ACE inhibitor. J Biol Chem. 2005;280:37644–50. https://doi.org/10.1074/jbc.M508460200.
129. Zou K, et al. Angiotensin-converting enzyme converts amyloid beta-protein 1-42 (Abeta(1-42)) to Abeta(1-40), and its inhibition enhances brain Abeta deposition. J Neurosci. 2007;27:8628–35. https://doi.org/10.1523/JNEUROSCI.1549-07.2007.
130. Lehmann DJ, et al. Large meta-analysis establishes the ACE insertion-deletion polymorphism as a marker of Alzheimer's disease. Am J Epidemiol. 2005;162:305–17. https://doi.org/10.1093/aje/kwi202.
131. Bertram L, McQueen MB, Mullin K, Blacker D, Tanzi RE. Systematic meta-analyses of Alzheimer disease genetic association studies: the AlzGene database. Nat Genet. 2007;39:17–23. https://doi.org/10.1038/ng1934.
132. Bernstein KE, et al. Angiotensin-converting enzyme overexpression in myelomonocytes prevents Alzheimer's-like cognitive decline. J Clin Invest. 2014;124:1000–12. https://doi.org/10.1172/JCI66541.
133. Eckman EA, Reed DK, Eckman CB. Degradation of the Alzheimer's amyloid beta peptide by endothelin-converting enzyme. J Biol Chem. 2001;276:24540–8. https://doi.org/10.1074/jbc.M007579200.
134. Barker R, Love S, Kehoe PG. Plasminogen and plasmin in Alzheimer's disease. Brain Res. 2010;1355:7–15. https://doi.org/10.1016/j.brainres.2010.08.025.
135. Humpel C. Organotypic vibrosections from whole brain adult Alzheimer mice (overexpressing amyloid-precursor-protein with the Swedish-Dutch-Iowa mutations) as a model to study clearance of beta-amyloid plaques. Front Aging Neurosci. 2015;7:47. https://doi.org/10.3389/fnagi.2015.00047.

136. Yan P, et al. Matrix metalloproteinase-9 degrades amyloid-beta fibrils in vitro and compact plaques in situ. J Biol Chem. 2006;281:24566–74. https://doi.org/10.1074/jbc.M602440200.
137. Rogers J, et al. Peripheral clearance of amyloid beta peptide by complement C3-dependent adherence to erythrocytes. Neurobiol Aging. 2006;27:1733–9.
138. Brubaker WD, et al. Peripheral complement interactions with amyloid beta peptide: Erythrocyte clearance mechanisms. Alzheimers Dement. 2017;13:1397–409. https://doi.org/10.1016/j.jalz.2017.03.010.
139. Johansson JU, et al. Peripheral complement interactions with amyloid beta peptide in Alzheimer's disease: Polymorphisms, structure, and function of complement receptor 1. Alzheimers Dement. 2018;14:1438–49. https://doi.org/10.1016/j.jalz.2018.04.003.
140. Jansen IE, et al. Genome-wide meta-analysis identifies new loci and functional pathways influencing Alzheimer's disease risk. Nat Genet. 2019;51:404–13. https://doi.org/10.1038/s41588-018-0311-9.
141. Crane A, et al. Peripheral complement interactions with amyloid beta peptide in Alzheimer's disease: 2. Relationship to amyloid beta immunotherapy. Alzheimers Dement. 2018;14:243–52. https://doi.org/10.1016/j.jalz.2017.04.015.
142. Chen SH, et al. Altered peripheral profile of blood cells in Alzheimer disease: A hospital-based case-control study. Medicine. 2017;96:e6843. https://doi.org/10.1097/MD.0000000000006843.
143. Tamaki C, et al. Major involvement of low-density lipoprotein receptor-related protein 1 in the clearance of plasma free amyloid beta-peptide by the liver. Pharm Res. 2006;23:1407–16. https://doi.org/10.1007/s11095-006-0208-7.
144. Oliveira SM, Ribeiro CA, Cardoso I, Saraiva MJ. Gender-dependent transthyretin modulation of brain amyloid-beta levels: evidence from a mouse model of Alzheimer's disease. J Alzheimer's Dis. 2011;27:429–39. https://doi.org/10.3233/JAD-2011-110488.
145. Schwarzman AL, et al. Transthyretin sequesters amyloid beta protein and prevents amyloid formation. Proc Natl Acad Sci USA. 1994;91:8368–72. https://doi.org/10.1073/pnas.91.18.8368.
146. Martel CL, et al. Isoform-specific effects of apolipoproteins E2, E3, and E4 on cerebral capillary sequestration and blood-brain barrier transport of circulating Alzheimer's amyloid beta. J Neurochem. 1997;69:1995–2004. https://doi.org/10.1046/j.1471-4159.1997.69051995.x.
147. Zlokovic BV, et al. Glycoprotein 330/megalin: probable role in receptor-mediated transport of apolipoprotein J alone and in a complex with Alzheimer disease amyloid beta at the blood-brain and blood-cerebrospinal fluid barriers. Proc Natl Acad Sci USA. 1996;93:4229–34. https://doi.org/10.1073/pnas.93.9.4229.
148. Sagare A, et al. Clearance of amyloid-beta by circulating lipoprotein receptors. Nat Med. 2007;13:1029–31. https://doi.org/10.1038/nm1635.
149. Sehgal N, et al. Withania somnifera reverses Alzheimer's disease pathology by enhancing low-density lipoprotein receptor-related protein in liver. Proc Natl Acad Sci USA. 2012;109:3510–5. https://doi.org/10.1073/pnas.1112209109.
150. Shinohara M, Tachibana M, Kanekiyo T, Bu G. Role of LRP1 in the pathogenesis of Alzheimer's disease: evidence from clinical and preclinical studies. J Lipid Res. 2017;58:1267–81. https://doi.org/10.1194/jlr.R075796.
151. Nielsen R, Christensen EI, Birn H. Megalin and cubilin in proximal tubule protein reabsorption: from experimental models to human disease. Kidney Int. 2016;89:58–67. https://doi.org/10.1016/j.kint.2015.11.007.
152. Ghiso J, et al. Alzheimer's soluble amyloid beta is a normal component of human urine. FEBS Lett. 1997;408:105–8. https://doi.org/10.1016/s0014-5793(97)00400-6.
153. Swirski FK, et al. Identification of splenic reservoir monocytes and their deployment to inflammatory sites. Science. 2009;325:612–6. https://doi.org/10.1126/science.1175202.
154. Gu BJ, et al. Innate phagocytosis by peripheral blood monocytes is altered in Alzheimer's disease. Acta Neuropathol. 2016;132:377–89. https://doi.org/10.1007/s00401-016-1596-3.

155. Wei Y, et al. Brain-spleen axis in health and diseases: A review and future perspective. Brain Res Bull. 2022;182:130–40. https://doi.org/10.1016/j.brainresbull.2022.02.008.
156. Tani Y, et al. Amyloid deposits in the gastrointestinal tract of aging dogs. Vet Pathol. 1997;34:415–20. https://doi.org/10.1177/030098589703400505.
157. March ME, et al. NAC blocks Cystatin C amyloid complex aggregation in a cell system and in skin of HCCAA patients. Nat Commun. 2021;12:1827. https://doi.org/10.1038/s41467-021-22120-4.
158. Akerman SC, et al. Neurodegenerative disease-related proteins within the epidermal layer of the human skin. J Alzheimer's Dis. 2019;69:463–78. https://doi.org/10.3233/JAD-181191.
159. Kummer C, Wehner S, Quast T, Werner S, Herzog V. Expression and potential function of beta-amyloid precursor proteins during cutaneous wound repair. Exp Cell Res. 2002;280:222–32. https://doi.org/10.1006/excr.2002.5631.
160. Hoffmann J, Twiesselmann C, Kummer MP, Romagnoli P, Herzog V. A possible role for the Alzheimer amyloid precursor protein in the regulation of epidermal basal cell proliferation. Eur J Cell Biol. 2000;79:905–14. https://doi.org/10.1078/0171-9335-00117.
161. Zhuang ZQ, et al. Gut microbiota is altered in patients with Alzheimer's disease. J Alzheimer's Dis. 2018;63:1337–46. https://doi.org/10.3233/JAD-180176.
162. Li B, et al. Mild cognitive impairment has similar alterations as Alzheimer's disease in gut microbiota. Alzheimers Dement. 2019;15:1357–66. https://doi.org/10.1016/j.jalz.2019.07.002.
163. Pils M, et al. Elevated Aβ aggregates in feces from Alzheimer's disease patients: a proof-of-concept study. Alzheimer's Res Ther. 2024;16:223. https://doi.org/10.1186/s13195-024-01597-3.
164. Villeda SA, et al. Young blood reverses age-related impairments in cognitive function and synaptic plasticity in mice. Nat Med. 2014;20:659–63. https://doi.org/10.1038/nm.3569.
165. Middeldorp J, et al. Preclinical assessment of young blood plasma for Alzheimer disease. JAMA Neurol. 2016;73:1325–33. https://doi.org/10.1001/jamaneurol.2016.3185.
166. Wang J, et al. Physiological clearance of tau in the periphery and its therapeutic potential for tauopathies. Acta Neuropathol. 2018;136:525–36. https://doi.org/10.1007/s00401-018-1891-2.
167. Satizabal CL, et al. Incidence of dementia over three decades in the Framingham Heart Study. N Engl J Med. 2016;374:523–32. https://doi.org/10.1056/NEJMoa1504327.
168. Osorio RS, et al. Sleep-disordered breathing advances cognitive decline in the elderly. Neurology. 2015;84:1964–71. https://doi.org/10.1212/wnl.0000000000001566.
169. Ancoli-Israel S, et al. Cognitive effects of treating obstructive sleep apnea in Alzheimer's disease: a randomized controlled study. J Am Geriatr Soc. 2008;56:2076–81. https://doi.org/10.1111/j.1532-5415.2008.01934.x.
170. Haag MD, Hofman A, Koudstaal PJ, Stricker BH, Breteler MM. Statins are associated with a reduced risk of Alzheimer disease regardless of lipophilicity. The Rotterdam Study. J Neurol Neurosurg Psychiatry. 2009;80:13–7. https://doi.org/10.1136/jnnp.2008.150433.
171. Bradshaw EM, et al. CD33 Alzheimer's disease locus: altered monocyte function and amyloid biology. Nat Neurosci. 2013;16:848–50. https://doi.org/10.1038/nn.3435.
172. Koronyo-Hamaoui M, et al. Peripherally derived angiotensin converting enzyme-enhanced macrophages alleviate Alzheimer-related disease. Brain. 2020;143:336–58. https://doi.org/10.1093/brain/awz364.
173. Ma M, et al. Self-protecting biomimetic nanozyme for selective and synergistic clearance of peripheral amyloid-β in an Alzheimer's disease model. J Am Chem Soc. 2020;142:21702–11. https://doi.org/10.1021/jacs.0c08395.
174. Brambilla D, et al. PEGylated nanoparticles bind to and alter amyloid-beta peptide conformation: toward engineering of functional nanomedicines for Alzheimer's disease. ACS Nano. 2012;6:5897–908. https://doi.org/10.1021/nn300489k.

175. Kim D, Kwon HJ, Hyeon T. Magnetite/ceria nanoparticle assemblies for extracorporeal cleansing of amyloid-β in Alzheimer's disease. Adv Mater. 2019;31:e1807965. https://doi.org/10.1002/adma.201807965.
176. Ettcheto M, et al. Peripheral and central effects of memantine in a mixed preclinical mice model of obesity and familial Alzheimer's disease. Mol Neurobiol. 2018;55:7327–39. https://doi.org/10.1007/s12035-018-0868-4.
177. Moreno-Gonzalez I, et al. Molecular interaction between type 2 diabetes and Alzheimer's disease through cross-seeding of protein misfolding. Mol Psychiatry. 2017;22:1327–34. https://doi.org/10.1038/mp.2016.230.
178. Xu W, et al. Meta-analysis of modifiable risk factors for Alzheimer's disease. J Neurol Neurosurg Psychiatry. 2015;86:1299–306. https://doi.org/10.1136/jnnp-2015-310548.
179. Velayudhan L, et al. Risk of developing dementia in people with diabetes and mild cognitive impairment. Br J Psychiatry. 2010;196:36–40. https://doi.org/10.1192/bjp.bp.109.067942.
180. Biessels GJ, Kappelle LJ. Increased risk of Alzheimer's disease in Type II diabetes: insulin resistance of the brain or insulin-induced amyloid pathology? Biochem Soc Trans. 2005;33:1041–4. https://doi.org/10.1042/bst0331041.
181. Milone M. Mitochondria, diabetes, and Alzheimer's disease. Diabetes. 2012;61:991–2. https://doi.org/10.2337/db12-0209.
182. Gasparini L, et al. Stimulation of beta-amyloid precursor protein trafficking by insulin reduces intraneuronal beta-amyloid and requires mitogen-activated protein kinase signaling. J Neurosci. 2001;21:2561–70. https://doi.org/10.1523/jneurosci.21-08-02561.2001.
183. Vekrellis K, et al. Neurons regulate extracellular levels of amyloid beta-protein via proteolysis by insulin-degrading enzyme. J Neurosci. 2000;20:1657–65. https://doi.org/10.1523/jneurosci.20-05-01657.2000.
184. Kang S, Lee YH, Lee JE. Metabolism-centric overview of the pathogenesis of Alzheimer's disease. Yonsei Med J. 2017;58:479–88. https://doi.org/10.3349/ymj.2017.58.3.479.
185. Bharadwaj P, et al. The link between type 2 diabetes and neurodegeneration: roles for Amyloid-β, Amylin, and Tau proteins. J Alzheimer's Dis. 2017;59:421–32. https://doi.org/10.3233/jad-161192.
186. Wang Y, et al. Blood-brain barrier disruption and perivascular beta-amyloid accumulation in the brain of aged rats with spontaneous hypertension: evaluation with dynamic contrast-enhanced magnetic resonance imaging. Korean J Radiol. 2018;19:498–507. https://doi.org/10.3348/kjr.2018.19.3.498.
187. Salameh TS, Shah GN, Price TO, Hayden MR, Banks WA. Blood–brain barrier disruption and neurovascular unit dysfunction in diabetic mice: protection with the mitochondrial carbonic anhydrase inhibitor topiramate. J Pharmacol Exp Ther. 2016;359:452–9. https://doi.org/10.1124/jpet.116.237057.
188. Mascitelli L, Seneff S, Goldstein MR. Association of Alzheimer disease pathology with abnormal lipid metabolism: the Hisayama study. Neurology. 2012;78:151; author reply 151–152. https://doi.org/10.1212/WNL.0b013e318242b283.
189. Lesser GT. Association of Alzheimer disease pathology with abnormal lipid metabolism: the Hisayama study. Neurology. 2012;78:1280. https://doi.org/10.1212/WNL.0b013e318254f6ad.
190. Sato N, Morishita R. The roles of lipid and glucose metabolism in modulation of β-amyloid, tau, and neurodegeneration in the pathogenesis of Alzheimer disease. Front Aging Neurosci. 2015;7:199. https://doi.org/10.3389/fnagi.2015.00199.
191. Yu JT, Tan L, Hardy J. Apolipoprotein E in Alzheimer's disease: an update. Annu Rev Neurosci. 2014;37:79–100. https://doi.org/10.1146/annurev-neuro-071013-014300.
192. Jiang Q, et al. ApoE promotes the proteolytic degradation of Abeta. Neuron. 2008;58:681–93. https://doi.org/10.1016/j.neuron.2008.04.010.
193. Li J, et al. Differential regulation of amyloid-β endocytic trafficking and lysosomal degradation by apolipoprotein E isoforms. J Biol Chem. 2012;287:44593–601. https://doi.org/10.1074/jbc.M112.420224.

194. Zissimopoulos JM, Barthold D, Brinton RD, Joyce G. Sex and race differences in the association between statin use and the incidence of Alzheimer disease. JAMA Neurol. 2016;74:225–32. https://doi.org/10.1001/jamaneurol.2016.37832591317[pii].
195. Reed B, et al. Associations between serum cholesterol levels and cerebral amyloidosis. JAMA Neurol. 2014;71:195–200. https://doi.org/10.1001/jamaneurol.2013.5390.
196. Fassbender K, et al. Simvastatin strongly reduces levels of Alzheimer's disease beta -amyloid peptides Abeta 42 and Abeta 40 in vitro and in vivo. Proc Natl Acad Sci USA. 2001;98:5856–61. https://doi.org/10.1073/pnas.081620098.
197. Liu Q, Zhang J. Lipid metabolism in Alzheimer's disease. Neurosci Bull. 2014;30:331–45. https://doi.org/10.1007/s12264-013-1410-3.
198. Zubenko GS, et al. Platelet membrane fluidity in Alzheimer's disease and major depression. Am J Psychiatry. 1987;144:860–8. https://doi.org/10.1176/ajp.144.7.860.
199. Collins JM, Scott RB, McClish DK, Taylor JR, Grogan WM. Altered membrane anisotropy gradients of plasma membranes of living peripheral blood leukocytes in aging and Alzheimer's disease. Mech Ageing Dev. 1991;59:153–62, doi: 10.1016/0047-6374(91)90081-a
200. Zubenko GS, Howland R. Markedly increased platelet membrane fluidity in Down syndrome with a (14q, 21q) translocation. J Geriatr Psychiatry Neurol. 1988;1:218–9.
201. Scott RB, Collins JM, Hunt PA. Alzheimer's disease and Down syndrome: leukocyte membrane fluidity alterations. Mech Ageing Dev. 1994;75:1–10, doi:0047-6374(94)90023-X [pii].
202. Yassine HN, et al. Association of serum docosahexaenoic acid with cerebral amyloidosis. JAMA Neurol. 2016;73:1208–16. https://doi.org/10.1001/jamaneurol.2016.1924.
203. Nishihira J, et al. Associations between serum omega-3 fatty acid levels and cognitive functions among community-dwelling octogenarians in Okinawa, Japan: the KOCOA study. J Alzheimer's Dis. 2016;51:857–66. https://doi.org/10.3233/JAD-150910.
204. Hollingworth P, et al. Common variants at ABCA7, MS4A6A/MS4A4E, EPHA1, CD33 and CD2AP are associated with Alzheimer's disease. Nat Genet. 2011;43:429–35. https://doi.org/10.1038/ng.803.
205. Jonsson T, et al. Variant of TREM2 associated with the risk of Alzheimer's disease. N Engl J Med. 2013;368:107–16. https://doi.org/10.1056/NEJMoa1211103.
206. Jay TR, et al. TREM2 deficiency eliminates TREM2+ inflammatory macrophages and ameliorates pathology in Alzheimer's disease mouse models. J Exp Med. 2015;212:287–95. https://doi.org/10.1084/jem.20142322.
207. Cao W, Zheng H. Peripheral immune system in aging and Alzheimer's disease. Mol Neurodegener. 2018;13:51. https://doi.org/10.1186/s13024-018-0284-2.
208. Zaghi J, et al. Alzheimer disease macrophages shuttle amyloid-beta from neurons to vessels, contributing to amyloid angiopathy. Acta Neuropathol. 2009;117:111–24. https://doi.org/10.1007/s00401-008-0481-0.
209. Frenkel D, et al. Scara1 deficiency impairs clearance of soluble amyloid-beta by mononuclear phagocytes and accelerates Alzheimer's-like disease progression. Nat Commun. 2013;4:2030. https://doi.org/10.1038/ncomms3030.
210. Zenaro E, et al. Neutrophils promote Alzheimer's disease-like pathology and cognitive decline via LFA-1 integrin. Nat Med. 2015;21:880–6. https://doi.org/10.1038/nm.3913.
211. Marsh SE, et al. The adaptive immune system restrains Alzheimer's disease pathogenesis by modulating microglial function. Proc Natl Acad Sci USA. 2016;113:E1316–25. https://doi.org/10.1073/pnas.1525466113.
212. Baruch K, et al. Breaking immune tolerance by targeting Foxp3(+) regulatory T cells mitigates Alzheimer's disease pathology. Nat Commun. 2015;6:7967. https://doi.org/10.1038/ncomms8967.
213. Yousefzadeh MJ, et al. An aged immune system drives senescence and ageing of solid organs. Nature. 2021;594:100–5. https://doi.org/10.1038/s41586-021-03547-7.
214. Cancro MP. Age-associated B cells. Annu Rev Immunol. 2020;38:315–40. https://doi.org/10.1146/annurev-immunol-092419-031130.

215. Rusanen M, et al. Heart diseases and long-term risk of dementia and Alzheimer's disease: a population-based CAIDE study. J Alzheimer's Dis. 2014;42:183–91. https://doi.org/10.3233/JAD-132363.
216. Qiu C, et al. Heart failure and risk of dementia and Alzheimer disease: a population-based cohort study. Arch Intern Med. 2006;166:1003–8. https://doi.org/10.1001/archinte.166.9.1003.
217. Jefferson AL, et al. Low cardiac index is associated with incident dementia and Alzheimer disease: the Framingham Heart Study. Circulation. 2015;131:1333–9. https://doi.org/10.1161/CIRCULATIONAHA.114.012438.
218. Luchsinger JA, et al. Aggregation of vascular risk factors and risk of incident Alzheimer disease. Neurology. 2005;65:545–51. https://doi.org/10.1212/01.wnl.0000172914.08967.dc.
219. Li J, et al. Vascular risk factors promote conversion from mild cognitive impairment to Alzheimer disease. Neurology. 2011;76:1485–91, WNL.0b013e318217e7a4 [pii]. https://doi.org/10.1212/WNL.0b013e318217e7a4.
220. Dickstein DL, et al. Role of vascular risk factors and vascular dysfunction in Alzheimer's disease. Mt Sinai J Med. 2010;77:82–102. https://doi.org/10.1002/msj.20155.
221. Leszek J, Sochocka M, Gąsiorowski K. Vascular factors and epigenetic modifications in the pathogenesis of Alzheimer's disease. J Neurol Sci. 2012;323:25–32. https://doi.org/10.1016/j.jns.2012.09.010.
222. Prins ND, et al. Cerebral small-vessel disease and decline in information processing speed, executive function and memory. Brain. 2005;128:2034–41. https://doi.org/10.1093/brain/awh553.
223. Thorin E. Hypertension and Alzheimer disease: another brick in the wall of awareness. Hypertension. 2015;65:36–8. https://doi.org/10.1161/hypertensionaha.114.04257.
224. Vogels RL, et al. Brain magnetic resonance imaging abnormalities in patients with heart failure. Eur J Heart Fail. 2007;9:1003–9. https://doi.org/10.1016/j.ejheart.2007.07.006.
225. Hoth KF, Poppas A, Moser DJ, Paul RH, Cohen RA. Cardiac dysfunction and cognition in older adults with heart failure. Cogn Behav Neurol. 2008;21:65–72. https://doi.org/10.1097/WNN.0b013e3181799dc8.
226. Kumar R, et al. Brain axonal and myelin evaluation in heart failure. J Neurol Sci. 2011;307:106–13. https://doi.org/10.1016/j.jns.2011.04.028.
227. Li D, et al. Mutations of presenilin genes in dilated cardiomyopathy and heart failure. Am J Hum Genet. 2006;79:1030–9. https://doi.org/10.1086/509900.
228. Ihara M, Washida K. Linking atrial fibrillation with Alzheimer's disease: epidemiological, pathological, and mechanistic evidence. J Alzheimer's Dis. 2018;62:61–72. https://doi.org/10.3233/jad-170970.
229. Okamoto Y, et al. Cerebral hypoperfusion accelerates cerebral amyloid angiopathy and promotes cortical microinfarcts. Acta Neuropathol. 2012;123:381–94. https://doi.org/10.1007/s00401-011-0925-9.
230. Zetterberg H, et al. Hypoxia due to cardiac arrest induces a time-dependent increase in serum amyloid beta levels in humans. PLoS One. 2011;6:e28263. https://doi.org/10.1371/journal.pone.0028263.
231. Wang L, et al. Chronic cerebral hypoperfusion induces memory deficits and facilitates Aβ generation in C57BL/6J mice. Exp Neurol. 2016;283:353–64.
232. Mattsson N, et al. Association of brain amyloid-β with cerebral perfusion and structure in Alzheimer's disease and mild cognitive impairment. Brain. 2014;137:1550–61.
233. Leeuwis AE, et al. Lower cerebral blood flow is associated with impairment in multiple cognitive domains in Alzheimer's disease. Alzheimers Dement. 2017;13:531–40. https://doi.org/10.1016/j.jalz.2016.08.013.
234. Marnane M, Hsiung GY. Could better phenotyping small vessel disease provide new insights into Alzheimer disease and improve clinical trial outcomes? Curr Alzheimer Res. 2016;13:750–63.

235. Kester MI, et al. Associations between cerebral small-vessel disease and Alzheimer disease pathology as measured by cerebrospinal fluid biomarkers. JAMA Neurol. 2014;71:855–62. https://doi.org/10.1001/jamaneurol.2014.754.
236. Jin WS, et al. Reduced cardiovascular functions in patients with Alzheimer's disease. J Alzheimer's Dis. 2017; https://doi.org/10.3233/JAD-170088.
237. Ghiso J, et al. Systemic catabolism of Alzheimer's Abeta40 and Abeta42. J Biol Chem. 2004;279:45897–908. https://doi.org/10.1074/jbc.M407668200.
238. Mohamed LA, Kaddoumi A. In vitro investigation of amyloid-β hepatobiliary disposition in sandwich-cultured primary rat hepatocytes. Drug Metab Dispos. 2013;41:1787–96. https://doi.org/10.1124/dmd.113.052514.
239. Wang YR, et al. Associations between hepatic functions and plasma amyloid-beta levels—implications for the capacity of liver in peripheral amyloid-beta clearance. Mol Neurobiol. 2017;54:2338–44. https://doi.org/10.1007/s12035-016-9826-1.
240. Nho K, et al. Association of altered liver enzymes with Alzheimer disease diagnosis, cognition, neuroimaging measures, and cerebrospinal fluid biomarkers. JAMA Netw Open. 2019;2:e197978. https://doi.org/10.1001/jamanetworkopen.2019.7978.
241. Seo SW, et al. Nonalcoholic fatty liver disease is associated with cognitive function in adults. Neurology. 2016;86:1136–42. https://doi.org/10.1212/wnl.0000000000002498.
242. Yamazaki Y, Zhao N, Caulfield TR, Liu CC, Bu G. Apolipoprotein E and Alzheimer disease: pathobiology and targeting strategies. Nat Rev Neurol. 2019;15:501–18. https://doi.org/10.1038/s41582-019-0228-7.
243. Kress GJ, et al. Regulation of amyloid-beta dynamics and pathology by the circadian clock. J Exp Med. 2018;215:1059–68. https://doi.org/10.1084/jem.20172347.
244. Chauhan R, Chen KF, Kent BA, Crowther DC. Central and peripheral circadian clocks and their role in Alzheimer's disease. Dis Model Mech. 2017;10:1187–99. https://doi.org/10.1242/dmm.030627.
245. Tamaki C, Ohtsuki S, Terasaki T. Insulin facilitates the hepatic clearance of plasma amyloid beta-peptide (1 40) by intracellular translocation of low-density lipoprotein receptor-related protein 1 (LRP-1) to the plasma membrane in hepatocytes. Mol Pharmacol. 2007;72:850–5. https://doi.org/10.1124/mol.107.036913.
246. Deckers K, et al. Dementia risk in renal dysfunction: a systematic review and meta-analysis of prospective studies. Neurology. 2017;88:198–208. https://doi.org/10.1212/wnl.0000000000003482.
247. Arvanitakis Z, Lucas JA, Younkin LH, Younkin SG, Graff-Radford NR. Serum creatinine levels correlate with plasma amyloid Beta protein. Alzheimer Dis Assoc Disord. 2002;16:187–90.
248. Liu YH, et al. Association between serum amyloid-beta and renal functions: implications for roles of kidney in amyloid-beta clearance. Mol Neurobiol. 2015;52:115–9. https://doi.org/10.1007/s12035-014-8854-y.
249. Sakai K, et al. Patients that have undergone hemodialysis exhibit lower amyloid deposition in the brain: evidence supporting a therapeutic strategy for Alzheimer's disease by removal of blood amyloid. J Alzheimer's Dis. 2016;51:997–1002. https://doi.org/10.3233/JAD-151139.
250. Etgen T, Chonchol M, Forstl H, Sander D. Chronic kidney disease and cognitive impairment: a systematic review and meta-analysis. Am J Nephrol. 2012;35:474–82. https://doi.org/10.1159/000338135.
251. Guo Z, et al. Common 1H-MRS characteristics in patients with Alzheimer's disease and vascular dementia diagnosed with kidney essence deficiency syndrome: a preliminary study. Altern Ther Health Med. 2017;23:12–8.
252. Radic J, et al. Kidney transplantation improves cognitive and psychomotor functions in adult hemodialysis patients. Am J Nephrol. 2011;34:399–406. https://doi.org/10.1159/000330849.
253. Gronewold J, et al. Factors responsible for plasma β-Amyloid accumulation in chronic kidney disease. Mol Neurobiol. 2016;53:3136–45. https://doi.org/10.1007/s12035-015-9218-y.

254. Chuang YF, et al. Use of diuretics is associated with reduced risk of Alzheimer's disease: the Cache County Study. Neurobiol Aging. 2014;35:2429–35. https://doi.org/10.1016/j.neurobiolaging.2014.05.002.
255. Kang JE, et al. Amyloid-beta dynamics are regulated by orexin and the sleep-wake cycle. Science. 2009;326:1005–7. https://doi.org/10.1126/science.1180962.
256. Yulug B, Hanoglu L, Kilic E. Does sleep disturbance affect the amyloid clearance mechanisms in Alzheimer's disease? Psychiatry Clin Neurosci. 2017;71:673–7. https://doi.org/10.1111/pcn.12539.
257. Dubois B, et al. Preclinical Alzheimer's disease: Definition, natural history, and diagnostic criteria. Alzheimers Dement. 2016;12:292–323. https://doi.org/10.1016/j.jalz.2016.02.002.
258. Spira AP, et al. Self-reported sleep and β-amyloid deposition in community-dwelling older adults. JAMA Neurol. 2013;70:1537–43. https://doi.org/10.1001/jamaneurol.2013.4258.
259. Spira AP, et al. Sleep duration and subsequent cortical thinning in cognitively normal older adults. Sleep. 2016;39:1121–8. https://doi.org/10.5665/sleep.5768.
260. Sabia S, et al. Association of sleep duration in middle and old age with incidence of dementia. Nat Commun. 2021;12:2289. https://doi.org/10.1038/s41467-021-22354-2.
261. Musiek ES, Holtzman DM. Mechanisms linking circadian clocks, sleep, and neurodegeneration. Science. 2016;354:1004–8. https://doi.org/10.1126/science.aah4968.
262. Cedernaes J, et al. Candidate mechanisms underlying the association between sleep-wake disruptions and Alzheimer's disease. Sleep Med Rev. 2017;31:102–11. https://doi.org/10.1016/j.smrv.2016.02.002.
263. Djonlagic I, et al. Associations between quantitative sleep EEG and subsequent cognitive decline in older women. J Sleep Res. 2019;28:e12666. https://doi.org/10.1111/jsr.12666.
264. Gareau M. Microbiota-gut-brain axis and cognitive function. Adv Exp Med Biol. 2014;817:357–71.
265. Dowling LR, Strazzari MR, Keely S, Kaiko GE. Enteric nervous system and intestinal epithelial regulation of the gut-brain axis. J Allergy Clin Immunol. 2022;150:513–22. https://doi.org/10.1016/j.jaci.2022.07.015.
266. Generoso JS, Giridharan VV, Lee J, Macedo D, Barichello T. The role of the microbiota-gut-brain axis in neuropsychiatric disorders. Braz J Psychiatry. 2021;43:293–305. https://doi.org/10.1590/1516-4446-2020-0987.
267. Zhan X, et al. Gram-negative bacterial molecules associate with Alzheimer disease pathology. Neurology. 2016;87:2324–32. https://doi.org/10.1212/WNL.0000000000003391.
268. Akbari E, et al. Effect of probiotic supplementation on cognitive function and metabolic status in Alzheimer's disease: A randomized, double-blind and controlled trial. Front Aging Neurosci. 2016;8:256. https://doi.org/10.3389/fnagi.2016.00256.
269. Dodiya HB, et al. Sex-specific effects of microbiome perturbations on cerebral Aβ amyloidosis and microglia phenotypes. J Exp Med. 2019;216:1542–60. https://doi.org/10.1084/jem.20182386.
270. Cuervo-Zanatta D, et al. Dietary fiber modulates the release of gut bacterial products preventing cognitive decline in an Alzheimer's mouse model. Cell Mol Neurobiol. 2023;43:1595–618. https://doi.org/10.1007/s10571-022-01268-7.
271. Li M, et al. Application of dominant gut microbiota promises to replace fecal microbiota transplantation as a new treatment for Alzheimer's disease. Microorganisms. 2023;11 https://doi.org/10.3390/microorganisms11122854.
272. Unda SR, Antoniazzi AM, Altschul DJ, Marongiu R. Peripheral leukocytosis predicts cognitive decline but not behavioral disturbances: a nationwide study of Alzheimer's and Parkinson's disease patients. Dement Geriatr Cogn Disord. 2021;50:143–52. https://doi.org/10.1159/000516340.
273. Xue W, Li J, Fu K, Teng W. Differential expression of mRNAs in peripheral blood related to prodrome and progression of Alzheimer's disease. Biomed Res Int. 2020;2020:4505720. https://doi.org/10.1155/2020/4505720.

274. Rosenberg RN, et al. Altered amyloid protein processing in platelets of patients with Alzheimer disease. Arch Neurol. 1997;54:139–44.
275. Di Luca M, et al. Abnormal pattern of platelet APP isoforms in Alzheimer disease and Down syndrome. Arch Neurol. 1996;53:1162–6.
276. Srisawat C, et al. The platelet amyloid precursor protein ratio as a diagnostic marker for Alzheimer's disease in Thai patients. J Clin Neurosci. 2013;20:644–8. https://doi.org/10.1016/j.jocn.2012.06.008.
277. Doecke JD, et al. Blood-based protein biomarkers for diagnosis of Alzheimer disease. Arch Neurol. 2012;69:1318–25. https://doi.org/10.1001/archneurol.2012.1282.
278. Liu Z, et al. Characterization of insulin degrading enzyme and other amyloid-β degrading proteases in human serum: a role in Alzheimer's disease? J Alzheimer's Dis. 2012;29:329–40. https://doi.org/10.3233/JAD-2011-111472.
279. Bu XL, et al. A study on the association between infectious burden and Alzheimer's disease. Eur J Neurol. 2015;22:1519–25. https://doi.org/10.1111/ene.12477.
280. Harris SA, Harris EA. Herpes simplex virus type 1 and other pathogens are key causative factors in sporadic Alzheimer's disease. J Alzheimer's Dis. 2015;48:319–53. https://doi.org/10.3233/JAD-142853.
281. Devanand DP. Viral hypothesis and antiviral treatment in Alzheimer's disease. Curr Neurol Neurosci Rep. 2018;18:55. https://doi.org/10.1007/s11910-018-0863-1.
282. Fulop T, et al. Can an infection hypothesis explain the beta amyloid hypothesis of Alzheimer's disease? Front Aging Neurosci. 2018;10:224. https://doi.org/10.3389/fnagi.2018.00224.
283. Bu XL, Wang YJ. Should infectious diseases be targeted to prevent dementias? Lancet Infect Dis. 2021;21:1477–8. https://doi.org/10.1016/s1473-3099(21)00258-9.
284. Sochocka M, Zwolińska K, Leszek J. The infectious etiology of Alzheimer's disease. Curr Neuropharmacol. 2017;15:996–1009. https://doi.org/10.2174/1570159x15666170313122937.
285. Lin WR, Shang D, Wilcock GK, Itzhaki RF. Alzheimer's disease, herpes simplex virus type 1, cold sores and apolipoprotein E4. Biochem Soc Trans. 1995;23:594s. https://doi.org/10.1042/bst023594s.
286. Itzhaki RF, et al. Herpes simplex virus type 1 in brain and risk of Alzheimer's disease. Lancet (London, England). 1997;349:241–4. https://doi.org/10.1016/s0140-6736(96)10149-5.
287. Itzhaki RF, Wozniak MA. Could antivirals be used to treat Alzheimer's disease? Future Microbiol. 2012;7:307–9. https://doi.org/10.2217/fmb.12.10.
288. Lövheim H, et al. Herpes simplex infection and the risk of Alzheimer's disease: A nested case-control study. Alzheimers Dement. 2015;11:587–92. https://doi.org/10.1016/j.jalz.2014.07.157.
289. Britschgi M, Wyss-Coray T. Systemic and acquired immune responses in Alzheimer's disease. Int Rev Neurobiol. 2007;82:205–33. https://doi.org/10.1016/s0074-7742(07)82011-3.
290. Gupta P, Sil S, Ghosh R, Ghosh A, Ghosh T. Intracerebroventricular Aβ-Induced Neuroinflammation Alters Peripheral Immune Responses in Rats. J Mol Neurosci. 2018;66:572–86. https://doi.org/10.1007/s12031-018-1189-9.
291. Guerrero-Carrasco M, Targett I, Olmos-Alonso A, Vargas-Caballero M, Gomez-Nicola D. Low-grade systemic inflammation stimulates microglial turnover and accelerates the onset of Alzheimer's-like pathology. Glia. 2024;72:1340–55. https://doi.org/10.1002/glia.24532.
292. Kamer AR, et al. Inflammation and Alzheimer's disease: possible role of periodontal diseases. Alzheimers Dement. 2008;4:242–50. https://doi.org/10.1016/j.jalz.2007.08.004.
293. Abbayya K, Puthanakar NY, Naduwinmani S, Chidambar YS. Association between periodontitis and Alzheimer's disease. N Am J Med Sci. 2015;7:241–6. https://doi.org/10.4103/1947-2714.159325.
294. Shaik MM, et al. How do periodontal infections affect the onset and progression of Alzheimer's disease? CNS Neurol Disord Drug Targets. 2014;13:460–6. https://doi.org/10.2174/1871527311312666015 2.

295. Wallin K, et al. Midlife rheumatoid arthritis increases the risk of cognitive impairment two decades later: a population-based study. J Alzheimer's Dis. 2012;31:669–76. https://doi.org/10.3233/jad-2012-111736.
296. Rivest S. Regulation of innate immune responses in the brain. Nat Rev Immunol. 2009;9:429–39. https://doi.org/10.1038/nri2565.
297. Gao HM, Hong JS. Why neurodegenerative diseases are progressive: uncontrolled inflammation drives disease progression. Trends Immunol. 2008;29:357–65. https://doi.org/10.1016/j.it.2008.05.002.
298. Etminan M, Gill S, Samii A. Effect of non-steroidal anti-inflammatory drugs on risk of Alzheimer's disease: systematic review and meta-analysis of observational studies. BMJ. 2003;327:128. https://doi.org/10.1136/bmj.327.7407.128.
299. Baruch K, et al. PD-1 immune checkpoint blockade reduces pathology and improves memory in mouse models of Alzheimer's disease. Nat Med. 2016;22:135–7. https://doi.org/10.1038/nm.4022.
300. Tan ZS, et al. Bone mineral density and the risk of Alzheimer disease. Arch Neurol. 2005;62:107–11. https://doi.org/10.1001/archneur.62.1.107.
301. Kostev K, Hadji P, Jacob L. Impact of osteoporosis on the risk of dementia in almost 60,000 patients followed in general practices in Germany. J Alzheimer's Dis. 2018;65:401–7. https://doi.org/10.3233/jad-180569.
302. Kwon MJ, et al. The occurrence of Alzheimer's disease and Parkinson's disease in individuals with osteoporosis: A longitudinal follow-up study using a national health screening database in Korea. Front Aging Neurosci. 2021;13:786337. https://doi.org/10.3389/fnagi.2021.786337.
303. Zhou R, Deng J, Zhang M, Zhou HD, Wang YJ. Association between bone mineral density and the risk of Alzheimer's disease. J Alzheimer's Dis. 2011;24:101–8. https://doi.org/10.3233/jad-2010-101467.
304. Lin SF, Fan YC, Pan WH, Bai CH. Bone and lean mass loss and cognitive impairment for healthy elder adults: analysis of the nutrition and health survey in Taiwan 2013–2016 and a validation study with structural equation modeling. Front Nutr. 2021;8:747877. https://doi.org/10.3389/fnut.2021.747877.
305. Zhao Y, Chen H, Qiu F, He J, Chen J. Cognitive impairment and risks of osteoporosis: A systematic review and meta-analysis. Arch Gerontol Geriatr. 2023;106:104879. https://doi.org/10.1016/j.archger.2022.104879.
306. Wang HK, et al. Increased risk of hip fractures in patients with dementia: a nationwide population-based study. BMC Neurol. 2014;14:175. https://doi.org/10.1186/s12883-014-0175-2.
307. Loskutova N, Honea RA, Vidoni ED, Brooks WM, Burns JM. Bone density and brain atrophy in early Alzheimer's disease. J Alzheimer's Dis. 2009;18:777–85. https://doi.org/10.3233/jad-2009-1185.
308. Kalc P, Dahnke R, Hoffstaedter F, Gaser C. Low bone mineral density is associated with gray matter volume decrease in UK Biobank. Front Aging Neurosci. 2023;15:1287304. https://doi.org/10.3389/fnagi.2023.1287304.
309. Gao F, Pan R, Fan T, Liu L, Pan H. Identification of heel bone mineral density as a risk factor of Alzheimer's disease by analyzing large-scale genome-wide association studies datasets. Front Cell Dev Biol. 2023;11:1247067. https://doi.org/10.3389/fcell.2023.1247067.
310. Weber A, et al. Association between osteoarthritis and increased risk of dementia: A systemic review and meta-analysis. Medicine (Baltimore). 2019;98:e14355. https://doi.org/10.1097/md.0000000000014355.
311. Guo R, et al. The association between osteoarthritis with risk of dementia and cognitive impairment: a meta-analysis and systematic review. J Alzheimer's Dis. 2022;89:1159–72. https://doi.org/10.3233/Jad-220568.
312. Lary CW, et al. Bone mineral density and the risk of incident dementia: A meta-analysis. J Am Geriatr Soc. 2024;72:194–200. https://doi.org/10.1111/jgs.18638.

313. Du J, et al. Association of APOE-ε4, osteoarthritis, β-Amyloid, and tau accumulation in primary motor and somatosensory regions in Alzheimer disease. Neurology. 2023;101:e40–9. https://doi.org/10.1212/wnl.0000000000207369.
314. Liu J, et al. The altered hippocampal functional connectivity and serum brain-derived neurotrophic factor level predict cognitive decline in patients with knee osteoarthritis. Cereb Cortex. 2023;33:10584–94. https://doi.org/10.1093/cercor/bhad305.
315. Roberts BR, et al. Biochemically-defined pools of amyloid-β in sporadic Alzheimer's disease: correlation with amyloid PET. Brain. 2017; https://doi.org/10.1093/brain/awx057.
316. Bush AI, et al. The amyloid precursor protein of Alzheimer's disease is released by human platelets. J Biol Chem. 1990;265:15977–83.
317. Li QX, et al. Secretion of Alzheimer's disease Abeta amyloid peptide by activated human platelets. Lab Invest. 1998;78:461–9.
318. Citron M, et al. Excessive production of amyloid beta-protein by peripheral cells of symptomatic and presymptomatic patients carrying the Swedish familial Alzheimer disease mutation. Proc Natl Acad Sci USA. 1994;91:11993–7.

# Chapter 8
# Alerting to Behavioral and Psychological Symptoms of Dementia Using Machine Learning and Wearable Devices

**Oscar Tai-Yuan Chen, Bo-Wei Yao, Vincent S. Tseng, and Yuan-Han Yang**

**Abstract** *Behavioral and Psychological Symptoms of Dementia* (BPSD) significantly impact dementia care, presenting challenges for both patients and caregivers. Recognizing the occurrence of BPSD at an early stage and effectively managing BPSD is critical for alleviating caregiver burden and reducing strain on healthcare systems. While utilizing machine learning technologies has enhanced the performance of BPSD prediction, there is still a lack of an integrated system for BPSD prediction and alerting. In this study, a smart wearable device-based BPSD Alerting System was developed to present a real-world clinical application. This system can send alert notifications to users when the predicted BPSD probability is higher than the user-specific threshold. We also introduced two BPSD prediction studies and their methodologies. Besides, we offered insights into their approaches to personalized and generalized modeling and their binary and ternary (fine-grained) classification strategies. This review highlights the strengths and limitations of each framework and provides valuable guidance for developing an effective BPSD

---

O. T.-Y. Chen
Institute of Computer Science and Engineering, National Yang Ming Chiao Tung University, Hsinchu, Taiwan

B.-W. Yao
Institute of Artificial Intelligence Innovation, National Yang Ming Chiao Tung University, Hsinchu, Taiwan

V. S. Tseng (✉)
Institute of Computer Science and Engineering, National Yang Ming Chiao Tung University, Hsinchu, Taiwan

Institute of Artificial Intelligence Innovation, National Yang Ming Chiao Tung University, Hsinchu, Taiwan

Department of Computer Science, National Yang Ming Chiao Tung University, Hsinchu, Taiwan
e-mail: vtseng@cs.nycu.edu.tw

Y.-H. Yang
Neuroscience Research Center, Kaohsiung Medical University, Kaohsiung, Taiwan

Department of Neurology, Kaohsiung Medical University Hospital, Kaohsiung, Taiwan



Y.-H. Yang (ed.), *Management of Dementia from the Preclinical Stage*,
https://doi.org/10.1007/978-981-95-5222-1_8

Alerting System. To the best of our knowledge, this is the first work to mention the integrated system based on smart wearable devices to implement machine learning applications of BPSD Alerting in a clinical environment, laying the foundation for further innovations in personalized dementia care in geriatric healthcare.

**Keywords** Behavioral and Psychological Symptoms of Dementia · Wearable Devices · Machine Learning · Predictive Models · Artificial Intelligence · Alerting System

## 8.1 Introduction

Dementia is often accompanied by a diverse range of non-cognitive symptoms, collectively referred to as *Behavioral and Psychological Symptoms of Dementia* (BPSD). These symptoms are commonly observed in individuals with dementia and include aberrant motor behavior, agitation or aggression, anxiety, apathy or indifference, appetite and eating abnormalities, delusions, depression or dysphoria, disinhibition, elation or euphoria, hallucinations, irritability, as well as sleep and nighttime behavior disruptions. BPSD can emerge at any stage of the disease and constitute a critical clinical aspect of dementia [19, 22, 26]. Caring for and managing BPSD patients presents considerable challenges in clinical practices, especially for caregivers, as it not only affects patients' well-being and quality of life but also causes elder mistreatment, heightened caregiver burden, and the rapid deterioration of functional abilities in individuals with dementia [5, 8, 13, 15]. Furthermore, BPSD is linked to several negative outcomes, such as higher risks of hospitalization, reduced ability to perform daily activities, diminished quality of life, and an increased likelihood of rapid progression to severe dementia [2, 10, 24]. Therefore, recognizing the occurrence of BPSD at an early stage is crucial for implementing timely interventions, providing necessary support, and ensuring proper care [22]. These efforts can contribute to better patient outcomes and help ease the burden on caregivers and healthcare systems. To pursue this objective, highly accurate BPSD prediction models based on machine learning and integrated alerting systems are needed. Although rare, some studies are still on machine learning-based BPSD prediction models. The machine learning study on next-day BPSD prediction used demographics, cognitive status, personality type, and acceleration signals, demonstrating the effectiveness of these factors [11]. Nevertheless, the prediction time window (next day) limits its practicality for timely interventions, as it fails to provide a precise timeframe for early medical treatment in real-world applications. In contrast, the study of next-four-hour BPSD prediction machine learning models based on the physiological signal collected from smart wearable devices was proposed [21]. They defined the workflow of this prediction problem, as shown in Fig. 8.1. In addition to shortening the prediction time window, this study also proposed generalized and personalized model training strategies to explore the ability of individualized prediction.

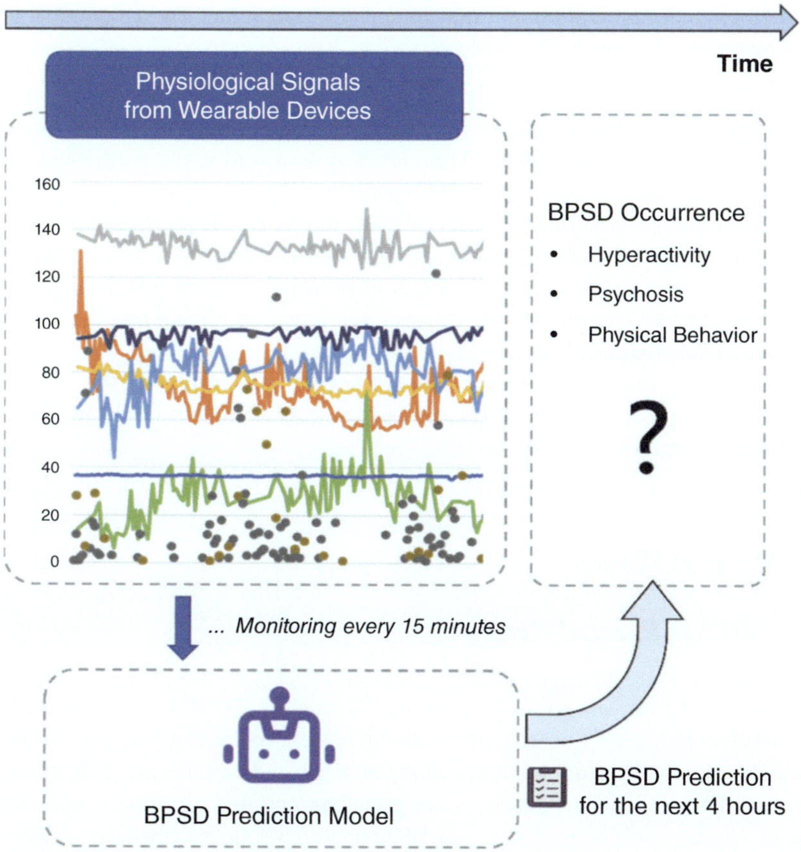


**Fig. 8.1** Overview of the next-4-hours BPSD prediction defined in [21]

However, although there are some studies related to BPSD prediction models, to the best of our knowledge, no prior research has mentioned the integrated system based on smart wearable devices to implement machine learning applications of BPSD Alerting in a clinical environment. To address the aforementioned problems, this study developed an integrated system, the BPSD Alerting System, to provide a comprehensive clinical application solution for smart wearable device-based machine learning BPSD prediction. We designed an extensible Model Inference Module in this system to allow developers to put in other related machine learning models. In this study, to achieve the demand for BPSD-related healthcare clinical applications, we prioritize utilizing the works of BPSD prediction [21, 22] to become applied models in our system. We will also introduce those two works in this chapter.

By introducing a comprehensive BPSD Alerting System, this study has made a valuable contribution to dementia care, aiming to enhance patient outcomes and provide a clinical application solution in geriatric medicine. The key contributions of this study can be outlined as follows:

- We have developed a novel integrated BPSD Alerting System based on smart wearable devices and machine learning BPSD prediction models to present a real-world clinical application. This novel system will assist caregivers in providing proper care to potential BPSD patients.
- We have conducted a comprehensive review of two BPSD prediction studies [21, 22] and incorporated their models into our BPSD Alerting System. This review enabled us to examine the applications of personalized and generalized prediction models and investigate the distinctions between binary and ternary (fine-grained) classification frameworks.
- We compared the datasets, experimental setups, and results of the two BPSD prediction studies [21, 22], providing key insights to inform future research and clinical applications.

## 8.2 Related Works

### *8.2.1 BPSD-Related Research*

*Behavioral and Psychological Symptoms of Dementia* (BPSD) represent a diverse and complex range of non-cognitive disturbances, including but not limited to aggression, apathy, agitation, depression, anxiety, hallucinations, delusions, and sleep disturbances. These symptoms are prevalent among individuals with dementia, with studies indicating that up to 91% of nursing home residents experience clinically significant BPSD during their illness. Among these, depression (43.9%), apathy (43.1%), and agitation (31.2%) are identified as the most common [18]. BPSD significantly exacerbates the challenges of dementia care, as these symptoms often lead to heightened emotional distress, increased functional decline, and reduced quality of life for patients.

From a caregiving perspective, BPSD imposes a profound psychological and physical burden. The unpredictable nature of symptoms, such as sudden outbursts of aggression or persistent apathy, complicates care routines and requires caregivers to adapt their strategies constantly. This property can lead to caregiver burnout, emotional exhaustion, and even physical health issues. Studies have shown that caregivers frequently experience heightened levels of stress, anxiety, and depression, with some ultimately feeling incapable of providing adequate care [25].

#### 8.2.1.1 Current Management Strategies for BPSD

Person-centered and multidisciplinary approaches have been widely advocated as the gold standard for managing BPSD [4, 7, 33]. These strategies emphasize understanding patients' individual needs, preferences, and histories to identify underlying causes of symptoms. Interventions often involve a combination of pharmacological treatments, non-pharmacological therapies (e.g., music therapy, reminiscence therapy, or physical activities), and environmental modifications to reduce stressors or triggers.

However, despite their theoretical benefits, these strategies exhibit significant limitations in practice. One of the most critical challenges is the heavy reliance on subjective assessments conducted by caregivers or healthcare professionals [12]. These evaluations are inherently inconsistent, influenced by personal biases, varying levels of expertise, and the emotional state of the assessors. For instance, a caregiver's perception of a patient's aggression may differ significantly depending on their stress levels, leading to discrepancies in symptom severity ratings.

Another key limitation lies in the static nature of traditional data collection methods [23]. Care plans are often formulated based on sporadic observations or periodic assessments, which fail to capture the dynamic and fluctuating characteristics of BPSD. Symptoms may vary significantly over short periods, influenced by varied factors such as time of day, environmental changes, or interactions with others. This lack of real-time monitoring hinders the ability to provide timely interventions, resulting in missed opportunities to address symptoms before they escalate.

Furthermore, the absence of structured and standardized observation methods represents a critical gap in current BPSD management. Care teams frequently resort to reactive measures, such as removing immediate triggers or isolating patients who exhibit disruptive behaviors. While these actions may provide short-term relief, they do not address the root causes of symptoms, leading to recurring issues that compromise long-term care efficacy.

The fragmented nature of communication between multidisciplinary team members further exacerbates these challenges. For example, a patient's behavioral changes may not be promptly relayed to all relevant stakeholders, such as psychologists, occupational therapists, or nursing staff. This lack of coordination undermines the holistic nature of person-centered care and reduces the overall effectiveness of interventions.

There is a growing need for innovative, real-time monitoring and predictive systems that leverage technological advancements to overcome these barriers. Such systems can enhance the accuracy and consistency of symptom assessment by integrating continuous data streams from wearable devices, environmental sensors, and other monitoring tools. Machine learning algorithms can analyze these data, identifying patterns and predicting symptoms with high precision. This proactive approach can revolutionize BPSD management, enabling timely interventions that alleviate symptoms and improve the overall quality of life for both patients and caregivers.

## 8.2.2 *Machine Learning Applications for Dementia*

In recent years, the application of advanced machine learning and data analytics techniques in the medical domain has gained significant attention [34]. Dementia research, a critical area within the medical field, has experienced a notable increase in studies employing machine learning (ML) methodologies to enhance diagnostic precision, predict disease progression, and support clinical decision-making [23].

Machine learning techniques have demonstrated exceptional capabilities in identifying patterns and relationships within complex, high-dimensional datasets that are often challenging to analyze using traditional statistical approaches. In the context of dementia research, these techniques have been applied to predict the onset and progression of dementia by utilizing diverse types of input data, including neuroimaging modalities such as magnetic resonance imaging (MRI) [1, 6] and positron emission tomography (PET) scans [14], cognitive test scores [30], genetic information [28], and medical records [35].

### 8.2.2.1 Machine Learning Applications for Dementia Prediction

Neuroimaging data, particularly from MRI and PET scans, have been a cornerstone in Alzheimer's disease (AD) research and related dementia studies. By extracting and analyzing structural and functional features of the brain, ML algorithms have demonstrated high accuracy in classifying dementia subtypes and predicting disease progression [1, 6]. For instance, advanced deep learning models, such as convolutional neural networks (CNNs), have been employed to automatically identify biomarkers of AD in brain images, achieving robust performance in both sensitivity and specificity. These models capture intricate spatial features, making them particularly effective for neuroimaging-based analyses.

Cognitive test data, including widely used assessments such as the Mini-Mental State Examination (MMSE) or more detailed cognitive function scales, have also been extensively utilized [11]. ML models applied to these datasets often utilize algorithms like support vector machines (SVMs), random forests (RFs), and ensemble methods to predict dementia onset. These models provide interpretable insights into how specific test results correlate with disease risk, making them valuable for clinicians seeking evidence-based tools to support early diagnosis.

Genetic information represents another critical data source for dementia research [28]. ML approaches have been used to analyze genome-wide association studies (GWAS) and identify genetic markers associated with dementia. These methods often integrate genetic data with other modalities, such as neuroimaging or cognitive tests, to enhance prediction accuracy. For example, multimodal learning frameworks have shown promise in uncovering complex interactions between genetic factors and phenotypic manifestations of dementia.

#### 8.2.2.2 Comparison of Methods in Terms of Data Requirements, Timeliness, and Accuracy

While the diversity of input data types enriches ML-based dementia prediction research, each method has strengths and limitations regarding data requirements, timeliness, and accuracy.

**Data Requirements**
Neuroimaging techniques such as MRI and PET scans require access to specialized equipment, significant financial resources, and expert interpretation [1, 6]. These high costs and logistical challenges limit their widespread applicability, particularly in resource-constrained settings. Conversely, cognitive test data and structured medical records are more readily available and cost-effective, making them practical for large-scale applications. Genetic data, while powerful, requires sequencing technologies and bioinformatics expertise, which can also be resource-intensive.

**Timeliness**
The timeliness of predictions depends heavily on the nature of the data and the computational requirements of the ML models. For instance, models based on neuroimaging data often require substantial preprocessing steps, such as segmentation and feature extraction, which can delay predictions. Cognitive tests, on the other hand, provide faster results since they rely on straightforward numerical data. Advances in wearable technology and real-time monitoring tools are bridging this gap, enabling continuous data collection that supports more timely predictions.

**Accuracy**
Regarding accuracy, deep learning models trained on neuroimaging data generally outperform traditional ML algorithms because they can learn non-linear relationships. However, these models are often criticized for their "black box" nature, which limits interpretability. Simpler models applied to cognitive test data or structured medical records may sacrifice some predictive power for transparency and ease of use. Multimodal approaches, combining data sources such as imaging, genetics, and clinical tests, have been shown to yield the highest accuracy by leveraging complementary information from different modalities.

Overall, the choice of ML approach depends on the specific research or clinical objectives and the availability of data and resources. While neuroimaging-based methods provide high accuracy and rich diagnostic insights, their cost and resource demand often restrict their use to specialized centers. Conversely, methods relying on cognitive tests or medical records offer broader accessibility and timeliness, despite their potentially lower predictive performance.

### *8.2.3 Wearable Devices for Health Monitoring and Prediction*

The rapid development and adoption of wearable health monitoring devices provide unprecedented opportunities for continuous, real-time physiological and behavioral data collection [32], revolutionizing healthcare-related applications. These devices, equipped with advanced sensors such as accelerometers, gyroscopes, heart rate monitors, and temperature sensors, offer a non-invasive, user-friendly means to track various health parameters over extended periods. This technological evolution has been particularly impactful in dementia care, where wearables enable early detection of subtle physiological and behavioral changes that may indicate disease progression or emerging symptoms [32].

In dementia care, wearable devices have proven effective in capturing data such as sleep quality and heart rate variability. These factors are often disrupted in individuals with cognitive decline [29]. For instance, decreases in physical activity, changes in gait stability, and irregular sleep-wake cycles are recognized as early indicators of dementia. Wearables not only allow for the detection of these changes but also enable caregivers and clinicians to monitor their progression in real-time.

Furthermore, these devices offer an innovative approach to Behavioral and Psychological Symptoms of Dementia (BPSD) prediction by identifying patterns and triggers that may precede episodes of aggression, agitation, or apathy. Research such as that by Cho et al. [11] highlights the potential of accelerometer-based data to predict BPSD occurrences. However, challenges such as limited predictive time windows remain to be addressed. Besides, a generalized and personalized training framework for BPSD prediction was proposed [21]. In addition to shortening the predictive time window, they emphasized a personalized modeling strategy for capturing individual information by using each patient's specific physiological signal data from smart wearable devices to give personalized analysis. Moreover, a fine-grained BPSD prediction model [22] was proposed to enhance the model, enabling it not only to predict the occurrence of BPSD but also to identify the specific type of BPSD. These works show the effectiveness of using data from smart wearable devices to predict BPSD that occurs for the following hours.

## 8.3 The BPSD Alerting System

### *8.3.1 System Architecture*

In this study, we developed an integrated system based on smart wearable devices to implement machine learning applications of BPSD Alerting in a clinical environment. The developed system architecture, named BPSD Alerting System, is illustrated in Fig. 8.2. This system allows users (e.g., patients) to get the risk probability of BPSD occurrences for the following hours by wearing a physiological signal monitoring smart device, and it sends alert notifications when the risk probability is

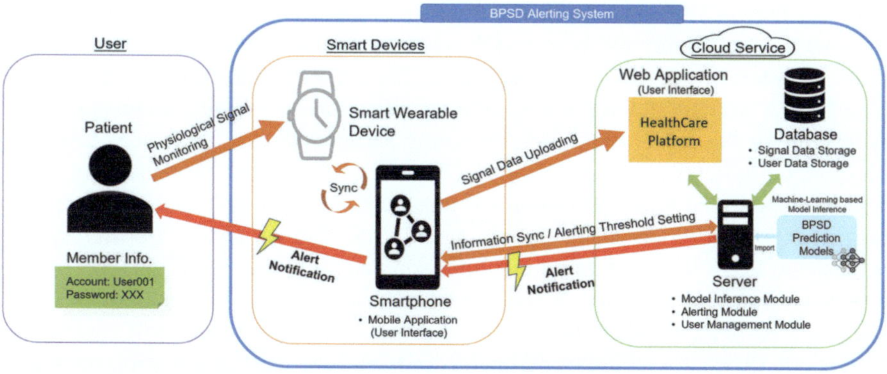


**Fig. 8.2** The overall architecture of our developed Behavioral and Psychological Symptoms of Dementia (BPSD) Alerting System

higher than the user-specific threshold. Clinicians can use this system to monitor the health status of dementia patients and perform related analyses. This system consists of two main components: the "Smart Devices" and the "Cloud Service." The following sections will introduce these in detail.

**System Components: Smart Devices**

Our developed BPSD Alerting System is based on smart devices. These devices allow us to collect signal data or become the user's operation interface. We can divide the devices into "Smart Wearable Device" and "Smartphone."

Smart wearable devices are responsible for collecting physiological signal data from patients. We use smart watches in our implementation. Each patient must wear a specific smart watch equipped with multi-sensors such as Electricalgraphy, PPG (photoplethysmography), infrared, temperature, and activity sensors. This watch will record the varied signal data, including the variables we used in this study, and promptly synchronize with the connected mobile application. Mobile applications are installed on smartphones. This application will be one of the user interfaces in this system. The user (could be the patient or clinicians) can use that to adjust the alerting threshold to control the sensitivity level of the alerting system. In addition, the main core of this application is to regularly upload the signal data into the HealthCare platform in the cloud service. With this strategy, data from the cache on the smart watch can be released to reduce memory usage. Simultaneously, that data will be sent to the server for further predictions. Users will receive alert notifications with this mobile application if there are any risks of BPSD occurrences predicted through the models. In our practical implementation, we let the patients use the ASUS VivoWatch 5, which contains all the sensors we mentioned above.

**System Components: Cloud Service**

The main computing device in our BPSD Alerting System is in the cloud. The online server is responsible for handling the process of model inference, alert notifications, and user management. Through the HealthCare platform, the web interface between the mobile application and cloud service, the physiological signal data recorded from the smart watch will be gathered into the server and storage units. Besides, this platform provides a graphical interface for users to retrieve the historical data. Also, the user can get the complete analysis results on this platform. After getting the signal data, the computing server will call the Model Inference Module to predict the risk probability of BPSD occurrences in the following hours. This extensible module can contain various machine learning-based BPSD prediction models. In addition, more models can be applied in our BPSD Alerting System if these models follow our unified Application Programming Interface (API). After model inference computing, if the predicted probability is higher than the user-specific threshold, another module, named the Alerting Module, will resume the connection process to the mobile device and send the alert notification to related users. The clinicians can adopt corresponding medical strategies according to the prediction results. To improve the model tuning strategy, the clinicians can also record any BPSD-related anomalies on the HealthCare platform and comment on predicted results. Apart from what has been mentioned above, the server will also have the User Management Module to manage the permissions of different user roles. This module allows us to assign different roles to users, such as patients, clinicians, or system administrators. Also, it has a Member Management Mechanism for future use cases to help service providers establish the membership system. In our practical implementation, we utilized the ASUS OmniCare platform as the web application (web-based user interface).

In the following two sections, we will introduce two machine learning models that are compatible with our BPSD Alerting System.

### 8.3.2 Generalized and Personalized BPSD Prediction Model

Recently, many medical studies have been utilizing machine learning technologies to develop prediction models. The field of dementia is no exception. However, there are still scarce studies about machine learning-based BPSD prediction models. The work of next-day BPSD prediction [11] showed the effectiveness of considering demographics, cognitive status, and personality type and adopting acceleration signals. Nevertheless, the time range of the prediction window (next day) is too long to give the user an accurate time period to make the early medical treatment. For a BPSD Alerting System, timeliness is essential and matches real-world applications. Besides, because the physiological signal data distribution may vary among users, this problem will decrease performance. Therefore, the personalized prediction model is another key point of a BPSD Alerting System.

The work of the next four-hour BPSD prediction framework with generalized and personalized models [21] is suitable for our BPSD Alerting System. In the

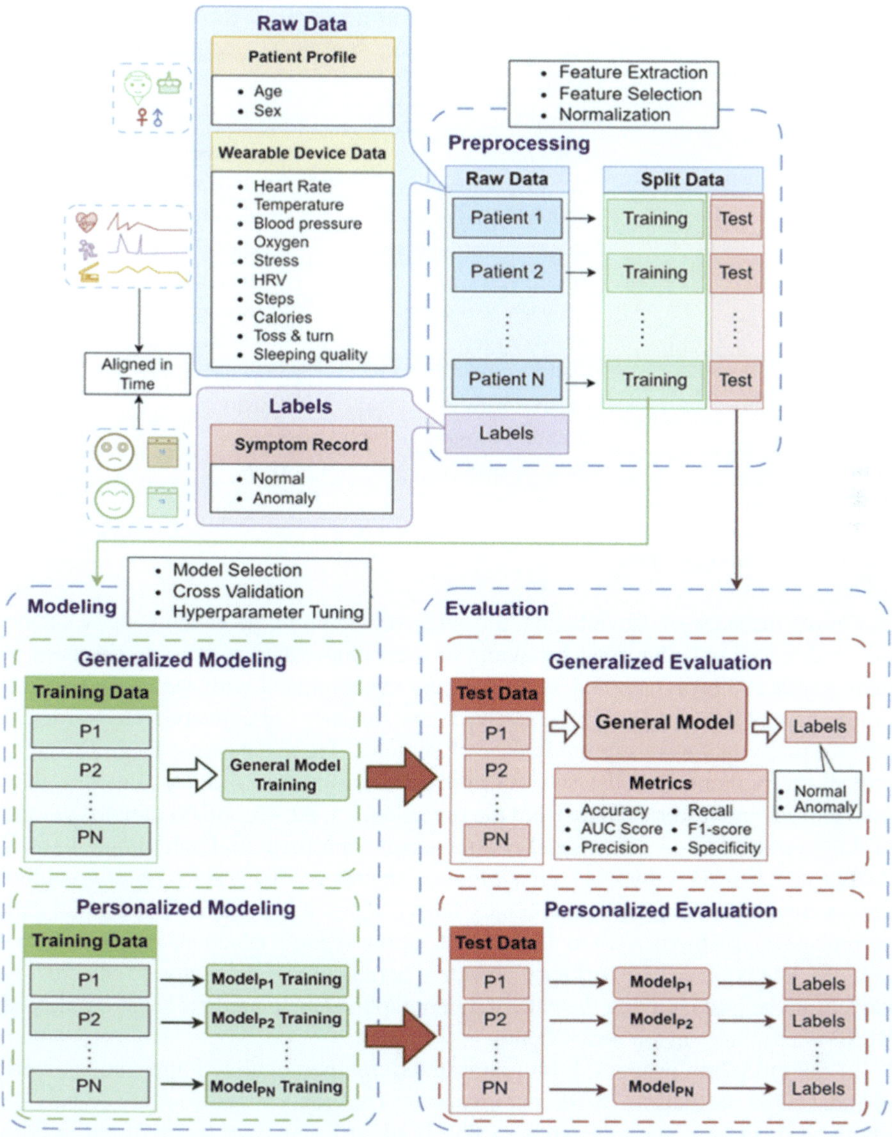


**Fig. 8.3** Overview of the generalized and personalized BPSD prediction models proposed in Hsu et al. [21]

following, we describe the framework and approaches of their work briefly. Their proposed framework is illustrated in Fig. 8.3. Their proposed models adopt various types of physiological signals from smart wearable devices. Table 8.1 presents the data composition and corresponding description.

**Table 8.1** Description of the variables used in Hsu et al. [21]

| Variable | Description | Measurement Occasion |
|---|---|---|
| Age | Patient age | – |
| Sex | Patient sex | – |
| HR | Heart rate | Continuous[a] |
| HRV | Heart rate variability | Continuous |
| SYS | Systolic blood pressure | Continuous |
| DIA | Diastolic blood pressure | Continuous |
| Stress | Stress index | Continuous |
| Temp | Body temperature | Continuous |
| Oxygen | Blood oxygen | Continuous |
| Steps | Steps | Activity[b] |
| Calories | Calories burned | Activity |
| Toss & Turn | Number of tosses and turns | Sleep[c] |
| Sleeping Quality | Sleeping quality | Sleep |

[a]Passive measurement while wearing
[b]Measurement during activity
[c]Measurement during sleeping

During the stage of data labeling, the caregivers monitor the patients' daily behaviors and record any abnormal behaviors or dementia-related symptoms observed in their routines. Those recorded symptoms are synchronized with the corresponding timestamps of data collected by smart wearable devices. For collecting physiological signals, these data were captured every 15 minutes. These data were then utilized to predict the probability of BPSD occurrence within the next 4 hours. Besides, they used current and historical data from the preceding 15, 30, 45, and 60 minutes (a total of 5 time points) to give the model comprehensive information. Each sample in their dataset contains 55 values (11 physiological signals recorded across 5 consecutive time points) with a corresponding binary label ("Normal" or "BPSD"). Standard data preprocessing methods such as feature extraction, feature selection, and normalization are then adopted. The primary objective here is to use the features collected by devices in the past hour and the patient demographic data to predict the probability of BPSD occurrences in the next 4 hours.

In the modeling process, both generalized and personalized approaches were proposed for predicting BPSD occurrences. The generalized model focuses on identifying shared characteristics of BPSD by utilizing data from all patients to create a unified model. In contrast, the personalized model considers individual features by constructing a separate model for each patient using their specific data. The modeling algorithms they chose are tree-based methods, such as

Decision Tree [27], Random Forest [20], and Extremely Randomized Trees [17], as well as gradient-boosting-based methods, such as Gradient Boosting Classifier [16], Extreme Gradient Boosting [9], and Categorical Boosting Classifier [31]. They used a split strategy to divide the personal data into the training dataset (70%) and the testing dataset (30%) for each patient due to the limited amount of data available. For generalized model training, they used 5fold cross-validation to evaluate the model performance. Next, the best model algorithm based on the performance evaluation of generalized models, Extremely Randomized Trees [17], is used to train personalized models using each patient's data.

With the approaches of personalized and generalized modeling, we adopted these technologies as one of our main cores in the Model Inference Module of the BPSD Alerting System to improve the performance of BPSD prediction.

### *8.3.3 Fine-Grained BPSD Prediction Model*

The binary BPSD prediction model has already given caregivers direction in deciding whether they need to add medical intervention; however, if the model can provide fine-grained prediction results, more information can be considered to help clinicians make more accurate decisions.

This section describes briefly fine-grained BPSD prediction model approaches proposed by Hsu et al. [22]. Their proposed framework is illustrated in Fig. 8.4. In comparison with the work of Hsu et al. [21], the data also consist of physiological signals collected from dementia patients' smart wearable devices. They also adopted demographic data and the variables mentioned in Table 8.1. Notably, they additionally considered the variable of education level in the demographic data. To train the fine-grained BPSD prediction models, each sample can be labeled as Normal, Hyperactivity, Psychosis, or Physical Behavior symptoms. Except for normal data, others are defined as abnormal (BPSD). The goal here is to predict the probability of BPSD occurrences and provide fine-grained results within the next 4 hours using features gathered by devices over the past hour, combined with patient demographic data.

After standard data preprocessing, the collected data is used to train the personalized and generalized model. In contrast to the previous work from Hsu et al. [21], they utilized two-stage architecture to build up the fine-grained personalized model because patients do not all exhibit the same types of BPSD,

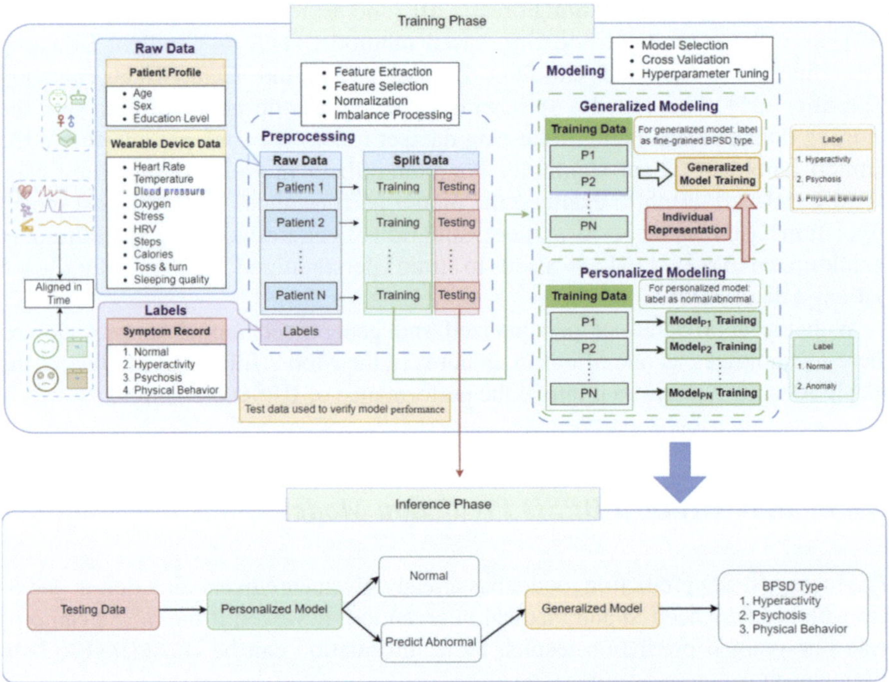


**Fig. 8.4** Overview of the fine-grained BPSD prediction model proposed in Hsu et al. [22]

constructing a multiclass BPSD model tailored to each individual is impractical. The personalized model will be responsible for giving binary predicted results by using personal information to distinguish normal or abnormal (BPSD). If the predicted result in the first stage is abnormal, the generalized model will provide a fine-grained prediction result to show the user more information. For the personalized model, they adopted Extremely Randomized Trees [17] to train each personalized model. In addition, for the generalized model, they utilized ensemble methods to aggregate three different models. The workflow of the generalized model training process is illustrated in Fig. 8.5. First, all patient records are combined to train a generalized model, referred to as the Raw-Data-based Generalized model. To evaluate the performance of the backbone models, three machine learning algorithms: Extremely Randomized Trees [17], Random Forest [20], and Logistic Regression, are applied. Second, they utilized a Temporal Convolutional Network [3] to develop a generalized model for extracting temporal features from raw data. Third, an Individual Representation-based Generalized model is implemented, which integrates each patient's unique features during training, emphasizing refined information derived from personalized models. After training these three generalized models, an ensemble approach is employed to consider diverse perspectives, improving performance in predicting BPSD occurrences.

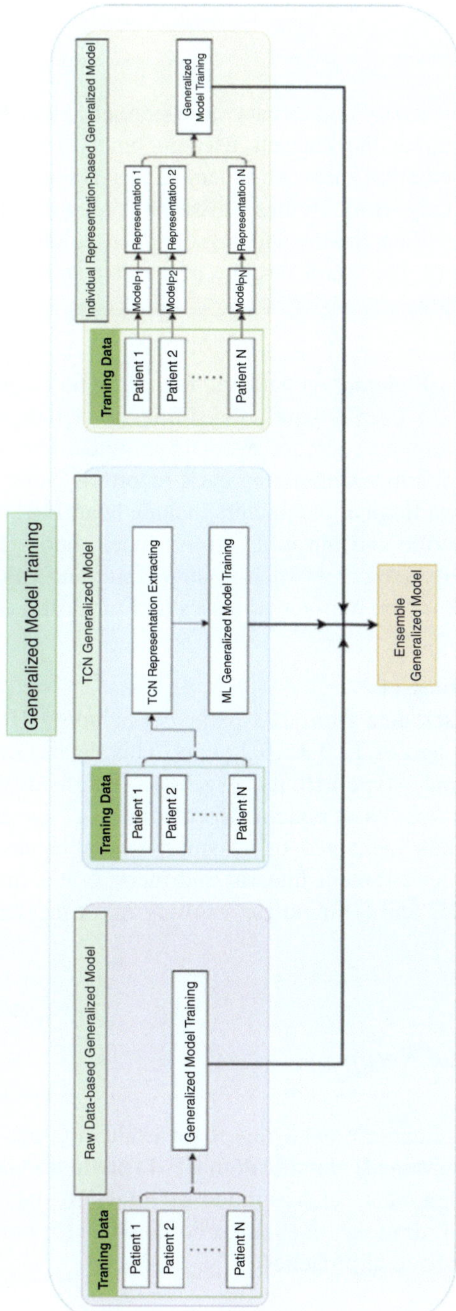


**Fig. 8.5** Workflow of the generalized model training process proposed in Hsu et al. [22]

## 8.4 Experiments and Results

### 8.4.1 Datasets

This section presents the binary and ternary (fine-grained) classification datasets of BPSD prediction. We name the datasets used in binary [21] and ternary (fine-grained) [22] BPSD prediction tasks as Binary_Class_Dataset and Fine-grained_Class_Dataset, respectively. Both studies utilize physiological signals from smart wearable devices to facilitate timely and personalized behavioral predictions for individuals with dementia. The characteristics of the data and the method of collection are summarized below.

**Binary_Class_Dataset**
This dataset comprises 100 dementia patients, including 66 females and 34 males, with an average age of 75.1 ± 9.9 years. Physiological signals were collected for 2–4 weeks, with measurements recorded every 15 minutes. This study focuses on a binary classification problem, categorizing each record as usual or exhibiting any form of BPSD. Key physiological parameters include heart rate, heart rate variability, blood pressure (systolic and diastolic), stress index, body temperature, blood oxygen level, and activity indicators such as step count and calorie consumption. Sleep-related data, such as the number of tosses and turns and sleep quality, were included.

**Fine-grained_Class_Dataset**
This dataset encompasses data from 183 patients, including 101 females and 82 males, with an average age of 77.9 ± 10.2 years. This dataset categorizes records into four classes: Normal, Hyperactivity, Psychosis, or Physical Behavior symptoms. Each record comprises basic patient information (e.g., age and gender) alongside physiological signals measured using smart wearable devices. The dataset employs a 15-minute measurement interval and incorporates historical data from the preceding 15, 30, 45, and 60 minutes, resulting in a time-series input with 55 features.

### 8.4.2 Experimental Setup

This section presents the experimental setups for evaluating the methodologies of binary and ternary (fine-grained) classification BPSD prediction models. The experiments emphasized key elements such as model architecture, data partitioning strategies, and training configurations, enabling a comprehensive comparison between personalized and generalized approaches.

**Model Architectures**

The study [21, 22] employed tree-based ensemble methods and gradient-boosting techniques as the primary model architectures for the generalized models, owing to their proven effectiveness in handling structured data and imbalanced distributions. The key algorithms utilized for the generalized models included Decision Tree (DT) [27], Random Forest (RF) [20], Extremely Randomized Trees (ET) [17], Gradient Boosting Classifier (GBC) [16], Extreme Gradient Boosting (XGB) [9], and Categorical Boosting Classifier (CBC) [31]. These models were chosen to capture complex patterns in the data and address the challenges posed by class imbalance, each offering distinct advantages regarding generalization and predictive accuracy.

**Data Partitioning**

*Personalized Models*: Each patient's data was split into training sets (70%) and testing sets (30%). Personalized models were constructed only for patients with labeled BPSD occurrences. Data from patients without BPSD records were excluded from personalized model training.

*Generalized Models*: The data from all patients were aggregated into a single dataset for training and testing generalized models. A 5fold cross-validation strategy was applied to ensure robust evaluation.

**Training Configurations**

Hyperparameter tuning was performed for all models to achieve optimal performance. The process involved applying grid search to explore various configurations, including the number of estimators, tree depth, and learning rate. Weighted loss functions addressed the class imbalance issue, particularly in the ternary classification task. Additionally, early stopping mechanisms were utilized during training to prevent overfitting and ensure more generalized model performance.

**Evaluation Metrics**

Model performance was evaluated using accuracy, AUC, sensitivity, specificity, precision, and F1-score. These metrics comprehensively assessed the classification capabilities of models, highlighting their effectiveness in distinguishing between classes and balancing predictive performance.

### 8.4.3 *Results and Discussion*

This section presents the experimental results, comparing personalized and generalized models for BPSD prediction in binary and ternary (fine-grained) classification tasks. It also discusses the impact of various backbone models on personalized frameworks and the outcomes of ablation studies conducted on generalized models.

#### 8.4.3.1 Performance Comparison of Personalized and Generalized Models

**Binary Classification**

Table 8.2 presents the performance of various generalized models for binary classification using the Binary_Class_Dataset. The ensemble method achieved the best performance among the models evaluated, with an AUC of 0.936, sensitivity of 0.761, and an F1-score of 0.828. Other tree-based ensemble methods, such as Extremely Randomized Trees (ET) and Random Forest (RF), also demonstrated strong results, with AUC values of 0.932 and 0.925, respectively. These findings underscore the effectiveness of ensemble-based approaches in handling binary classification tasks, particularly in scenarios with imbalanced datasets.

Table 8.3 shows the average performance of personalized models across all patients. The average results indicate an AUC of 0.823, sensitivity of 0.843, and specificity of 0.800. The accuracy was found to be 0.799, with an F1-score of 0.736. Additionally, the standard deviations across these metrics highlight the variation within the dataset, with standard deviations of 0.138 for AUC, 0.211 for sensitivity, and 0.172 for specificity. These figures suggest that while personalized models generally provide strong predictive performance, a notable variation exists among individual patient data.

**Ternary (Fine-Grained) Classification**

Table 8.4 compares personalized and generalized models for ternary (fine-grained) classification using the Fine-grained_Class_Dataset. The personalized models outperformed the generalized approach across all metrics. The generalized model achieved an AUC of 0.701, a sensitivity of 0.472, and an F1-score of 0.441, which indicates limited effectiveness in addressing the class imbalance, where normal samples dominate.

In contrast, the personalized method achieved an AUC of 0.813 ± 0.129, a sensitivity of 0.741 ± 0.152, and an F1-score of 0.661 ± 0.153. This demonstrates a

**Table 8.2** Performance comparison of various generalized models for binary classification

| Models | AUC | Sensitivity | Specificity | Accuracy | F1-score |
|---|---|---|---|---|---|
| DT | 0.800 | 0.659 | 0.844 | 0.816 | 0.705 |
| RF | 0.925 | 0.799 | 0.900 | 0.885 | 0.805 |
| ET | 0.932 | **0.817** | 0.909 | 0.895 | 0.821 |
| GBC | 0.931 | 0.710 | 0.937 | 0.902 | 0.812 |
| XGB | 0.925 | 0.694 | 0.936 | 0.898 | 0.809 |
| CBC | 0.928 | 0.698 | **0.943** | **0.906** | 0.819 |
| Ensemble | **0.936** | 0.761 | 0.932 | **0.906** | **0.828** |

**Table 8.3** Average performance for personalized models of all patients

| | AUC | Sensitivity | Specificity | Accuracy | F1-score |
|---|---|---|---|---|---|
| Average | 0.823 | 0.843 | 0.800 | 0.799 | 0.736 |
| Std. Dev. | 0.138 | 0.211 | 0.172 | 0.132 | 0.146 |

**Table 8.4** Performance comparison between personalized and generalized models

| Method | AUC | Sensitivity | Specificity | Accuracy | Precision | F1-score |
|---|---|---|---|---|---|---|
| Conventional Generalized Method | 0.701 | 0.472 | 0.647 | 0.744 | 0.484 | 0.441 |
| Personalized Method | **0.813 ± 0.129** | **0.741 ± 0.152** | **0.858 ± 0.085** | **0.771 ± 0.144** | **0.685 ± 0.150** | **0.661 ± 0.153** |

**Table 8.5** Performance comparison of conventional classifiers with preprocessing approaches

| Model | AUC | Sensitivity | Specificity | Accuracy | Precision | F1-score |
|---|---|---|---|---|---|---|
| LR | 0.740 ± 0.145 | 0.615 ± 0.174 | 0.852 ± 0.097 | 0.706 ± 0.176 | 0.582 ± 0.148 | 0.549 ± 0.155 |
| RF | **0.775 ± 0.141** | **0.706 ± 0.159** | 0.833 ± 0.089 | **0.741 ± 0.150** | **0.627 ± 0.141** | **0.607 ± 0.147** |

**Table 8.6** Performance comparison of backbone classifiers with and without the proposed personalized framework

| Backbone | AUC | Sensitivity | Specificity | Accuracy | Precision | F1-score |
|---|---|---|---|---|---|---|
| LR | 0.793 ± 0.130 | 0.690 ± 0.145 | **0.857 ± 0.092** | 0.733 ± 0.159 | 0.655 ± 0.141 | 0.620 ± 0.142 |
| RF | **0.818 ± 0.120** | **0.739 ± 0.149** | 0.855 ± 0.092 | **0.764 ± 0.149** | **0.675 ± 0.137** | **0.654 ± 0.146** |

superior ability to capture individual variations in patient data. With a specificity of 0.858 ± 0.085, the personalized model also showed enhanced precision in distinguishing between normal and abnormal behaviors. These results highlight the significant advantage of personalized models in predicting fine-grained BPSD symptoms, such as hyperactivity and psychosis, which are often underrepresented in generalized models.

#### 8.4.3.2 Analysis of Personalized Model with Various Backbone Models

To explore the flexibility of the personalized framework, several machine learning algorithms were tested as backbone models and compared in performance. The results, as shown in Tables 8.5 and 8.6, highlight the differences in performance between conventional classifiers and models utilizing the proposed preprocessing approaches.

Table 8.5 presents the performance of conventional classifiers, including Logistic Regression (LR) and Random Forest (RF). Logistic Regression (LR) showed an AUC of 0.740, with a sensitivity of 0.615, revealing its inadequacy in modeling the intricate and non-linear patterns present in patient data. Additionally, its precision and F1-score were also relatively low. On the other hand, Random Forest (RF) exhibited stronger performance with an AUC of 0.775 and a sensitivity of 0.706, making it more effective at handling imbalanced datasets. However, while it showed improved performance over LR, its results were still not as high as those of more advanced models in subsequent experiments.

Table 8.6 demonstrates the performance of the backbone classifiers when integrated with the proposed personalized framework. The results reveal improvements across the board. Specifically, the AUC for Random Forest (RF) increased to 0.818, and sensitivity rose to 0.739, showing better dataset handling after incorporating personalized approaches. Similarly, Logistic Regression (LR) improved its AUC to 0.793 and sensitivity to 0.690, highlighting the benefits of personalized preprocessing in enhancing the ability to capture relevant patterns in the data.

These results underscore the effectiveness of the personalized framework in boosting model performance, especially in terms of sensitivity and AUC, when applied to both conventional and backbone classifiers.

#### 8.4.3.3 Ablation Study on Generalized Model

Ablation studies were presented to evaluate the effects of individual components in the generalized model using the Fine-grained_Class_Dataset. Table 8.7 presents the results of various model configurations, beginning with the Raw-Data-based Generalized model (RDG) as the baseline. The RDG model achieved an AUC of 0.795. When the Temporal Convolutional Network (TCN) was incorporated into the RDG model (RDG + TCN), the model experienced a slight performance decline, with an AUC of 0.779. This degradation can be attributed to overfitting to time-series patterns, which hindered its overall effectiveness.

Next, when the Individual Representation-based Generalized (IRG) model was added to the RDG framework (RDG + IRG), the performance improved significantly, with an AUC of 0.808. This result highlighted the importance of personalized information, even within a generalized model. The final configuration, combining RDG, IRG, and TCN (RDG + IRG + TCN), achieved the best overall performance, with an AUC of 0.813, sensitivity of 0.741, and specificity of 0.858. This model demonstrated the power of integrating both temporal context and individual-specific features, which allowed it to capture finer details of BPSD prediction more accurately.

These findings underscore the significance of combining multiple components—temporal context and individual representations—to improve the ability of the model to predict diverse types of BPSD. The integrated approach resulted in a robust model, balancing key performance metrics and pushing the boundaries of current methodologies in BPSD prediction.

**Table 8.7** Overall performance with ablation studies on generalized models

| Combination | AUC | Sensitivity | Specificity | Accuracy | Precision | F1-score |
|---|---|---|---|---|---|---|
| RDG | 0.795 ± 0.129 | 0.734 ± 0.156 | 0.842 ± 0.090 | 0.760 ± 0.149 | 0.643 ± 0.141 | 0.626 ± 0.153 |
| RDG + TCN | 0.779 ± 0.143 | 0.559 ± 0.140 | 0.850 ± 0.101 | 0.544 ± 0.199 | 0.645 ± 0.213 | 0.484 ± 0.157 |
| RDG + IRG | 0.808 ± 0.129 | 0.733 ± 0.164 | 0.846 ± 0.090 | 0.762 ± 0.147 | 0.642 ± 0.140 | 0.629 ± 0.150 |
| RDG + IRG + TCN | **0.813 ± 0.129** | **0.741 ± 0.152** | **0.858 ± 0.085** | **0.771 ± 0.144** | **0.685 ± 0.150** | **0.661 ± 0.153** |

## 8.5 Conclusion

This study developed a novel smart wearable device-based BPSD Alerting System that incorporates BPSD prediction-related machine learning models, addressing a critical gap in developing comprehensive solutions to meet the demand for BPSD-related healthcare clinical applications. We examined the potential of personalized and generalized modeling approaches by analyzing and comparing two BPSD prediction studies [21, 22]. This work also introduced effective modeling methodologies and detailed experimental evaluation results, providing valuable insights into binary and ternary (fine-grained) classification frameworks. Our review highlights the strengths and limitations of existing approaches, offering practical guidance for developing robust solutions for BPSD management in clinical practice.

Future directions include the enhancement of the accuracy and generalization of the system by incorporating diverse datasets, refining model architectures, and addressing real-world challenges. By bridging the gap between research studies and practical applications, this BPSD Alerting System represents a transformative step in improving dementia care and reducing caregiver burden, laying a strong foundation for future innovations in personalized healthcare for geriatric patients.

**Acknowledgments** This study was supported by the National Health Research Institutes, Taiwan, under grant no. NHRI-11A1-CG-CO-06-2225-1, NHRI-12A1-CG-CO-06-2225-1, and NHRI-13A1-CG-CO-06-2225-1.

## References

1. Acharya UR, Fernandes SL, WeiKoh JE, et al. Automated detection of Alzheimer's disease using brain MRI images—a study with various feature extraction techniques. J Med Syst. 2019;43 https://doi.org/10.1007/s10916-019-1428-9.
2. Baharudin AD, Din NC, Subramaniam P, Razali R. The associations between behavioral-psychological symptoms of dementia (BPSD) and coping strategy, burden of care and personality style among low-income caregivers of patients with dementia. BMC Public Health. 2019;19(Suppl 4):447. https://doi.org/10.1186/s12889-019-6868-0.
3. Bai S, Kolter JZ, Koltun V. An empirical evaluation of generic convolutional and recurrent networks for sequence modeling. arXiv preprint arXiv:1803.01271. 2018.

4. Berkovic D, Macrae A, Gulline H, et al. The delivery of person-centered care for people living with dementia in residential aged care: a systematic review and meta-analysis. Gerontologist. 2024;64:gnad052. https://doi.org/10.1093/geront/gnad052.
5. Bessey LJ, Walaszek A. Management of behavioral and psychological symptoms of dementia. Curr Psychiatry Rep. 2019;21:66. https://doi.org/10.1007/s11920-019-1049-5.
6. Bron EE, Klein S, Papma JM, et al. Cross-cohort generalizability of deep and conventional machine learning for MRI-based diagnosis and prediction of Alzheimer's disease. Neuroimage Clin. 2021;31:102712. https://doi.org/10.1016/j.nicl.2021.102712.
7. Carparelli C, Jones C, Oyebode JR, et al. A systematic review of the effectiveness of educational interventions in promoting person-centred care in dementia services. Clin Gerontol. 2024;47:665–83. https://doi.org/10.1080/07317115.2022.2152515.
8. Cerejeira J, Lagarto L, Mukaetova-Ladinska EB. Behavioral and psychological symptoms of dementia. Front Neurol. 2012;3:73.
9. Chen T, Guestrin C. XGBoost: a scalable tree boosting system. In: Proceedings of the 22nd ACM SIGKDD international conference on knowledge discovery and data mining (KDD'16). New York: Association for Computing Machinery; 2016. p. 785–94. https://doi.org/10.1145/2939672.2939785.
10. Cheng S-T. Dementia caregiver burden: a research update and critical analysis. Curr Psychiatry Rep. 2017;19:64. https://doi.org/10.1007/s11920-017-0818-2.
11. Cho E, Kim S, Heo S-J, et al. Machine learning-based predictive models for the occurrence of behavioral and psychological symptoms of dementia: model development and validation. Sci Rep. 2023;13:8073.
12. Davidsson R, Baker D, Chintakrindi S, et al. Exploring the multidimensionality of home-based dementia caregiving and related challenges based on digital journaling and interviews. Int J Older People Nurs. 2024;19:e12600. https://doi.org/10.1111/opn.12600.
13. Deardorff WJ, Grossberg GT. Behavioral and psychological symptoms in Alzheimer's dementia and vascular dementia. Handb Clin Neurol. 2019;165:5–32.
14. Ding Y, Sohn JH, Kawczynski MG, et al. A deep learning model to predict a diagnosis of Alzheimer disease by using 18 F-FDG PET of the brain. Radiology. 2019;290:456–64. https://doi.org/10.1148/radiol.2018180958.
15. Feast A, Moniz-Cook E, Stoner C, et al. A systematic review of the relationship between behavioral and psychological symptoms (BPSD) and caregiver well-being. Int Psychogeriatr. 2016;28:1761–74. https://doi.org/10.1017/S1041610216000922.
16. Friedman JH. Greedy function approximation: a gradient boosting machine. Ann Stat. 2001:1189–232.
17. Geurts P, Ernst D, Wehenkel L. Extremely randomized trees. Mach Learn. 2006;63:3–42.
18. Grootscholten E, Poslawsky I, Bakker T. Nursing staff's observations of BPSD amongst older adults with dementia living in a nursing home: a qualitative study. Nurs Rep. 2023;13:166–78. https://doi.org/10.3390/nursrep13010018.
19. Hjetland GJ, Pallesen S, Thun E, et al. Light interventions and sleep, circadian, behavioral, and psychological disturbances in dementia: a systematic review of methods and outcomes. Sleep Med Rev. 2020;52:101310. https://doi.org/10.1016/j.smrv.2020.101310.
20. Ho TK. Random decision forests. In: Proceedings of 3rd international conference on document analysis and recognition; 1995. p. 278–82.
21. Hsu BW-Y, Chen Y-M, Lin T-Y, et al. Predicting behavioral and psychological symptoms of dementia using machine learning and smart wearable devices. In: Joint Conference on Medical Informatics in Taiwan; 2023.
22. Hsu BW-Y, Chen Y-M, Yang Y-H, Tseng VS. Predicting fine-grained behavioral and psychological symptoms of dementia based on machine learning and smart wearable devices. arXiv preprint arXiv:2410.18091. 2024.
23. Javeed A, Dallora AL, Berglund JS, et al. Machine learning for dementia prediction: a systematic review and future research directions. J Med Syst. 2023;47 https://doi.org/10.1007/s10916-023-01906-7.

24. Kales HC, Gitlin LN, Lyketsos CG. Assessment and management of behavioral and psychological symptoms of dementia. BMJ. 2015;350:h369. https://doi.org/10.1136/bmj.h369.
25. Kallmyer BA, Bass D, Baumgart M, et al. Dementia care navigation: building toward a common definition, key principles, and outcomes. Alzheimers Dement. 2023;9:e12408.
26. Kim B, Noh GO, Kim K. Behavioural and psychological symptoms of dementia in patients with Alzheimer's disease and family caregiver burden: a path analysis. BMC Geriatr. 2021;21:1–12.
27. Li B, Friedman J, Olshen R, Stone C. Classification and regression trees (CART). Biometrics. 1984;40:358–61.
28. Mirabnahrazam G, Ma D, Lee S, et al. Machine learning based multimodal neuroimaging genomics dementia score for predicting future conversion to Alzheimer's disease. J Alzheimers Dis. 2022;87:1345–65. https://doi.org/10.3233/JAD-220021.
29. Palmese F, Druda Y, Benintende V, et al. Wearable sensors for monitoring caregivers of people with dementia: a scoping review. Eur Geriatr Med. 2024;16:1–11.
30. Pellegrini E, Ballerini L, Hernandez M d CV, et al. Machine learning of neuroimaging for assisted diagnosis of cognitive impairment and dementia: a systematic review. Alzheimers Dement Diagn Assess Dis Monit. 2018;10:519–35. https://doi.org/10.1016/j.dadm.2018.07.004.
31. Prokhorenkova L, Gusev G, Vorobev A, et al. CatBoost: unbiased boosting with categorical features. Adv Neural Inf Process Syst. 2018;31
32. Rocha IC, Arantes M, Moreira A, et al. Monitoring wearable devices for elderly people with dementia: a review. Designs. 2024;8(4)
33. Saragih ID, Suarilah I, Saragih IS, et al. A meta-analysis of person-centered care interventions for improving health outcomes in persons living with dementia. Worldviews Evid-Based Nurs. 2025;22(1):e12746. https://doi.org/10.1111/wvn.12746.
34. Shehab M, Abualigah L, Shambour Q, et al. Machine learning in medical applications: a review of state-of-the-art methods. Comput Biol Med. 2022;145:105458.
35. Vyas A, Aisopos F, Vidal ME, et al. Identifying the presence and severity of dementia by applying interpretable machine learning techniques on structured clinical records. BMC Med Inform Decis Mak. 2022;22 https://doi.org/10.1186/s12911-022-02004-3.

# Chapter 9
# Pharmacological Precision Medicine to Treat Dementia

**Kang-Po Lee, Po-Yu Lin, Meng-Ju Wu, and Pi-Shan Sung**

**Abstract** This chapter provides an in-depth exploration of pharmacological precision medicine strategies for addressing diverse forms of dementia. It delves into the nuanced treatments available for Alzheimer's disease (AD), encompassing symptomatic relief through cholinesterase inhibitors and N-methyl-D-aspartate (NMDA) receptor antagonists, as well as anti-amyloid therapies. Moreover, it delves into potential disease-modifying avenues like cell and gene therapy, anti-tau interventions, and repurposing medications originally intended for metabolic disorders. In the realm of vascular dementia (VaD), the focus remains on alleviating symptoms via cholinesterase inhibitors and NMDA receptor antagonists, complemented by repurposing cardiovascular drugs to target underlying vascular factors.

The chapter also navigates through treatment approaches for dementia with Lewy bodies (DLB) and Parkinson's disease dementia (PDD), addressing symptomatic management, repurposing of other medications, and emerging disease-modifying options that target alpha-synuclein pathology. Furthermore, it delves into the evolving landscape of frontotemporal dementia (FTD) treatment, exploring potential interventions aimed at modifying the disease course by targeting tau and TDP-43 proteinopathies.

Emphasizing the pivotal role of personalized medicine in dementia care, this comprehensive review underscores current strategies while also projecting toward future advancements. By tailoring treatments to individual patient profiles and leveraging cutting-edge therapeutic modalities, this paradigm aims not only to improve immediate outcomes but also to enhance overall patient well-being and quality of life in the long term.

---

K.-P. Lee
Department of Neurology, Kaohsiung Show Chwan Memorial Hospital, Kaohsiung, Taiwan
e-mail: I54984033@gs.ncku.edu.tw

P.-Y. Lin · M.-J. Wu · P.-S. Sung (✉)
Department of Neurology, National Cheng Kung University Hospital, College of Medicine, National Cheng Kung University, Tainan, Taiwan



Y.-H. Yang (ed.), *Management of Dementia from the Preclinical Stage*,
https://doi.org/10.1007/978-981-95-5222-1_9

**Keywords** Dementia treatment · Alzheimer's disease · Vascular dementia · Dementia with Lewy body · Parkinson disease dementia · Frontotemporal dementia · Personalized precision medicine

Dementia is a progressive disorder that significantly impacts cognitive functions, leading to substantial consequences for individuals, caregivers, and society. This condition has driven a concerted effort among neurologists and neuroscientists to discover effective treatments. Consequently, a broad spectrum of established and emerging treatments for various types of dementia are under investigation, highlighting a collective effort to address the challenges posed by this complex condition.

## 9.1 Treatments for Alzheimer's Disease

### *9.1.1 Symptomatic Treatments*

#### 9.1.1.1 Cholinesterase Inhibitors and NMDA Receptor Antagonist

In Alzheimer's disease, the degeneration of cholinergic neurons is believed to be a primary cause of cognitive impairment [1]. As a result, cholinesterase inhibitors (CHEis), which inhibit the breakdown of acetylcholine, form the cornerstone of symptomatic treatment for Alzheimer's disease. While these drugs do not modify the disease course, they have gained approval from the US Food and Drug Administration (FDA) based on randomized, placebo-controlled trials. Tacrine, the first CHEi developed, is no longer widely used due to its hepatotoxicity and potential for drug–drug interactions.

Currently, three CHEis—donepezil [2, 3], rivastigmine [4, 5], and galantamine [6, 7]—are commonly prescribed for Alzheimer's disease. Additionally, memantine, an activity-dependent N-methyl-D-aspartate (NMDA) receptor antagonist, has been approved for moderate to severe Alzheimer's disease [8]. Table 9.1 summarizes the current FDA-approved CHEis and NMDA receptor antagonist for AD patients.

Current evidence suggests that all three CHEis can decelerate the progression of Alzheimer's Disease Assessment Scale–Cognitive Subscale (ADAS-cog) scores in patients with mild-to-moderate Alzheimer's disease, although there is significant heterogeneity in the response to rivastigmine [13]. Short-term follow-up studies indicate that donepezil may provide superior outcomes in cognitive function and activities of daily living (ADLs) compared to galantamine and is comparably effective to rivastigmine [14, 15]. However, long-term efficacy between donepezil, galantamine, and rivastigmine shows no significant differences [16, 17].

**Table 9.1** FDA-approved CHEis and NMDA receptor antagonist for Alzheimer's Disease

| Drug | Indication | | Initial dose | Maximum dose | Suggested titration schedule |
|---|---|---|---|---|---|
| Donepezil [9] | Mild to moderate | | 5 mg once daily | 10 mg once daily | Titrate after 4–6 weeks |
| | Moderate to severe | | 10 mg once daily | 23 mg once daily | Titrate after 3 months |
| Rivastigmine [10] | Mild to moderate | Oral | 1.5 mg twice daily | 6 mg twice daily | 3 mg → 4.5 mg → 6 mg in 2 weeks interval |
| | | Patch | 4.6 mg/24 h once daily | 9.5 mg/24 h once daily | Titrate after 4 weeks |
| Galantamine [11] | Mild to moderate | | 8 mg once daily | 24 mg once daily | 8 mg → 16 mg → 24 mg in 4 weeks interval |
| Memantine [12] | Moderate to severe | | 5 mg once daily | 10 mg twice daily | Titrate after 1 week |
| | | | | 5 mg twice daily[a] | |

[a]Patients with severe renal impairment

In everyday practice, neurologists frequently encounter variability in patient responses to different CHEis. Studies indicate that the clinical response rate to CHEis ranges from 30% to 60% [18]. Developing potential biomarkers for treatment response could help clarify these individual differences. For instance, patients with hippocampal-sparing or minimal atrophy subtypes might respond better to donepezil in early amnestic mild cognitive impairment (aMCI) [19]. This highlights the importance of research into subtype stratification for disease prognosis and treatment response. Genetic factors also play a significant role; donepezil is metabolized by CYP enzymes, specifically CYP2D6, CYP3A4, and CYP1A2. Patients with extensive (*1/*1, *1/*10) and intermediate metabolizer (*1/*3, *1/*5, *1/*6, *7/*10) genotypes exhibit better responses compared to poor (*4/*4) and ultra-rapid (*1×N/*1) metabolizers [20].

Research indicates that rivastigmine is more effective in individuals with higher education levels and those exhibiting rapid initial progression, but less effective in non-carriers of the apolipoprotein E (APOE) ε4 allele [21, 22]. Although fewer studies discuss serial biomarkers for galantamine and memantine, one study suggested that memantine responders with decreased heart rates (HR) experienced better outcomes compared to those with increased HR [23].

### 9.1.2 *Anti-Amyloid Treatments*

Amyloid beta (Aβ) plaques are a hallmark of Alzheimer's disease and are believed to play a critical role in its pathogenesis. Consequently, Aβ-targeted therapies are essential in the development of disease-modifying treatments. Several strategies target Aβ, including inhibiting β- and γ-secretase, preventing oligomerization, and enhancing clearance. However, the primary focus of current anti-amyloid therapies is the reduction in amyloid plaques through immune mechanisms. As of 2025, three anti-amyloid therapies have been approved by the US FDA. Lecanemab and Donanemab have received full approval, while Aducanumab was approved via an accelerated pathway for drugs addressing serious illnesses and impacting a biomarker likely to predict clinical response.

A detailed guide to using anti-amyloid therapy is beyond the scope of this chapter. For an in-depth understanding, readers can refer to the review articles titled "Appropriate Use Recommendation" by the Alzheimer's Disease and Related Disorders Therapeutics Work Group [25, 26]. To provide foundational knowledge of their efficacy, a summary of phase 3 clinical trials is presented below.

#### 9.1.2.1 Lecanemab

Lecanemab is a recombinant humanized immunoglobulin gamma 1 monoclonal antibody specifically designed to target Aβ pathology. It exhibits binding affinity to amyloid oligomers, protofibrils, and insoluble fibrils, with a particular high affinity for Aβ soluble protofibrils. The phase 3 clinical trial, CLARITY AD (NCT03887455), enrolled patients who met the diagnostic criteria for mild cognitive impairment due to Alzheimer's disease or mild Alzheimer's disease dementia, as defined by the National Institute on Aging-Alzheimer's Association (NIA-AA). Inclusion in the study required confirmation of amyloid pathology, ensuring that all participants met the necessary biological criteria for Alzheimer's disease [27, 28]. Additional inclusion criteria for the CLARITY AD trial stipulated that participants be aged between 50 and 90 years and possess a Mini-Mental State Examination (MMSE) score ranging from 22 to 30. The presence of amyloid pathology was verified through amyloid positron emission tomography (PET) or cerebrospinal fluid (CSF) biomarkers.

Lecanemab was administered intravenously at a dose of 10 mg/kg of body weight biweekly, over a treatment period of 18 months [29]. The main outcome measure, the Clinical Dementia Rating–Sum of Boxes (CDR-SB), demonstrated a mean change from baseline to 18 months of 1.21 with lecanemab and 1.66 with placebo. The difference between the two groups was −0.45 (95% confidence interval [CI], −0.67 to −0.23; $P < 0.001$), indicating a significant effect favoring lecanemab. Common adverse events included infusion-related reactions in 26.4% of participants and amyloid-related imaging abnormalities with edema or effusions in 12.6% of participants.

#### 9.1.2.2 Aducanumab

Aducanumab is a human monoclonal antibody that exhibits high affinity for both soluble and insoluble forms of amyloid plaque. Two clinical trials, EMERGE (NCT02484547) and ENGAGE (NCT02477800), have evaluated this medication [30]. The inclusion criteria were similar to those in the trial of lecanemab, with minor differences in the patient's age range (50–85 years) and MMSE score (24–30). Aducanumab was administered once every 4 weeks for a total of 76 weeks [30]. Unlike lecanemab, aducanumab involved a dose titration phase, and the target dose varied depending on the patient's ApoE ε4 carrier status at the beginning of the trials. This protocol was later revised to a fixed target dose of 10 mg/kg.

The primary outcome measure was the CDR-SB at 78 weeks. Both trials were halted based on a futility analysis conducted at approximately 50% enrollment. The EMERGE trial demonstrated a reduced CDR-SB increment (difference −0.39, 95% CI, −0.69 to −0.09; $P = 0.012$), whereas the ENGAGE trial did not show a significant difference (difference of 0.03, 95% CI, −0.26 to 0.33; $P = 0.833$). Amyloid-related imaging abnormalities with edema or effusions were observed in 35% of patients receiving a 10 mg/kg dose.

#### 9.1.2.3 Donanemab

Donanemab is an immunoglobulin gamma 1 monoclonal antibody targeting insoluble, modified, N-terminal truncated form of β-amyloid, which is specifically present in brain amyloid plaques. The phase 3 clinical trial, TRAILBLAZER-ALZ 2 (NCT04437511), enrolled patients with mild cognitive impairment of mild dementia due to Alzheimer's disease [31]. In contrast to the inclusion criteria of the phase 3 trials of lecanemab and aducanumab, the TRAILBLAZER-ALZ 2 trial included criteria such as the amount of amyloid (≥37 Centiloids) in amyloid PET, the presence of tau pathology, the patient's age (60–85 years old), and MMSE score (20–30).

Donanemab is administered intravenously every 4 weeks, with a dosing regimen of 700 mg in the first three doses, and 1400 mg in subsequent doses. The intervention lasted for 72 weeks, but patients whose amyloid plaque level reduced to a predefined threshold in subsequent amyloid PET scans were switched to placebo early. The primary outcome, the least-squares mean change in the integrated Alzheimer Disease Rating Scale from baseline to 76 weeks, was −10.2 (95% CI, −11.22 to −9.16) with donanemab and −13.1 (95% CI, −14.10 to −12.13) with placebo (difference, 2.92 [95% CI, 1.51–4.33]; $P < 0.001$) in the study population.

Common side effects included infusion-related reactions in 8.7% of participants and amyloid-related imaging abnormalities with edema or effusions in 24.0% of participants.

#### 9.1.2.4 Diagnosis of Alzheimer's Disease in Clinical Trials

Accurate patient selection was the most important aspect of utilizing anti-amyloid therapy. The selection was primarily based on the inclusion and exclusion criteria of the phase 3 clinical trials, with some modifications made to make it more practical [25, 26]. Here we summarize the diagnostic criteria used in clinical trials.

Clinically, patients with mild cognitive impairment due to Alzheimer's disease were defined as having objective impairment in at least 1 cognitive domain, which had an onset and progressed gradually for at least 1 year [27]. The patient's clinical dementia rating (CDR) score was 0.5, with a CDR Memory Box score of 0.5 [29]. Patients with mild Alzheimer's disease dementia were defined as having cognitive impairment in at least 2 domains, and the symptoms should have interfered with the ability to function at work or perform usual activities, showing a decline from the previous level of functioning [28]. The CDR score should have been between 0.5 and 1.0, and a CDR Memory Box score should have been at least 0.5 [29]. In addition to the above criteria, the MMSE score should have been 22–30 for lecanemab and 24–30 for aducanumab, respectively [29, 30]. In order to fulfill the biomarker aspect of diagnosis, an amyloid PET or total-tau/A$\beta_{1-42}$ ratio in CSF should be measured for lecanemab. The trial of Aducanumab used amyloid PET as the only method of patient inclusion, and it did not include any CSF biomarkers. It is worth noting that in May 2025, the FDA had approved its 1st blood biomarker, the Lumipulse G pTau217/ß-Amyloid 1-42 Plasma Ratio, for diagnosing Alzheimer's disease [32].

#### 9.1.2.5 Side Effects of Anti-Amyloid Therapy

Anti-amyloid therapy is associated with two major side effects: Amyloid-related Imaging Abnormalities (ARIA) and infusion reactions.

##### 9.1.2.5.1 Amyloid-Related Imaging Abnormalities (ARIA)

ARIA includes signal hyperintensities and sulcal effusion observed in fluid attenuation inversion recovery sequences, depicting "vasogenic edema" (referred to as ARIA-E), and signal hypointensities in T2* sequences indicating hemosiderin deposits (ARIA-H), representing microhemorrhage or superficial siderosis [33]. The risk stratification of ARIA depends largely on the APOE ε4 carrier status. In clinical trial data for lecanemab and aducanumab, the incidence of ARIA, symptomatic ARIA, and recurrent ARIA significantly increased in APOE ε4 carriers compared to non-carriers, with homozygous carriers showing an even higher incidence than heterozygous carriers (Table 9.2). And aducanumab had an even higher incidence of ARIA compared to lecanemab.

**Table 9.2** Incidence of amyloid-related imaging abnormalities with difference APOE ε4 carrier status

| | Non-carrier | Heterozygous carrier | Homozygous carrier |
|---|---|---|---|
| Lecanemab [29] | | | |
| ARIA-E | 5.4% (15/278) | 10.9% (52/479) | 32.6% (46/141) |
| Symptomatic ARIA-E | 1.4% (4/278) | 1.7% (8/479) | 9.2% (13/141) |
| ARIA-H | 11.9% (33/278) | 14.0% (67/479) | 39% (55/141) |
| Symptomatic ARIA-H | 0.4% (1/278) | 1.0% (5/479) | 0% (0/141) |
| Aducanumab [30] | | | |
| ARIA-E | 20.3% (72/355) | 35.9% (185/515) | 66% (105/159) |

The table was modified from trial data in reference [29, 30]

*ARIA-E* amyloid-related imaging abnormalities-edema, *ARIA-H* amyloid-related imaging abnormalities-hemorrhage

Monitoring of ARIA includes regular magnetic resonance imaging (MRI) follow-ups and additional safety MRIs based on symptoms. For lecanemab, the regular MRI was arranged prior to the 5th, 7th, and 14th medication infusions in the trial, and an additional regular MRI before the 26th infusion [25, 29]. According to trial data, 71% of ARIA occurred in the first regular MRI and 81% of the ARIA resolved within 4 months of detection. After the first two regular MRIs, the risk of ARIA for APOE ε4 non-carriers became very low, while APOE ε4 carriers still had a relatively high risk. Aducanumab had higher incidence of ARIA comparing to lecanemab, and regular MRI follow-ups was recommended before the 5th, 7th, 9th, and the 12th doses [26, 30]. As for symptom-based safety MRIs, symptoms including seizure, encephalopathy, consciousness disturbance, and focal neurologic signs may prompt additional safety MRIs. This proactive approach aids in promptly addressing emerging issues related to ARIA.

Once ARIAs have manifested, the management hinges upon the severity grading of both symptoms and imaging findings. Symptoms are categorized from none to severe based on their impact on daily activities and work ability. Meanwhile, MRI findings are stratified from mild to severe, with distinct criteria for ARIA-E and ARIA-H subtypes [25]. Table 9.3 summarizes the detail grading criteria.

The treatment strategy predominantly revolves around the severity of symptoms and MRI abnormalities. Irrespective of the severity grade, all patients diagnosed with ARIA should undergo monthly MRI scans until resolution of imaging abnormalities is achieved. The prognosis for ARIA varies widely, ranging from fully reversible outcomes to potentially life-threatening situations, particularly in severe cases.

In instances of severe symptoms or MRI findings indicative of ARIA, prompt intervention is crucial. This may involve initiating pulse steroid therapy, such as intravenous methylprednisolone at 1 g per day for 5 days, followed by a gradual tapering regimen of oral steroids to address cerebral edema. Additionally, an electroencephalogram should be conducted, and anti-seizure medication administered if seizure activity is detected. Regarding the continuation of anti-amyloid therapy infusion, only patients with none to mild symptoms and mild MRI abnormalities can

**Table 9.3** Treatment plan for amyloid-related imaging abnormalities, based on their severity

| | Mild | Moderate | Severe |
|---|---|---|---|
| Symptom | Discomfort noted; no disruption of daily activity | Discomfort sufficient to reduce or affect normal daily activity | Incapacitating, with inability to work or to perform normal daily activity |
| ARIA-E | FLAIR hyperintensity confined to sulcus and/or cortex/subcortex white matter in one location <5 cm | FLAIR hyperintensity 5–10 cm in single greatest dimension, or more than 1 site of involvement, each measuring <10 cm | FLAIR hyperintensity >10 cm with associated gyral swelling and sulcal effacement. One or more separate/independent sites of involvement may be noted |
| ARIA-H microhemorrhage | ≤ 4 new incident microhemorrhages | 5–9 new incident microhemorrhages | 10 or more new incident microhemorrhages |
| ARIA-H Superficial Siderosis | 1 focal area of superficial siderosis | 2 focal areas of superficial siderosis | > 2 areas of superficial siderosis |

| | | Symptom severity | | | |
|---|---|---|---|---|---|
| | | None | Mild | Moderate | Severe |
| MRI severity | Mild | Continue dosing | | | |
| | Moderate | Suspend dosing | | | |
| | Severe | Discontinue dosing | | | |

The table was modified from trial data in reference [25]
*ARIA-E* Amyloid-Related Imaging Abnormalities-Edema, *ARIA-H* Amyloid-Related Imaging Abnormalities-Hemorrhage, *FLAIR* Fluid Attenuation Inversion Recovery sequences of MRI

safely proceed with the original treatment schedule. However, if a patient exhibits severe symptoms or MRI abnormalities, experiences microhemorrhage, or undergoes recurrent episodes of ARIA, discontinuation of the anti-amyloid therapy is warranted. Patients falling into other severity grading categories necessitate a temporary suspension of dosing, with re-initiation contingent upon complete remission of ARIA, following a comprehensive reassessment of potential risks and benefits.

##### 9.1.2.5.2 Infusion Reactions

Infusion reactions were noted in 26.4% of patients treated with lecanemab. These reactions exhibited a spectrum of severity, ranging from mild symptoms such as fever, chills, headache, nausea, vomiting, abdominal discomfort, elevated blood pressure, and skin rash, to more severe manifestations including disturbances in consciousness, neck stiffness, and focal neurologic signs suggestive of meningoencephalitis. Typically, these reactions were mild to moderate and resolved within 24 h, commonly occurring during the initial treatment sessions.

The management of infusion reactions is tailored based on their severity. Mild reactions can often be alleviated with medications such as 25–50 mg of diphenhydramine and 650–1000 mg of acetaminophen administered every 4–6 h until symptoms abate. Moderate reactions may necessitate the use of 0.75 mg per day of oral dexamethasone or 80 mg of oral methylprednisolone administered twice daily for 2–3 days. For future infusions, prophylactic measures may be employed, including administering 25–50 mg of diphenhydramine, 650–1000 mg of acetaminophen 30 min before infusion, and possibly incorporating steroids such as 0.75 mg of dexamethasone or 80 mg of methylprednisolone 6 h before infusion if the initial preventive measures prove inadequate. Additionally, preparations should be made to address potential respiratory distress with the use of a bronchodilator, oxygen therapy, and epinephrine if required.

Patients experiencing infusion reactions of grade 3 severity or higher, according to the National Cancer Institute—Common Terminology Criteria for Adverse Events, characterized by prolonged recurrence of symptoms lasting more than 24 h following initial improvement, should not undergo further infusion sessions. Clinical symptoms indicative of meningoencephalitis or tissue injury, such as arthritis, glomerulonephritis, or mononeuritis multiplex, warrant careful consideration and evaluation for discontinuation of treatment.

#### 9.1.2.6 Other Disease-Modifying Treatment for Alzheimer's Disease

In the modern era of Alzheimer's disease research, five prominent categories of mechanisms have emerged as the focal points of numerous clinical trials: amyloid, neurotransmitter receptors, inflammation/immunity, synaptic plasticity/neuroprotection, and tau [34]. In the subsequent sections, we will provide a brief overview of the ongoing developments in anti-tau therapy as well as cell and gene therapy.

##### 9.1.2.6.1 Anti-Tau Therapy

The amyloid cascade theory underscores the aggregation of tau protein into neurofibrillary tangles, a hallmark of Alzheimer's disease pathology. Tau pathology not only signifies neurodegeneration but also contributes to neurotoxicity processes.

Current disease-modifying therapies targeting tau protein in Alzheimer's disease are detailed in Table 9.4. These therapies span across 11 clinical trials, employing various strategies: 7 utilize anti-tau antibodies to clear tau protein, 2 leverage antisense oligonucleotides to reduce tau mRNA translation, 1 trial focuses on an O-GlcNAcase enzyme inhibitor to enhance O-GlcNAcylation (thereby countering phosphorylation and reducing aggregation), and the remaining trial targets the inhibition of tau protein self-aggregation. Among these trials, 2 focus on autosomal dominant Alzheimer's disease, while the other 5 studies target mild cognitive impairment due to Alzheimer's disease or early Alzheimer's disease dementia, each with nuanced inclusion criteria.

**Table 9.4** Current clinical trials targeting tau protein

| Trial stage | Agent | Mechanism of action | Clinical trial ID | Target population | Start date | Estimated primary completion | Key published findings (as of 2025) |
|---|---|---|---|---|---|---|---|
| Phase 3 | E2814 | Anti-tau monoclonal antibody | NCT01760005 | ADAD | Dec-12 | Oct-27 | Plasma MTBR-tau243 significantly reduced; FDA Fast-Track designation. No definitive clinical outcomes yet. |
| Phase 3 | E2814 | Anti-tau monoclonal antibody | NCT05269394 | ADAD | Dec-21 | Jul-27 | |
| Phase 2 | Bepranemab | Anti-tau monoclonal antibody | NCT04867616 | MCI due to AD or mild AD dementia | Jun-21 | May-24 | Phase 2 "TOGETHER" trial: slowed tau accumulation (33–58% by tau-PET). Primary cognitive endpoint (CDR-SB) not met; ADAS-Cog showed improvement trend. |
| Phase 2 | BIIB080 | ASO | NCT05399888 | MCI due to AD or mild AD dementia | Aug-22 | Nov-27 | Dose-dependent reduction in CSF total tau and p-tau181; tau-PET reduction; cognitive trends favorable. Phase 2 ongoing. |
| Phase 2 | E2814 | Anti-tau monoclonal antibody | NCT04971733 | ADAD | Jun-21 | Jul-25 | Demonstrated target engagement and reduction of MTBR-tau species. |
| Phase 2 | JNJ-63733657 | Anti-tau monoclonal antibody | NCT04619420 | Early AD | Jan-21 | Mar-25 | |
| Phase 2 | LY3372689 | O-GlcNAcase enzyme inhibitor | NCT05063539 | Early AD | Sep-21 | Jul-24 | |
| Phase 2 | Methylene Blue (TRx0237) | Tau protein aggregation inhibitor | NCT02380573 | MCI due to AD or mild AD dementia | Jul-15 | Apr-22 | Did not demonstrate clinical cognitive benefit; no significant slowing of progression. |
| Phase 1 | APNmAb005 | Anti-tau monoclonal antibody | NCT05344989 | — | May-22 | Mar-24 | |
| Phase 1 | MK-2214 | Anti-tau monoclonal antibody | NCT05466422 | — | Sep-22 | May-25 | |
| Phase 1 | NIO752 | ASO | NCT05469360 | — | Feb-23 | Oct-24 | |
| Phase 1 | OLX-07010 | Inhibits tau self-aggregation | NCT05696483 | — | Jan-23 | Dec-24 | |

*ADAD* autosomal dominant Alzheimer's disease, *MCI* mild cognitive impairment, *AD* Alzheimer's disease, *ASO* Antisense oligonucleotide

#### 9.1.2.6.2 Cell Therapy and Gene Therapy

Cell therapy and gene therapy represent promising and evolving treatment modalities in the context of Alzheimer's disease [34, 35]. Current clinical trials in these areas are summarized in Table 9.5 for cell therapy and Table 9.6 for gene therapy.

Advancements in cell therapy for Alzheimer's disease have progressed up to phase 2 trials with positive result from Lomecel. The primary focus involves the use of mesenchymal stem cells sourced from various origins. Additionally, studies are exploring the potential of regulatory T cells and autologous natural killer cells in therapeutic interventions. Patient cohorts targeted for these therapies predominantly comprise individuals with mild to moderate Alzheimer's disease. Notably, the disease severity within these cohorts tends to exceed that of previous trials involving anti-amyloid or anti-tau antibody treatments.

In the realm of gene therapy, ongoing trials encompass three distinct mechanisms: (1) Anti-tau Antisense Oligonucleotide: This approach targets the tau protein, a key player in Alzheimer's pathology, (2) Adeno-associated Virus Gene Transfer of APOE ε2: Specifically directed at individuals with APOE ε4 Homozygote and mild to moderate Alzheimer's disease, and (3) RNA Interference to Decrease Amyloid Precursor Protein: Addressing the amyloid cascade, another hallmark feature of Alzheimer's disease. While gene therapy trials have also advanced to phase 2, the focus remains on individuals with mild cognitive impairment due to Alzheimer's disease or early-stage Alzheimer's dementia. The objective is to initiate disease-modifying interventions at the earliest feasible stage. Noteworthy is the targeted modification of genetic risk factors, particularly through adeno-associated virus gene transfer of APOE ε2 in patients with specific genetic profiles.

In the foreseeable future, outcomes from these ongoing studies are poised to unveil the efficacy and viability of these mechanistically driven gene therapies for Alzheimer's disease.

### *9.1.3 Repurpose of Known Medications for Metabolic Disorders in Alzheimer's Disease Treatment*

The repurposing of medications originally developed for metabolic disorders has gained attention as a potential strategy for the treatment of AD. These medications, designed for conditions like diabetes mellitus (DM) and hypertension (HTN), are being explored due to their effects on underlying biological processes relevant to AD pathology. Leveraging existing drugs with established safety profiles offers a promising avenue for discovering effective treatments.

#### **9.1.3.1 Diabetes Mellitus Medications**

The well-documented increased risk of AD in patients with DM [36, 37] has led to investigations into DM medications as potential AD therapies. AD, often termed type 3 diabetes, implicates insulin in tau phosphorylation and amyloid plaque

**Table 9.5** List of cell therapy trial targeting Alzheimer's disease

| Trial stage | Agent | Mechanism of action | Clinical trial ID | Target population | Start date | Estimated primary completion date | Key findings (as of 2025) |
|---|---|---|---|---|---|---|---|
| Phase 2 | AstroStem | Autologous adipose tissue-derived mesenchymal stem cells | NCT04482413 | Mild AD | Feb-23 | Dec-24 | |
| Phase 2 | Lomecel-B (Lomecel) | Mesenchymal stem cells | NCT05233774 | Mild AD | Dec-21 | Sep-23 | |
| Phase 2 | hUC-MSCs | Human umbilical cord–derived mesenchymal stem cells | NCT02672306 | AD, mixed dementia | Oct-17 | Oct-19 | Safe; *no significant cognitive benefit* (ADAS-Cog/MMSE negative). |
| Phase 2 | Allogeneic MSCs | Allogeneic human mesenchymal stem cells | NCT02833792 | Mild to moderate AD | Jun-16 | Dec-24 | |
| Phase 2 | CB-AC-02 | Mesenchymal stem cells | NCT02899091 | Mild to moderate AD | Sep-16 | Dec-24 | |
| Phase 1/2 | GB301 | Regulatory T cells | NCT03865017 | Mild to moderate AD | Dec-20 | Dec-21 | |
| Phase 1 | Amniotic & umbilical cord tissue | Amniotic/umbilical cord tissue–derived cells | NCT03899298 | AD + other indications | Sep-19 | Mar-29 | |
| Phase 1 | Allogeneic MSCs | Allogeneic mesenchymal stem cells | NCT04040348 | Mild to moderate AD | Oct-19 | Apr-23 | Demonstrated safety; *no cognitive efficacy observed.* |
| Phase 1 | SNK01 | Autologous natural killer (NK) cells | NCT04678453 | AD | Jan-21 | Jan-24 | |
| Phase 1 | Amniotic & umbilical cord tissue | Amniotic/umbilical cord cells | NCT03899298 | AD + other diseases | Sep-19 | Mar-29 | |
| Phase 1 | Autologous adipose-derived stem cells | Autologous adipose-derived stem cells | NCT05667649 | Mild to moderate AD | Aug-23 | Mar-25 | |
| Phase 1 | VT301 | Regulatory T cells | NCT05016427 | Mild to moderate AD | Nov-21 | Apr-22 | |
| Not applicable | Bone marrow–derived stem cells | Bone marrow–derived stem cells | NCT03724136 | AD, autism | Oct-18 | Jul-25 | Safe; *no cognitive or behavioral improvement* demonstrated in AD subgroup. |

**Table 9.6** List of gene-related therapy trial targeting Alzheimer's disease

| Trial stage | Agent | Mechanism of action | Clinical trial ID | Target population | Start date | Estimated primary completion date | Key findings (as of 2025) |
|---|---|---|---|---|---|---|---|
| Phase 2 | BIIB080 | Anti-tau ASO | NCT05399888 | MCI due to AD or mild AD dementia | Aug-22 | Nov-27 | |
| Phase 2 | LX1001 | AAV gene transfer of APOE2 | NCT03634007 | Mild–moderate AD with APOE4 homozygotes | Nov-19 | Nov-24 | |
| Phase 1 | ALN-APP | RNAi to suppress APP | NCT05231785 | Early-onset AD | Feb-22 | Jul-25 | Reduced CSF sAPPα/sAPPβ (target engagement). No cognitive results yet |
| Phase 1 | LX1001 | AAV-APOE2 gene transfer | NCT05400330 | Mild–moderate AD with APOE4 homozygotes | May-23 | Nov-28 | |
| Phase 1 | NIO752 | Anti-tau ASO | NCT05469360 | Early AD | Feb-23 | Oct-24 | |

*ASO* antisense oligonucleotide, *MCI* mild cognitive impairment, *AD* Alzheimer's disease, *AAV* Adeno-associated virus, *APOE2* apolipoprotein ε2, *APOE4* apolipoprotein E ε4, *RNAi* RNA interference, *APP* amyloid precursor protein formation [38]. Consequently, medications used for type 2 DM are under consideration for AD treatment

#### 9.1.3.1.1 Insulin

Prescribed for advanced T2DM and T1DM, insulin usage is associated with a heightened risk of dementia due to hypoglycemia [39]. Intra-nasal insulin spray has shown cognitive function improvement in AD animal models [40–42]. Nonetheless, this effect seems less pronounced in individuals carrying the APOE ε4 allele [43].

#### 9.1.3.1.2 DPP-4 Inhibitor

These inhibitors offer neuroprotective benefits by elevating glucagon-like peptide 1 (GLP-1) levels, reducing inflammation, and providing antioxidative effects. While positive outcomes have been observed in animal models, human studies have shown variability.

Four types of Dipeptidyl Peptidase-4 inhibitors (DPP-4i) are currently available: saxagliptin, vildagliptin, linagliptin, and sitagliptin. These inhibitors offer neuroprotective benefits by elevating GLP-1 levels, reducing inflammation, and providing antioxidative effects [44, 45]. While sitagliptin and linagliptin have demonstrated positive outcomes in animal models [46–51], human studies have shown variability [52–55].

#### 9.1.3.1.3 PPAR-γ Agonists

PPAR-*γ* agonists, used in type 2 DM treatment, have shown promise in animal models but have conflicting outcomes in human studies [56, 57]. Early studies with rosiglitazone in AD patients showed improved cognitive function [58], but this effect was not consistent in individuals carrying the APOE ε4 allele [59]. Biomarkers such as Interleukin-6 and -10, C-reactive protein, Tumor Necrotic Factor α, Fatty Acid Binding Protein 3, and pancreatic polypeptide may aid clinicians in identifying potential responders [60].

#### 9.1.3.1.4 SGLT-2 Inhibitors

Sodium glucose cotransporter 2 inhibitors (SGLT2i) function as anti-diabetic agents by blocking glucose reabsorption in the proximal renal tubules, leading to increased urinary glucose excretion. However, these inhibitors may also affect the sodium glucose cotransporter 1 (SGLT1), particularly canagliflozin and sotagliflozin [61]. SGLT1 is found in hippocampal and cortical pyramidal cells [62]. These agents have shown neuroprotective potential in animal models of AD [63]. However, evidence from human studies is limited, necessitating further research [64, 65].

##### 9.1.3.1.5 GLP-1R Agonist

GLP-1 receptor (GLP-1R) agonists, a subset of the incretin hormone family, exert their antidiabetic effects by stimulating insulin release and reducing glucagon secretion [66]. Additionally, they have the ability to cross the blood-brain barrier, impacting cognitive function and providing neuroprotective advantages within the central nervous system [67]. These mechanisms encompass anti-inflammatory properties, mitigation of amyloid accumulation, inhibition of tau protein hyperphosphorylation, facilitation of neurogenesis and cell proliferation, enhancement of synaptic plasticity, and mitigation of oxidative stress [68]. Studies involving AD patients have shown that liraglutide can enhance connectivity among brain regions [69]; however, these improvements did not translate into observable cognitive differences between treatment groups. Notably, a phase II trial of ELAD demonstrated liraglutide's potential in slowing the progression of AD [70]. Moreover, a phase III trial of semaglutide in early AD is scheduled for publication in 2026 (NCT04777409), further highlighting the ongoing exploration of GLP-1R agonists in AD treatment.

#### 9.1.3.2 Hypertension Medication

Epidemiological data establish a correlation between hypertension and AD. Research involving postmortem brain tissues and in vivo studies suggests that hypertension can exacerbate the accumulation of Aβ plaques in the brain, a key feature of AD pathology [71–73]. A meta-analysis has indicated an 8% increase in the risk of developing AD due to hypertension [74]. Various classes of anti-hypertensive medications, particularly those targeting the renin-angiotensin system (RAS), such as angiotensin-receptor blockers (ARBs or sartans), angiotensin-converting enzyme inhibitors (ACE-inhibitors), and diuretics, have shown promise in reducing the risk of AD in individuals with normal cognitive function [75, 76]. However, conflicting findings exist. A 2020 meta-analysis suggested that while managing blood pressure in hypertensive individuals may lower the risk of dementia, there is insufficient evidence to determine the superiority of one class of antihypertensive agents over others [77]. This underscores the significance of comprehensive blood pressure management as a component of a holistic approach to brain health.

#### 9.1.3.3 Dyslipidemia Medications

Dyslipidemia medications play a significant role in AD management. Hypercholesterolemia is considered a risk factor for AD [78]. Autopsies have revealed that individuals taking statins, commonly used for dyslipidemia, exhibit fewer pathological changes associated with AD [79]. However, the effects of statins seem to vary depending on ethnicity and sex, with some studies suggesting a lower risk of AD among statin users, albeit with less pronounced effects in certain demographic groups [80]. In animal models of AD, statins such as simvastatin, fluvastatin, atorvastatin, and pitavastatin have demonstrated beneficial effects [81–86]. However, these benefits are less clear in human studies, with conflicting results regarding the impact of specific statins on AD progression. For example, simvastatin may slow AD progression in some patients [87]. Combining RAS-acting antihypertensive medications with certain statins like pravastatin or rosuvastatin has been suggested to be more effective in preventing AD compared to other statins, although this effect may not apply universally across all ethnicities [88]. Currently, there are no meta-analyses comparing the efficacy of statins in either preventing AD or delaying its progression.

Other dyslipidemia medications, such as fenofibrate, nicotinic acid, and ezetimibe, have shown protective effects in animal models of AD [89–91]. However, human data supporting these findings are currently lacking, indicating the need for further research. The emerging class of lipid-lowering agents known as Proprotein Convertase Subtilisin/Kexin Type 9 (PCSK9) inhibitors has shown mixed results regarding their impact on AD risk, with uncertain effects observed in different studies [92, 93]. Additional studies are required to clarify the potential effects of PCSK9 inhibitors and other dyslipidemia medications in the context of AD prevention and progression.

## 9.2 Treatments for Vascular Dementia

Treatments for vascular dementia are crucial given its prevalence, ranking second after Alzheimer's disease and affecting 10–30% of dementia cases [94]. Neurologists often categorize vascular dementia into three subtypes based on its etiology: strategic strokes, cerebral small vessel disease, and multi-infarct dementia. Unlike Alzheimer's disease, vascular dementia typically presents with a stepwise decline following a stroke and includes symptoms such as mood disturbances, apraxia, and gait abnormalities.

### *9.2.1 Symptomatic Treatments*

#### 9.2.1.1 Cholinesterase Inhibitors and NMDAR Antagonist

ChEIs have been explored for their potential in treating vascular dementia. A Cochrane review noted that in patients with vascular dementia or vascular cognitive impairment, higher doses of donepezil (10 mg) and galantamine (16–24 mg) were associated with more adverse events compared to placebo. However, rivastigmine's efficacy remains inconclusive due to inadequate dosing and limited sample sizes in certain trials [95].

Similarly, memantine, initially approved for moderate-to-severe Alzheimer's disease, has shown positive effects in vascular dementia patients. In mild-to-moderate vascular dementia, memantine improved cognitive function without worsening global function and behavior [96]. Vascular dementia patients treated with memantine showed better cognitive function compared to those on placebo, particularly those with severe dementia. Notably, individuals with a high burden of white matter hyperintensity (WMH) and subcortical vascular dementia responded more favorably to memantine [97–99].

### 9.2.2 *Repurpose of Other Known Medication for Vascular Dementia*

Given vascular dementia pathology involving infarcts and WMH, discussions have focused on treating metabolic disorders. Anti-thrombotic agents are commonly used in vascular dementia with ischemic events. However, studies like the Aspirin in Reducing Events in the Elderly (ASPREE) trial did not find a positive cognitive effect with aspirin [100].

A study from Taiwan demonstrated that cilostazol users with cerebrovascular disease had a reduced risk of dementia [101]. Retrospective studies also suggest that cilostazol may improve MMSE scores, especially in individuals with mild cognitive impairment or stroke [102, 103]. However, the results from randomized controlled trials are less convincing. For instance, the main analysis in the PreventIon of CArdiovascular events in iSchemic Stroke patients with high risk of cerebral hemOrrhage for reducing COGnitive decline (PICASSO-COG) trial found no significant difference between aspirin and cilostazol. Nevertheless, subgroup analysis revealed that patients with a baseline MMSE score of 24 or lower experienced less cognitive decline with cilostazol use [104]. It is worth noting that most cilostazol studies were conducted in Asia, potentially influencing results due to different ethnicities, which raises uncertainty about generalizing these findings globally.

Apart from the treatments mentioned earlier for vascular dementia, several other pharmaceutical options are being investigated, although they have not yet undergone large-scale studies. Piracetam, a cyclic derivative of the neurotransmitter GABA, is commonly used for cognitive impairment, myoclonus, and cortical aphasia. It has been reported to positively impact cognition in vascular dementia patients following cerebral infarction [105]. Pentoxifylline, a non-specific phosphodiesterase inhibitor and methylxanthine derivative, works by reducing plasma viscosity, fibrinogen levels, and erythrocyte aggregation, among other pathways. Systematic reviews suggest its potential therapeutic benefit in vascular dementia treatment [106, 107]. Ginkgo biloba, known for its antioxidant properties and ability to improve mitochondrial function, is widely used in Asia. A meta-analysis indicated that short-term use of Ginkgo biloba may prevent vascular cognitive impairment (VCI) from progressing into vascular dementia [108]. However, most studies included in these reviews had small sample sizes and methodological limitations, affecting the certainty of the evidence provided. Cerebrolysin, a commercially available mixture of neurotrophic factors like brain-derived neurotrophic factor (BDNF) and nerve growth factor (NGF), has shown promise in enhancing cognition and overall function in vascular dementia individuals, without apparent adverse effects. However, these findings are not conclusive due to heterogeneity and a high risk of bias in the studies included, impacting the reliability of the results [109].

Finally, medications that modulate nitric oxide, such as NO donors, PDE5 inhibitors, and guanylate cyclase activators, have also demonstrated potential in the treatment of vascular dementia [110].

## 9.3 Treatment for Dementia with Lewy Bodies and Parkinson Disease Dementia

Lewy body dementia (LBD), which includes Dementia with Lewy bodies (DLB) and Parkinson's disease dementia (PDD), involves similar neuropathological changes such as α-synuclein deposition and the loss of dopaminergic and cholinergic neurons. Both conditions present with progressive cognitive impairment, particularly affecting attention and consciousness, and are associated with parkinsonism and visual hallucinations. Despite the understanding of Lewy body deposition, there is currently no cure for LBD. The primary focus remains on symptomatic treatments to alleviate behavioral and psychiatric symptoms and to preserve cognitive function.

### *9.3.1 Symptomatic Treatments*

#### 9.3.1.1 Cholinesterase Inhibitors and NMDA Receptor Antagonist

Studies have shown some benefits of cholinesterase inhibitors (CHEi) in controlling neuropsychiatric symptoms in DLB [111–116]. Patients receiving CHEi at diagnosis had reduced usage of antipsychotics and anxiolytics [117]. Specific CHEi like donepezil improved cognitive function but not neuropsychiatric symptoms, and patients with impairment in specific cognitive domains, such as calculation/attention, object recall, and drawing may respond better to treatment than others [118–120]. Rivastigmine improved neuropsychiatric symptoms but not MMSE [114]. And there were only open-label studies or small-scale clinical trials for galantamine in DLB patients. Memantine showed positive effects in mild to moderate DLB in a phase IV study [121].

### 9.3.2 *Repurpose of Other Known Medication for DLB and PDD*

Armodafinil, a dopamine transporter inhibitor and wakefulness-promoting agent, has shown promise in improving hypersomnia and neuropsychiatric symptoms [122, 123]. Pimavanserin, acting as an antagonist/inverse agonist at the 5HT2A receptor, has demonstrated efficacy in reducing delusions and hallucinations [124, 125]. Zonisamide targets motor function by activating the dopaminergic pathway and inhibiting sodium and T-type calcium channels, leading to improvements in motor symptoms [126]. Mevidalen, a selective positive allosteric modulator at the D1 receptor, has shown some success in improving motor symptoms but fell short of the primary cognitive endpoint [127].

### 9.3.3 *Potential Disease-Modifying Treatment for DLB and PDD*

Potential disease-modifying treatments for DLB and PDD are currently under investigation. Advancements in genome-wide association studies have identified key genes associated with DLB, including SNCA, SNCB, SNCG, and GBA. SNCA (chr4q22) encodes α-synuclein, a hallmark protein in LBD pathogenesis [128]. SNCB and SNCG encode β-synuclein and γ-synuclein, respectively, with β-synuclein potentially acting as an antagonist to α-synuclein [128–130]. The GBA gene (chr1q22), encoding lysosomal glucosylceramidase, plays a role in degrading α-synuclein [131]. Additionally, the presence of APOE-ε4 has been linked to three times higher risk of LBD [131]. Targeted therapies aimed at abnormal genetic products, such as those implicated in LBD, are being actively pursued. Challenges in developing disease-modifying treatments for LBD stem from the intracellular deposition of α-synuclein, contrasting with the extracellular aggregation seen in β-amyloid-related diseases. Strategies to promote the genetic expression of GBA for α-synuclein clearance are being explored. However, specific disease-modifying treatments for LBD are not yet available.

## 9.4 Treatment for Frontotemporal Dementia

Frontotemporal Dementia (FTD) currently lacks a cure, similar to DLB and PDD. Despite advances in understanding tauopathy and TDP-43 pathology, developing disease-modifying treatments for FTD remains challenging [29–31, 132–134]. Several obstacles contribute to this difficulty, including delayed diagnosis, severe neuropsychiatric symptoms overshadowing cognitive impairment, low medical compliance, co-occurrence of different proteinopathies, and a lack of disease-specific biomarkers [135–137].

The cholinergic system, relatively intact in FTD [138] explains why cholinesterase inhibitors and memantine often have neutral or negative effects on cognition [139].

### 9.4.1 Potential Disease-Modifying Treatment for FTD

In the era of precision medicine, interventions targeting pathological genes and their derivatives show promise. Early intervention in individuals with a family history of FTD associated with MAPT or GRN mutations is a viable strategy. Biomarkers such as neurofilament light chain (NfL) and phosphorylated neurofilament heavy chain (pNfH) aid in selecting suitable candidates for clinical trials [140]. A study from the Genetic FTD Initiative (GENFI) cohort, which included 91 symptomatic and 179 asymptomatic subjects, showed that NfL levels increased at the conversion stage, while pNfH levels increased at the symptomatic stage. The dynamic changes in these biomarkers may assist in the staging of FTD.

Studies targeting microtubules, tau, and granulin aim to reduce abnormal protein aggregation and breakdown tau accumulation. Microtubule stabilizers (TPI-287 and Davunetide), anti-tau antibodies (C2N-8E12 and BMS-986168), and tau acetylation inhibitors (salsalate) have primarily been studied in progressive supranuclear palsy patients [141]. Immunotherapies targeting specific genetic products in FTD, such as TDP-43 accumulation secondary to VCP or TARDBP mutations, are also being explored [141, 142]. *Latozinemab, a monoclonal antibody increasing progranulin levels, has shown promise in phase 1 trials by successfully elevating progranulin levels in serum and CSF* [143, 144].

## 9.5 Summary

Precision medicine in dementia treatment continues to evolve, presenting a continuous journey for patients, clinicians, and researchers. While many clinical trials have yielded limited or unfavorable results, they have provided valuable insights into neuropathology, neuropharmacology, and disease-specific biomarkers. These advancements will fuel further research into disease-modifying therapies.

**Title of the Contribution** Kang-Po Lee drafted the initial manuscript for the Treatments for Alzheimer's Disease (excluding anti-amyloid and anti-Tau sections) and Treatments for Vascular Dementia. Lee also collaborated on the sections for Treatment for Dementia with Lewy Bodies, Parkinson's Disease Dementia, and Treatment for Frontotemporal Dementia, and conducted the initial editing for the entire chapter. Po-Yu Lin drafted the initial manuscript for the anti-amyloid and anti-Tau sections. Meng-Ju Wu drafted the initial manuscript for the Treatment for Dementia with Lewy Bodies, Parkinson's Disease Dementia, and Treatment for Frontotemporal Dementia. Pi-Shan Sung conceptualized and developed the framework of the chapter. Sung also performed the final editing for the entire chapter.

## References

1. Bartus RT, Dean RL 3rd, Beer B, Lippa AS. The cholinergic hypothesis of geriatric memory dysfunction. Science. 1982;217(4558):408–14. https://doi.org/10.1126/science.7046051.
2. Rogers SL, Friedhoff LT. The efficacy and safety of donepezil in patients with Alzheimer's disease: results of a US Multicentre, Randomized, Double-Blind, Placebo-Controlled Trial. The Donepezil Study Group. Dementia. 1996;7(6):293–303. https://doi.org/10.1159/000106895.
3. Rogers SL, Farlow MR, Doody RS, Mohs R, Friedhoff LT. A 24-week, double-blind, placebo-controlled trial of donepezil in patients with Alzheimer's disease. Donepezil Study Group. Neurology. 1998;50(1):136–45. https://doi.org/10.1212/wnl.50.1.136.
4. Farlow M, Anand R, Messina J Jr, Hartman R, Veach J. A 52-week study of the efficacy of rivastigmine in patients with mild to moderately severe Alzheimer's disease. Eur Neurol. 2000;44(4):236–41. https://doi.org/10.1159/000008243.
5. Rösler M, Anand R, Cicin-Sain A, Gauthier S, Agid Y, Dal-Bianco P, et al. Efficacy and safety of rivastigmine in patients with Alzheimer's disease: international randomised controlled trial. BMJ. 1999;318(7184):633–8. https://doi.org/10.1136/bmj.318.7184.633.
6. Wilkinson D, Murray J. Galantamine: a randomized, double-blind, dose comparison in patients with Alzheimer's disease. Int J Geriatr Psychiatry. 2001;16(9):852–7. https://doi.org/10.1002/gps.409.
7. Wilcock GK, Lilienfeld S, Gaens E. Efficacy and safety of galantamine in patients with mild to moderate Alzheimer's disease: multicentre randomised controlled trial. Galantamine International-1 Study Group. BMJ. 2000;321(7274):1445–9. https://doi.org/10.1136/bmj.321.7274.1445.
8. Reisberg B, Doody R, Stöffler A, Schmitt F, Ferris S, Möbius HJ. Memantine in moderate-to-severe Alzheimer's disease. N Engl J Med. 2003;348(14):1333–41. https://doi.org/10.1056/NEJMoa013128.
9. Birks JS, Harvey RJ. Donepezil for dementia due to Alzheimer's disease. Cochrane Database Syst Rev. 2018;6 https://doi.org/10.1002/14651858.CD001190.pub3.
10. Birks JS, Chong LY, Grimley Evans J. Rivastigmine for Alzheimer's disease. Cochrane Database Syst Rev. 2015;2015(9) https://doi.org/10.1002/14651858.CD001191.pub4.
11. Harvey AL. The pharmacology of galanthamine and its analogues. Pharmacol Ther. 1995;68(1):113–28. https://doi.org/10.1016/0163-7258(95)02002-0.
12. McShane R, Westby MJ, Roberts E, Minakaran N, Schneider L, Farrimond LE, et al. Memantine for dementia. Cochrane Database Syst Rev. 2019;3(3):Cd003154. https://doi.org/10.1002/14651858.CD003154.pub6.
13. Hansen RA, Gartlehner G, Webb AP, Morgan LC, Moore CG, Jonas DE. Efficacy and safety of donepezil, galantamine, and rivastigmine for the treatment of Alzheimer's disease: a systematic review and meta-analysis. Clin Interv Aging. 2008;3(2):211–25.
14. Jones RW, Soininen H, Hager K, Aarsland D, Passmore P, Murthy A, et al. A multinational, randomised, 12-week study comparing the effects of donepezil and galantamine in patients with mild to moderate Alzheimer's disease. Int J Geriatr Psychiatry. 2004;19(1):58–67. https://doi.org/10.1002/gps.1038.
15. Wilkinson DG, Passmore AP, Bullock R, Hopker SW, Smith R, Potocnik FC, et al. A multinational, randomised, 12-week, comparative study of donepezil and rivastigmine in patients with mild to moderate Alzheimer's disease. Int J Clin Pract. 2002;56(6):441–6.
16. Wilcock G, Howe I, Coles H, Lilienfeld S, Truyen L, Zhu Y, et al. A long-term comparison of galantamine and donepezil in the treatment of Alzheimer's disease. Drugs Aging. 2003;20(10):777–89. https://doi.org/10.2165/00002512-200320100-00006.
17. Bullock R, Touchon J, Bergman H, Gambina G, He Y, Rapatz G, et al. Rivastigmine and donepezil treatment in moderate to moderately-severe Alzheimer's disease over a 2-year period. Curr Med Res Opin. 2005;21(8):1317–27. https://doi.org/10.1185/030079905x56565.

18. Krall WJ, Sramek JJ, Cutler NR. Cholinesterase inhibitors: a therapeutic strategy for Alzheimer disease. Ann Pharmacother. 1999;33(4):441–50. https://doi.org/10.1345/aph.18211.
19. Diaz-Galvan P, Lorenzon G, Mohanty R, Mårtensson G, Cavedo E, Lista S, et al. Differential response to donepezil in MRI subtypes of mild cognitive impairment. Alzheimers Res Ther. 2023;15(1):117. https://doi.org/10.1186/s13195-023-01253-2.
20. Cacabelos R. Donepezil in Alzheimer's disease: from conventional trials to pharmacogenetics. Neuropsychiatr Dis Treat. 2007;3(3):303–33.
21. Chen T-H, Chou M-C, Lai C-L, Wu S-J, Hsu C-L, Yang Y-H. Factors affecting therapeutic response to Rivastigmine in Alzheimer's disease patients in Taiwan. Kaohsiung J Med Sci. 2017;33(6):277–83. https://doi.org/10.1016/j.kjms.2017.04.006.
22. Farlow MR, Hake A, Messina J, Hartman R, Veach J, Anand R. Response of patients with Alzheimer disease to Rivastigmine treatment is predicted by the rate of disease progression. Arch Neurol. 2001;58(3):417–22. https://doi.org/10.1001/archneur.58.3.417.
23. Swerdlow NR, Kotz JE, Joshi YB, Talledo J, Sprock J, Molina JL, et al. Using biomarkers to predict memantine effects in Alzheimer's disease: a proposal and proof-of-concept demonstration. J Alzheimer's Dis. 2021;84(4):1431–8. https://doi.org/10.3233/jad-215029.
24. Maheshwari S, Singh A, Ansari VA, Mahmood T, Wasim R, Akhtar J, et al. Navigating the dementia landscape: biomarkers and emerging therapies. Ageing Res Rev. 2024;94:102193. https://doi.org/10.1016/j.arr.2024.102193.
25. Cummings J, Apostolova L, Rabinovici GD, Atri A, Aisen P, Greenberg S, et al. Lecanemab: appropriate use recommendations. J Prev Alzheimers Dis. 2023;10(3):362–77. https://doi.org/10.14283/jpad.2023.30.
26. Cummings J, Rabinovici GD, Atri A, Aisen P, Apostolova LG, Hendrix S, et al. Aducanumab: appropriate use recommendations update. J Prev Alzheimers Dis. 2022;9(2):221–30. https://doi.org/10.14283/jpad.2022.34.
27. Albert MS, DeKosky ST, Dickson D, Dubois B, Feldman HH, Fox NC, et al. The diagnosis of mild cognitive impairment due to Alzheimer's disease: recommendations from the National Institute on Aging-Alzheimer's Association workgroups on diagnostic guidelines for Alzheimer's disease. Alzheimers Dement. 2011;7(3):270–9. https://doi.org/10.1016/j.jalz.2011.03.008.
28. McKhann GM, Knopman DS, Chertkow H, Hyman BT, Jack CR Jr, Kawas CH, et al. The diagnosis of dementia due to Alzheimer's disease: recommendations from the National Institute on Aging-Alzheimer's Association workgroups on diagnostic guidelines for Alzheimer's disease. Alzheimers Dement. 2011;7(3):263–9. https://doi.org/10.1016/j.jalz.2011.03.005.
29. van Dyck CH, Swanson CJ, Aisen P, Bateman RJ, Chen C, Gee M, et al. Lecanemab in early Alzheimer's disease. N Engl J Med. 2023;388(1):9–21. https://doi.org/10.1056/NEJMoa2212948.
30. Budd Haeberlein S, Aisen PS, Barkhof F, Chalkias S, Chen T, Cohen S, et al. Two randomized phase 3 studies of aducanumab in early Alzheimer's disease. J Prev Alzheimers Dis. 2022;9(2):197–210. https://doi.org/10.14283/jpad.2022.30.
31. Sims JR, Zimmer JA, Evans CD, Lu M, Ardayfio P, Sparks J, et al. Donanemab in early symptomatic Alzheimer disease: the TRAILBLAZER-ALZ 2 randomized clinical trial. JAMA. 2023;330(6):512–27. https://doi.org/10.1001/jama.2023.13239.
32. Hampel H, O'Bryant SE, Molinuevo JL, Zetterberg H, Masters CL, Lista S, et al. Blood-based biomarkers for Alzheimer disease: mapping the road to the clinic. Nat Rev Neurol. 2018;14(11):639–52. https://doi.org/10.1038/s41582-018-0079-7.
33. Sperling RA, Jack CR Jr, Black SE, Frosch MP, Greenberg SM, Hyman BT, et al. Amyloid-related imaging abnormalities in amyloid-modifying therapeutic trials: recommendations from the Alzheimer's Association Research Roundtable Workgroup. Alzheimers Dement. 2011;7(4):367–85. https://doi.org/10.1016/j.jalz.2011.05.2351.

34. Cummings J, Zhou Y, Lee G, Zhong K, Fonseca J, Cheng F. Alzheimer's disease drug development pipeline: 2024. Alzheimers Dement (N Y). 2024;10(2):e12465. https://doi.org/10.1002/trc2.12465.
35. Cummings J, Zhou Y, Lee G, Zhong K, Fonseca J, Cheng F. Alzheimer's disease drug development pipeline: 2023. Alzheimers Dement (N Y). 2023;9(2):e12385. https://doi.org/10.1002/trc2.12385.
36. Biessels GJ, Staekenborg S, Brunner E, Brayne C, Scheltens P. Risk of dementia in diabetes mellitus: a systematic review. Lancet Neurol. 2006;5(1):64–74. https://doi.org/10.1016/S1474-4422(05)70284-2.
37. Kopf D, Frölich L. Risk of incident Alzheimer's disease in diabetic patients: a systematic review of prospective trials. J Alzheimer's Dis. 2009;16(4):677–85. https://doi.org/10.3233/jad-2009-1011.
38. Kandimalla R, Thirumala V, Reddy PH. Is Alzheimer's disease a type 3 diabetes? A critical appraisal. Biochim Biophys Acta Mol basis Dis. 2017;1863(5):1078–89. https://doi.org/10.1016/j.bbadis.2016.08.018.
39. Weinstein G, Davis-Plourde KL, Conner S, Himali JJ, Beiser AS, Lee A, et al. Association of metformin, sulfonylurea and insulin use with brain structure and function and risk of dementia and Alzheimer's disease: pooled analysis from 5 cohorts. PLoS One. 2019;14(2):e0212293. https://doi.org/10.1371/journal.pone.0212293.
40. Lv H, Tang L, Guo C, Jiang Y, Gao C, Wang Y, et al. Intranasal insulin administration may be highly effective in improving cognitive function in mice with cognitive dysfunction by reversing brain insulin resistance. Cogn Neurodyn. 2020;14(3):323–38. https://doi.org/10.1007/s11571-020-09571-z.
41. Reger MA, Watson GS, Green PS, Wilkinson CW, Baker LD, Cholerton B, et al. Intranasal insulin improves cognition and modulates beta-amyloid in early AD. Neurology. 2008;70(6):440–8. https://doi.org/10.1212/01.Wnl.0000265401.62434.36.
42. Benedict C, Hallschmid M, Hatke A, Schultes B, Fehm HL, Born J, et al. Intranasal insulin improves memory in humans. Psychoneuroendocrinology. 2004;29(10):1326–34. https://doi.org/10.1016/j.psyneuen.2004.04.003.
43. Reger MA, Watson GS, Green PS, Baker LD, Cholerton B, Fishel MA, et al. Intranasal insulin administration dose-dependently modulates verbal memory and plasma amyloid-beta in memory-impaired older adults. J Alzheimer's Dis. 2008;13(3):323–31. https://doi.org/10.3233/jad-2008-13309.
44. Demuth HU, McIntosh CH, Pederson RA. Type 2 diabetes--therapy with dipeptidyl peptidase IV inhibitors. Biochim Biophys Acta. 2005;1751(1):33–44. https://doi.org/10.1016/j.bbapap.2005.05.010.
45. Wiciński M, Wódkiewicz E, Słupski M, Walczak M, Socha M, Malinowski B, et al. Neuroprotective activity of Sitagliptin via reduction of neuroinflammation beyond the incretin effect: focus on Alzheimer's disease. BioMed Res Int. 2018;2018:6091014. https://doi.org/10.1155/2018/6091014.
46. Siddiqui N, Ali J, Parvez S, Zameer S, Najmi AK, Akhtar M. Linagliptin, a DPP-4 inhibitor, ameliorates Aβ (1-42) peptides induced neurodegeneration and brain insulin resistance (BIR) via insulin receptor substrate-1 (IRS-1) in rat model of Alzheimer's disease. Neuropharmacology. 2021;195:108662. https://doi.org/10.1016/j.neuropharm.2021.108662.
47. Siddiqui N, Ali J, Parvez S, Najmi AK, Akhtar M. Neuroprotective role of DPP-4 inhibitor Linagliptin against neurodegeneration, neuronal insulin resistance and neuroinflammation induced by intracerebroventricular streptozotocin in rat model of Alzheimer's disease. Neurochem Res. 2023;48(9):2714–30. https://doi.org/10.1007/s11064-023-03924-w.
48. Ide M, Sonoda N, Inoue T, Kimura S, Minami Y, Makimura H, et al. The dipeptidyl peptidase-4 inhibitor, linagliptin, improves cognitive impairment in streptozotocin-induced diabetic mice by inhibiting oxidative stress and microglial activation. PLoS One. 2020;15(2):e0228750. https://doi.org/10.1371/journal.pone.0228750.

49. Dong Q, Teng S-W, Wang Y, Qin F, Li Y, Ai L-L, et al. Sitagliptin protects the cognition function of the Alzheimer's disease mice through activating glucagon-like peptide-1 and BDNF-TrkB signalings. Neurosci Lett. 2019;696:184–90. https://doi.org/10.1016/j.neulet.2018.12.041.
50. Kosaraju J, Gali CC, Khatwal RB, Dubala A, Chinni S, Holsinger RMD, et al. Saxagliptin: a dipeptidyl peptidase-4 inhibitor ameliorates streptozotocin induced Alzheimer's disease. Neuropharmacology. 2013;72:291–300. https://doi.org/10.1016/j.neuropharm.2013.04.008.
51. Ma QH, Jiang LF, Mao JL, Xu WX, Huang M. Vildagliptin prevents cognitive deficits and neuronal apoptosis in a rat model of Alzheimer's disease. Mol Med Rep. 2018;17(3):4113–9. https://doi.org/10.3892/mmr.2017.8289.
52. Jeong SH, Kim HR, Kim J, Kim H, Hong N, Jung JH, et al. Association of Dipeptidyl Peptidase-4 inhibitor use and amyloid burden in patients with diabetes and AD-related cognitive impairment. Neurology. 2021;97(11):e1110–e22. https://doi.org/10.1212/wnl.0000000000012534.
53. Isik AT, Soysal P, Yay A, Usarel C. The effects of sitagliptin, a DPP-4 inhibitor, on cognitive functions in elderly diabetic patients with or without Alzheimer's disease. Diabetes Res Clin Pract. 2017;123:192–8. https://doi.org/10.1016/j.diabres.2016.12.010.
54. Akimoto H, Negishi A, Oshima S, Wakiyama H, Okita M, Horii N, et al. Antidiabetic drugs for the risk of Alzheimer disease in patients with type 2 DM using FAERS. Am J Alzheimers Dis Other Demen. 2020;35:1533317519899546. https://doi.org/10.1177/1533317519899546.
55. Tseng C-H. Vildagliptin has a neutral association with dementia risk in type 2 diabetes patients. Front Endocrinol. 2021;12 https://doi.org/10.3389/fendo.2021.637392.
56. Lin H-C, Chung C-H, Chen L-C, Wang J-Y, Chen C-C, Huang K-Y, et al. Pioglitazone use increases risk of Alzheimer's disease in patients with type 2 diabetes receiving insulin. Sci Rep. 2023;13(1):6625. https://doi.org/10.1038/s41598-023-33674-2.
57. Cheng F, Fang J, Zhang P, Pieper AA, Cummings JL. Pioglitazone reduces the incidence of Alzheimer's disease: from genetics to population-based validation. Alzheimers Dement. 2021;17(S3):e051950. https://doi.org/10.1002/alz.051950.
58. Watson GS, Cholerton BA, Reger MA, Baker LD, Plymate SR, Asthana S, et al. Preserved cognition in patients with early Alzheimer disease and amnestic mild cognitive impairment during treatment with rosiglitazone: a preliminary study. Am J Geriatr Psychiatry. 2005;13(11):950–8. https://doi.org/10.1176/appi.ajgp.13.11.950.
59. Risner ME, Saunders AM, Altman JFB, Ormandy GC, Craft S, Foley IM, et al. Efficacy of rosiglitazone in a genetically defined population with mild-to-moderate Alzheimer's disease. Pharmacogenomics J. 2006;6(4):246–54. https://doi.org/10.1038/sj.tpj.6500369.
60. O'Bryant SE, Zhang F, Petersen M, Johnson L, Hall J, Rissman RA. A precision medicine approach to treating Alzheimer's disease using rosiglitazone therapy: a biomarker analysis of the REFLECT trials. J Alzheimer's Dis. 2021;81(2):557–68. https://doi.org/10.3233/jad-201610.
61. Cinti F, Moffa S, Impronta F, Cefalo C, Sun V, Sorice G, et al. Spotlight on ertugliflozin and its potential in the treatment of type 2 diabetes: evidence to date. Drug Des Devel Ther. 2017;11:2905–19. https://doi.org/10.2147/DDDT.S114932.
62. Poppe R, Karbach U, Gambaryan S, Wiesinger H, Lutzenburg M, Kraemer M, et al. Expression of the Na+-D-glucose cotransporter SGLT1 in neurons. J Neurochem. 1997;69(1):84–94. https://doi.org/10.1046/j.1471-4159.1997.69010084.x.
63. Huang J, Huang N, Cui D, Shi J, Qiu Y. Clinical antidiabetic medication used in Alzheimer's disease: from basic discovery to therapeutics development. Front Aging Neurosci. 2023;15 https://doi.org/10.3389/fnagi.2023.1122300.
64. Low S, Goh KS, Ng TP, Moh A, Ang SF, Wang J, et al. Association between use of sodium-glucose co-Transporter-2 (SGLT2) inhibitors and cognitive function in a longitudinal study of patients with type 2 diabetes. J Alzheimer's Dis. 2022;87(2):635–42. https://doi.org/10.3233/jad-215678.

65. Wium-Andersen IK, Osler M, Jørgensen MB, Rungby J, Wium-Andersen MK. Antidiabetic medication and risk of dementia in patients with type 2 diabetes: a nested case-control study. Eur J Endocrinol. 2019;181(5):499–507. https://doi.org/10.1530/eje-19-0259.
66. Holst JJ. The physiology of glucagon-like peptide 1. Physiol Rev. 2007;87(4):1409–39. https://doi.org/10.1152/physrev.00034.2006.
67. Yaribeygi H, Rashidy-Pour A, Atkin SL, Jamialahmadi T, Sahebkar A. GLP-1 mimetics and cognition. Life Sci. 2021;264:118645. https://doi.org/10.1016/j.lfs.2020.118645.
68. Du H, Meng X, Yao Y, Xu J. The mechanism and efficacy of GLP-1 receptor agonists in the treatment of Alzheimer's disease. Front Endocrinol. 2022;13 https://doi.org/10.3389/fendo.2022.1033479.
69. Watson KT, Wroolie TE, Tong G, Foland-Ross LC, Frangou S, Singh M, et al. Neural correlates of liraglutide effects in persons at risk for Alzheimer's disease. Behav Brain Res. 2019;356:271–8. https://doi.org/10.1016/j.bbr.2018.08.006.
70. Edison P, Femminella GD, Ritchie CW, Holmes C, Walker Z, Ridha BH, et al. Evaluation of liraglutide in the treatment of Alzheimer's disease. Alzheimers Dement. 2021;17(S9):e057848. https://doi.org/10.1002/alz.057848.
71. Sparks DL, Scheff SW, Liu H, Landers TM, Coyne CM, Hunsaker JC 3rd. Increased incidence of neurofibrillary tangles (NFT) in non-demented individuals with hypertension. J Neurol Sci. 1995;131(2):162–9. https://doi.org/10.1016/0022-510x(95)00105-b.
72. Ashby EL, Miners JS, Kehoe PG, Love S. Effects of hypertension and anti-hypertensive treatment on Amyloid-β (Aβ) plaque load and Aβ-synthesizing and Aβ-degrading enzymes in frontal cortex. J Alzheimer's Dis. 2016;50(4):1191–203. https://doi.org/10.3233/jad-150831.
73. Petrovitch H, White LR, Izmirilian G, Ross GW, Havlik RJ, Markesbery W, et al. Midlife blood pressure and neuritic plaques, neurofibrillary tangles, and brain weight at death: the HAAS. Honolulu-Asia aging Study. Neurobiol Aging. 2000;21(1):57–62. https://doi.org/10.1016/s0197-4580(00)00106-8.
74. Sáiz-Vazquez O, Puente-Martínez A, Pacheco-Bonrostro J, Ubillos-Landa S. Blood pressure and Alzheimer's disease: a review of meta-analysis. Front Neurol. 2022;13:1065335. https://doi.org/10.3389/fneur.2022.1065335.
75. Yasar S, Xia J, Yao W, Furberg CD, Xue QL, Mercado CI, et al. Antihypertensive drugs decrease risk of Alzheimer disease: Ginkgo Evaluation of Memory Study. Neurology. 2013;81(10):896–903. https://doi.org/10.1212/WNL.0b013e3182a35228.
76. Barthold D, Joyce G, Wharton W, Kehoe P, Zissimopoulos J. The association of multiple anti-hypertensive medication classes with Alzheimer's disease incidence across sex, race, and ethnicity. PLoS One. 2018;13(11):e0206705. https://doi.org/10.1371/journal.pone.0206705.
77. Ding J, Davis-Plourde KL, Sedaghat S, Tully PJ, Wang W, Phillips C, et al. Antihypertensive medications and risk for incident dementia and Alzheimer's disease: a meta-analysis of individual participant data from prospective cohort studies. Lancet Neurol. 2020;19(1):61–70. https://doi.org/10.1016/s1474-4422(19)30393-x.
78. Pappolla MA, Bryant-Thomas TK, Herbert D, Pacheco J, Fabra Garcia M, Manjon M, et al. Mild hypercholesterolemia is an early risk factor for the development of Alzheimer amyloid pathology. Neurology. 2003;61(2):199–205. https://doi.org/10.1212/01.wnl.0000070182.02537.84.
79. Li G, Larson EB, Sonnen JA, Shofer JB, Petrie EC, Schantz A, et al. Statin therapy is associated with reduced neuropathologic changes of Alzheimer disease. Neurology. 2007;69(9):878–85. https://doi.org/10.1212/01.wnl.0000277657.95487.1c.
80. Zissimopoulos JM, Barthold D, Brinton RD, Joyce G. Sex and race differences in the association between statin use and the incidence of Alzheimer disease. JAMA Neurol. 2017;74(2):225–32. https://doi.org/10.1001/jamaneurol.2016.3783.
81. Huang W, Li Z, Zhao L, Zhao W. Simvastatin ameliorate memory deficits and inflammation in clinical and mouse model of Alzheimer's disease via modulating the expression of miR-106b. Biomed Pharmacother. 2017;92:46–57. https://doi.org/10.1016/j.biopha.2017.05.060.

82. Yao D, Jing T, Niu L, Huang X, Wang Y, Deng X, et al. Amyloidogenesis induced by diet cholesterol and copper in a model mouse for Alzheimer's disease and protection effects of zinc and fluvastatin. Brain Res Bull. 2018;143:1–8. https://doi.org/10.1016/j.brainresbull.2018.09.003.
83. Kurinami H, Sato N, Shinohara M, Takeuchi D, Takeda S, Shimamura M, et al. Prevention of amyloid beta-induced memory impairment by fluvastatin, associated with the decrease in amyloid beta accumulation and oxidative stress in amyloid beta injection mouse model. Int J Mol Med. 2008;21(5):531–7.
84. Lu F, Li X, Suo A-Q, Zhang J-W. Inhibition of tau hyperphosphorylation and beta amyloid production in rat brain by oral administration of atorvastatin. Chin Med J. 2010;123(14)
85. Famer D, Wahlund LO, Crisby M. Rosuvastatin reduces microglia in the brain of wild type and ApoE knockout mice on a high cholesterol diet; implications for prevention of stroke and AD. Biochem Biophys Res Commun. 2010;402(2):367–72. https://doi.org/10.1016/j.bbrc.2010.10.035.
86. Kurata T, Miyazaki K, Kozuki M, Morimoto N, Ohta Y, Ikeda Y, et al. Atorvastatin and pitavastatin reduce senile plaques and inflammatory responses in a mouse model of Alzheimer's disease. Neurol Res. 2012;34(6):601–10. https://doi.org/10.1179/1743132812y.0000000054.
87. Petek B, Häbel H, Xu H, Villa-Lopez M, Kalar I, Hoang MT, et al. Statins and cognitive decline in patients with Alzheimer's and mixed dementia: a longitudinal registry-based cohort study. Alzheimers Res Ther. 2023;15(1):220. https://doi.org/10.1186/s13195-023-01360-0.
88. Barthold D, Joyce G, Diaz Brinton R, Wharton W, Kehoe PG, Zissimopoulos J. Association of combination statin and antihypertensive therapy with reduced Alzheimer's disease and related dementia risk. PLoS One. 2020;15(3):e0229541. https://doi.org/10.1371/journal.pone.0229541.
89. Lu Y, Fujioka H, Wang W, Zhu X. Bezafibrate confers neuroprotection in the 5xFAD mouse model of Alzheimer's disease. Biochim Biophys Acta Mol basis Dis. 2023;1869(8):166841. https://doi.org/10.1016/j.bbadis.2023.166841.
90. Wang Z, Zou Z, Li Q. Nicotinic acid supplementation contributes to the amelioration of Alzheimer's disease in mouse models. Ann Transl Med. 2022;10(19):1049. https://doi.org/10.21037/atm-22-1148.
91. Dalla Y, Singh N, Jaggi AS, Singh D, Ghulati P. Potential of ezetimibe in memory deficits associated with dementia of Alzheimer's type in mice. Indian J Pharmacol. 2009;41(6):262–7. https://doi.org/10.4103/0253-7613.59925.
92. Williams DM, Finan C, Schmidt AF, Burgess S, Hingorani AD. Lipid lowering and Alzheimer disease risk: a mendelian randomization study. Ann Neurol. 2020;87(1):30–9. https://doi.org/10.1002/ana.25642.
93. Mazura AD, Ohler A, Storck SE, Kurtyka M, Scharfenberg F, Weggen S, et al. PCSK9 acts as a key regulator of Aβ clearance across the blood-brain barrier. Cell Mol Life Sci. 2022;79(4):212. https://doi.org/10.1007/s00018-022-04237-x.
94. Wolters FJ, Ikram MA. Epidemiology of vascular dementia. Arterioscler Thromb Vasc Biol. 2019;39(8):1542–9. https://doi.org/10.1161/ATVBAHA.119.311908.
95. Battle CE, Abdul-Rahim AH, Shenkin SD, Hewitt J, Quinn TJ. Cholinesterase inhibitors for vascular dementia and other vascular cognitive impairments: a network meta-analysis. Cochrane Database Syst Rev. 2021;2(2):Cd013306. https://doi.org/10.1002/14651858.CD013306.pub2.
96. Orgogozo JM, Rigaud AS, Stöffler A, Möbius HJ, Forette F. Efficacy and safety of memantine in patients with mild to moderate vascular dementia: a randomized, placebo-controlled trial (MMM 300). Stroke. 2002;33(7):1834–9. https://doi.org/10.1161/01.str.0000020094.08790.49.
97. Möbius HJ, Stöffler A. Memantine in vascular dementia. Int Psychogeriatr. 2003;15(Suppl 1):207–13. https://doi.org/10.1017/s1041610203009219.
98. Wilcock G, Möbius HJ, Stöffler A. A double-blind, placebo-controlled multicentre study of memantine in mild to moderate vascular dementia (MMM500). Int Clin Psychopharmacol. 2002;17(6):297–305. https://doi.org/10.1097/00004850-200211000-00005.

99. Möbius HJ, Stöffler A. New approaches to clinical trials in vascular dementia: memantine in small vessel disease. Cerebrovasc Dis. 2002;13(Suppl. 2):61–6. https://doi.org/10.1159/000049153.
100. Ryan J, Storey E, Murray AM, Woods RL, Wolfe R, Reid CM, et al. Randomized placebo-controlled trial of the effects of aspirin on dementia and cognitive decline. Neurology. 2020;95(3):e320–e31. https://doi.org/10.1212/wnl.0000000000009277.
101. Tai SY, Chien CY, Chang YH, Yang YH. Cilostazol use is associated with reduced risk of dementia: a Nationwide Cohort Study. Neurotherapeutics. 2017;14(3):784–91. https://doi.org/10.1007/s13311-017-0512-4.
102. Taguchi A, Takata Y, Ihara M, Kasahara Y, Tsuji M, Nishino M, et al. Cilostazol improves cognitive function in patients with mild cognitive impairment: a retrospective analysis. Psychogeriatrics. 2013;13(3):164–9. https://doi.org/10.1111/psyg.12021.
103. Senda J, Ito K, Kotake T, Kanamori M, Kishimoto H, Kadono I, et al. Cilostazol use is associated with FIM cognitive improvement during convalescent rehabilitation in patients with ischemic stroke: a retrospective study. Nagoya J Med Sci. 2019;81(3):359–73. https://doi.org/10.18999/nagjms.81.3.359.
104. Lim JS, Kwon SU, Yu KH, Yu S, Park JH, Lee BC, et al. Cilostazol and Probucol for cognitive decline after stroke: a cognitive outcome substudy of the PICASSO trial. J Stroke. 2021;23(1):128–31. https://doi.org/10.5853/jos.2020.03650.
105. Zongfang Z, Wenjing L, Zhaomin C, Lei Z. Therapeutic effect of piracetam with nimodipine on vascular dementia after cerebral infarction. Pak J Pharm Sci. 2020;33(5(Special)):2405–11.
106. Zheng L, Jia J, Chen Y, Liu R, Cao R, Duan M, et al. Pentoxifylline alleviates ischemic white matter injury through up-regulating Mertk-mediated myelin clearance. J Neuroinflammation. 2022;19(1):128. https://doi.org/10.1186/s12974-022-02480-4.
107. Sha MC, Callahan CM. The efficacy of pentoxifylline in the treatment of vascular dementia: a systematic review. Alzheimer Dis Assoc Disord. 2003;17(1):46.
108. Zhan M, Sun L, Liu J, Zeng Z, Shen W, Li H, et al. EGb in the treatment for patients with VCI: a systematic review and meta-analysis. Oxid Med Cell Longev. 2021;2021:8787684. https://doi.org/10.1155/2021/8787684.
109. Cui S, Chen N, Yang M, Guo J, Zhou M, Zhu C, et al. Cerebrolysin for vascular dementia. Cochrane Database Syst Rev. 2019;2019(11) https://doi.org/10.1002/14651858.CD008900.pub3.
110. Hainsworth AH, Elahi FM, Corriveau RA. An introduction to therapeutic approaches to vascular cognitive impairment. Cereb Circ Cogn Behav. 2021;2:100033. https://doi.org/10.1016/j.cccb.2021.100033.
111. Wang HF, Yu JT, Tang SW, Jiang T, Tan CC, Meng XF, et al. Efficacy and safety of cholinesterase inhibitors and memantine in cognitive impairment in Parkinson's disease, Parkinson's disease dementia, and dementia with Lewy bodies: systematic review with meta-analysis and trial sequential analysis. J Neurol Neurosurg Psychiatry. 2015;86(2):135–43. https://doi.org/10.1136/jnnp-2014-307659.
112. Stinton C, McKeith I, Taylor JP, Lafortune L, Mioshi E, Mak E, et al. Pharmacological management of Lewy body dementia: a systematic review and meta-analysis. Am J Psychiatry. 2015;172(8):731–42. https://doi.org/10.1176/appi.ajp.2015.14121582.
113. Mori E, Ikeda M, Kosaka K, Donepezil DLBSI. Donepezil for dementia with Lewy bodies: a randomized, placebo-controlled trial. Ann Neurol. 2012;72(1):41–52. https://doi.org/10.1002/ana.23557.
114. McKeith I, Del Ser T, Spano P, Emre M, Wesnes K, Anand R, et al. Efficacy of rivastigmine in dementia with Lewy bodies: a randomised, double-blind, placebo-controlled international study. Lancet. 2000;356(9247):2031–6. https://doi.org/10.1016/s0140-6736(00)03399-7.
115. Edwards K, Royall D, Hershey L, Lichter D, Hake A, Farlow M, et al. Efficacy and safety of galantamine in patients with dementia with Lewy bodies: a 24-week open-label study. Dement Geriatr Cogn Disord. 2007;23(6):401–5. https://doi.org/10.1159/000101512.
116. Mori E, Ikeda M, Ohdake M. Donepezil for dementia with Lewy bodies: meta-analysis of multicentre, randomised, double-blind, placebo-controlled phase II, III, and, IV studies. Psychogeriatrics. 2024;24(3):589–96. https://doi.org/10.1111/psyg.13101.

117. Tan ECK, Johnell K, Bell JS, Garcia-Ptacek S, Fastbom J, Nordstrom P, et al. Do acetylcholinesterase inhibitors prevent or delay psychotropic prescribing in people with dementia? Analyses of the Swedish dementia registry. Am J Geriatr Psychiatry. 2020;28(1):108–17. https://doi.org/10.1016/j.jagp.2019.06.008.
118. Ikeda M, Mori E, Matsuo K, Nakagawa M, Kosaka K. Donepezil for dementia with Lewy bodies: a randomized, placebo-controlled, confirmatory phase III trial. Alzheimer's Res Ther. 2015;7(1):4. https://doi.org/10.1186/s13195-014-0083-0.
119. Mori E, Ikeda M, Nagai R, Matsuo K, Nakagawa M, Kosaka K. Long-term donepezil use for dementia with Lewy bodies: results from an open-label extension of phase III trial. Alzheimer's Res Ther. 2015;7(1):5. https://doi.org/10.1186/s13195-014-0081-2.
120. Mori E, Ikeda M, Nakagawa M, Miyagishi H, Kosaka K. Pretreatment cognitive profile likely to benefit from donepezil treatment in dementia with Lewy bodies: pooled analyses of two randomized controlled trials. Dement Geriatr Cogn Disord. 2016;42(1–2):58–68. https://doi.org/10.1159/000447586.
121. Sabbagh MN, Hake AM, Ahmed S, Farlow MR. The use of memantine in dementia with Lewy bodies. J Alzheimer's Dis. 2005;7(4):285–9. https://doi.org/10.3233/jad-2005-7403.
122. Lapid MI, Kuntz KM, Mason SS, Aakre JA, Lundt ES, Kremers W, et al. Efficacy, safety, and tolerability of armodafinil therapy for hypersomnia associated with dementia with Lewy bodies: a pilot study. Dement Geriatr Cogn Disord. 2017;43(5–6):269–80. https://doi.org/10.1159/000471507.
123. Wisor JP, Nishino S, Sora I, Uhl GH, Mignot E, Edgar DM. Dopaminergic role in stimulant-induced wakefulness. J Neurosci. 2001;21(5):1787–94. https://doi.org/10.1523/JNEUROSCI.21-05-01787.2001.
124. Tariot P, Foff EP, Cummings JL, Soto-Martin ME, McEvoy B, Stankovic S. Erratum to: HARMONY study: pimavanserin significantly prolongs time to relapse of dementia-related psychosis. Innov Aging. 2021;5(2):igab011. https://doi.org/10.1093/geroni/igab011.
125. Tariot P. HARMONY study: pimavanserin significantly prolongs time to relapse of dementia-related psychosis. Innov Aging. 2020;4(Suppl 1):163–4.
126. Odawara T, Hasegawa K, Kajiwara R, Takeuchi H, Tagawa M, Kosaka K, et al. Long-term efficacy and safety of Zonisamide for treatment of parkinsonism in patients with dementia with Lewy bodies: an open-label extension of a phase three randomized controlled trial. Am J Geriatr Psychiatry. 2022;30(3):314–28. https://doi.org/10.1016/j.jagp.2021.07.002.
127. Biglan K, Munsie L, Svensson KA, Ardayfio P, Pugh M, Sims J, et al. Safety and efficacy of Mevidalen in Lewy body dementia: a phase 2, randomized, placebo-controlled trial. Mov Disord. 2022;37(3):513–24. https://doi.org/10.1002/mds.28879.
128. Goddard TR, Brookes KJ, Sharma R, Moemeni A, Rajkumar AP. Dementia with Lewy bodies: genomics, transcriptomics, and its future with data science. Cells. 2024;13(3) https://doi.org/10.3390/cells13030223.
129. Kim TE, Newman AJ, Imberdis T, Brontesi L, Tripathi A, Ramalingam N, et al. Excess membrane binding of monomeric alpha-, beta- and gamma-synuclein is invariably associated with inclusion formation and toxicity. Hum Mol Genet. 2021;30(23):2332–46. https://doi.org/10.1093/hmg/ddab188.
130. Barba L, Paolini Paoletti F, Bellomo G, Gaetani L, Halbgebauer S, Oeckl P, et al. Alpha and Beta Synucleins: from pathophysiology to clinical application as biomarkers. Mov Disord. 2022;37(4):669–83. https://doi.org/10.1002/mds.28941.
131. Sanghvi H, Singh R, Morrin H, Rajkumar AP. Systematic review of genetic association studies in people with Lewy body dementia. Int J Geriatr Psychiatry. 2020;35(5):436–48. https://doi.org/10.1002/gps.5260.
132. Ning S, Jorfi M, Patel SR, Kim DY, Tanzi RE. Neurotechnological approaches to the diagnosis and treatment of Alzheimer's disease. Front Neurosci. 2022;16:854992. https://doi.org/10.3389/fnins.2022.854992.
133. Vogt AS, Jennings GT, Mohsen MO, Vogel M, Bachmann MF. Alzheimer's disease: a brief history of immunotherapies targeting amyloid beta. Int J Mol Sci. 2023;24(4) https://doi.org/10.3390/ijms24043895.

134. Xiao S, Chan P, Wang T, Hong Z, Wang S, Kuang W, et al. A 36-week multicenter, randomized, double-blind, placebo-controlled, parallel-group, phase 3 clinical trial of sodium oligomannate for mild-to-moderate Alzheimer's dementia. Alzheimers Res Ther. 2021;13(1):62. https://doi.org/10.1186/s13195-021-00795-7.
135. Patel B, Irwin DJ, Kaufer D, Boeve BF, Taylor A, Armstrong MJ. Outcome measures for dementia with Lewy body clinical trials: a review. Alzheimer Dis Assoc Disord. 2022;36(1):64–72. https://doi.org/10.1097/WAD.0000000000000473.
136. Agarwal K, Backler W, Bayram E, Bloom L, Boeve BF, Cha JH, et al. Lewy body dementia: overcoming barriers and identifying solutions. Alzheimers Dement. 2024;20(3):2298–308. https://doi.org/10.1002/alz.13674.
137. Baik K, Cha J, Park M, Lee Y, Chung SJ, Yoo HS, et al. Distinct amyloid-dependent patterns of nigra dopamine depletion in Lewy body diseases. Front Aging Neurosci. 2023;15:1196602. https://doi.org/10.3389/fnagi.2023.1196602.
138. Murley AG, Rowe JB. Neurotransmitter deficits from frontotemporal lobar degeneration. Brain. 2018;141(5):1263–85. https://doi.org/10.1093/brain/awx327.
139. Magrath Guimet N, Zapata-Restrepo LM, Miller BL. Advances in treatment of frontotemporal dementia. J Neuropsychiatry Clin Neurosci. 2022;34(4):316–27. https://doi.org/10.1176/appi.neuropsych.21060166.
140. Wilson KM, Katona E, Glaria I, Carcole M, Swift IJ, Sogorb-Esteve A, et al. Development of a sensitive trial-ready poly(GP) CSF biomarker assay for C9orf72-associated frontotemporal dementia and amyotrophic lateral sclerosis. J Neurol Neurosurg Psychiatry. 2022;93(7):761–71. https://doi.org/10.1136/jnnp-2021-328710.
141. Che XQ, Song N, Gao Y, Ren RJ, Wang G. Precision medicine of frontotemporal dementia: from genotype to phenotype. Front Biosci (Landmark Ed). 2018;23(6):1144–65. https://doi.org/10.2741/4637.
142. Silva MC, Haggarty SJ. Tauopathies: deciphering disease mechanisms to develop effective therapies. Int J Mol Sci. 2020;21(23) https://doi.org/10.3390/ijms21238948.
143. Ward M, Carter LP, Huang JY, Maslyar D, Budda B, Paul R, et al. Phase 1 study of latozinemab in progranulin-associated frontotemporal dementia. Alzheimers Dement (N Y). 2024;10(1):e12452. https://doi.org/10.1002/trc2.12452.
144. Kurnellas M, Mitra A, Schwabe T, Paul R, Arrant AE, Roberson ED, et al. Latozinemab, a novel progranulin-elevating therapy for frontotemporal dementia. J Transl Med. 2023;21(1):387. https://doi.org/10.1186/s12967-023-04251-y.

# Chapter 10
# Digital Medicines for the Management of Dementia with Its Related Disorder

**Yuan-Han Yang**

**Abstract** The increasing prevalence of dementia and its related disorders poses significant challenges for healthcare systems worldwide. Digital medicines, encompassing mobile health applications, wearable devices, artificial intelligence (AI)-driven diagnostics, telemedicine, and electronic health monitoring systems, offer innovative solutions for dementia management. These technologies enable early detection, personalized treatment, remote patient monitoring, and improved caregiver support. AI and machine learning algorithms enhance diagnostic accuracy by analyzing behavioral and cognitive patterns, while digital therapeutics provide cognitive training and behavioral interventions. Telemedicine facilitates access to specialist care, reducing the burden on patients and caregivers. Despite their potential, challenges such as data privacy, user accessibility, and regulatory compliance remain. This chapter will illustrate how to develop the AI model from clinical data, and explore the current landscape of digital medicines in dementia care and highlighting their benefits, limitations, and future directions for integration into clinical practice.

**Keywords** Digital medicine · Dementia management · Artificial intelligence · Telemedicine · Wearable devices · Cognition · Behavior

## 10.1 Introduction

In the face of the escalating burden of dementia on individuals, families, and healthcare systems worldwide, the advent of digital medicines presents a promising paradigm shift in the management of this complex condition. Digital medicines encompass a diverse range of technological innovations, spanning from mobile applications to wearable devices and telemedicine platforms. These tools are

---

Y.-H. Yang (✉)
Neuroscience Research Center, Kaohsiung Medical University, Kaohsiung, Taiwan
e-mail: endless@kmu.edu.tw



Y.-H. Yang (ed.), *Management of Dementia from the Preclinical Stage*,
https://doi.org/10.1007/978-981-95-5222-1_10

strategically designed to enhance various facets of dementia care, including diagnosis, monitoring, treatment, and support for patients and caregivers.

As the digital health landscape continues to evolve, the potential of these interventions to revolutionize dementia care becomes increasingly apparent. However, to fully harness this potential, ongoing research, collaboration, and integration into routine clinical practice are essential. For instance, one seminal study by Batsis et al. [1] delves into the emerging approaches in digital health for patients with dementia, shedding light on caregiver support and addressing neuropsychiatric symptoms. How to apply digital medicine scientifically and practically in dementia practice is becoming an important issue.

## 10.2 Digital Medicine

Digital medicine refers to the use of technology, particularly digital technologies like software, mobile apps, wearable devices, and sensors, to monitor, diagnose, treat, and manage medical conditions. It encompasses a wide range of applications aimed at improving healthcare delivery, patient outcomes, and the overall healthcare experience [2].

Here are some proposed examples of digital medicine:

- Remote Monitoring the Biomarkers: Digital tools enable the remote monitoring of patients' health parameters, such as heart rate, blood pressure, glucose levels, and activity levels [3]. This allows healthcare providers to track patients' progress and intervene as needed without requiring frequent in-person visits.
- Telemedicine: Telemedicine involves the use of digital communication technologies, such as video conferencing and messaging platforms, to provide healthcare services remotely [4]. It allows patients to consult with healthcare providers from the comfort of their homes, increasing access to care, especially for individuals in rural or underserved areas.
- Wearable Devices: Wearable devices, such as smartwatches, fitness trackers, and biosensors, can collect real-time health data and provide insights into patients' health and behavior patterns [2]. These devices can be used to monitor physical activity, sleep quality, heart rate variability, and even detect abnormalities or early signs of medical conditions.
- Digital Intervention: Digital therapeutics are software-based interventions designed to prevent, manage, or treat medical conditions [3]. They may include cognitive behavioral therapy programs for mental health disorders, digital platforms for chronic disease management, mobile apps for smoking cessation or weight loss, and physical intervention, light or sound, for mental health.
- Healthcare Apps: There is a growing number of mobile applications designed to support various aspects of healthcare [4]. These apps empower individuals to take a more active role in managing their health and well-being, including medication adherence, symptom tracking, health education, and lifestyle management.

- Artificial Intelligence (AI) and Machine Learning: AI and machine learning algorithms can analyze large datasets, including medical images, genomic data, and electronic health records, to identify patterns, predict outcomes, and assist healthcare providers in clinical decision-making [2].

## 10.3 Effectiveness of Digital Medicine

Overall, digital medicine holds the potential to revolutionize healthcare by making it more personalized, accessible, and efficient. However, it also raises important considerations related to data privacy, security, regulatory oversight, and equitable access to technology.

Digital medicine holds promise in enhancing dementia care through innovative interventions tailored to address cognitive, functional, and behavioral symptoms associated with the condition. Recent studies have highlighted the potential efficacy of digital interventions in dementia management, including cognitive training programs, virtual reality therapies, and telehealth services.

Research by Smith et al. [5] demonstrated the effectiveness of a smartphone-based cognitive training app in improving cognitive function and quality of life in individuals with mild cognitive impairment and early-stage dementia. The study found that participants who engaged with the app regularly showed significant improvements in memory, attention, and executive function compared to those in the control group.

Furthermore, virtual reality (VR) interventions have shown promise in alleviating behavioral and psychological symptoms of dementia (BPSD) and enhancing overall well-being in individuals with dementia. A meta-analysis by Jones et al. [6] revealed that VR-based interventions were associated with significant reductions in agitation, aggression, and anxiety among dementia patients, suggesting the potential of immersive technologies in managing BPSD.

Additionally, telehealth platforms have emerged as valuable tools for delivering remote dementia care and support services to individuals living in underserved areas or home settings. A systematic review by Brown et al. [7] highlighted the feasibility and acceptability of telehealth interventions in providing dementia assessments, caregiver support, and counseling services, indicating their potential to enhance access to dementia care and improve caregiver outcomes.

These findings underscore the promising role of digital medicine in supplementing traditional dementia care approaches and addressing unmet needs in dementia management. However, further research is needed to establish the long-term efficacy, cost-effectiveness, and scalability of digital interventions in real-world clinical settings.

## 10.4 Steps of Applying Artifical Intelligence in Dementia Outcomes

### 10.4.1 Getting Data Collection and Preprocessing

Gather diverse data sources, including electronic health records (EHR), imaging data, genetic data, and lifestyle information through digital measurement technologies. Clean and preprocess the data to handle missing values, normalize features, and create relevant input features for the model [8]. Digital measurement technologies can provide continuous, real-time data, enhancing traditional diagnostic methods, collecting data, and enabling proactive care, including:

- *Wearable Devices*: Devices such as smartwatches and fitness trackers can monitor physical activity, sleep patterns, heart rate variability, and other physiological parameters. These metrics can provide insights into the overall health and well-being of individuals with dementia.
- *Smartphone Applications*: Mobile apps can assess cognitive functions through gamified tasks and questionnaires, monitor daily activities, and track mood and behavior changes. These applications offer a user-friendly interface for both patients and caregivers.
- *Telehealth Platforms*: Telehealth services enable remote consultations with healthcare professionals, allowing for regular check-ins and adjustments to care plans based on real-time data.
- *Home Sensors*: In-home sensors can track movement patterns, detect falls, and monitor daily activities, providing valuable information on the patient's functional status and safety.

Digital measurement technologies generate vast amounts of data from various sources as mentioned above to sophisticated analysis. Data collected from these devices can include:

- *Physical Activity Data*: Monitoring steps taken, distance walked, and overall physical activity levels can help assess mobility and detect early signs of decline.
- *Sleep Data*: Tracking sleep patterns and disturbances can provide information on sleep quality and potential issues related to dementia.
- *Cognitive Data*: Cognitive assessment through apps can help identify early cognitive impairment and track changes over time.
- *Behavioral Data*: Monitoring mood, social interactions, and daily routines can offer insights into behavioral changes associated with dementia.

### 10.4.2 Feature Selection and Engineering

- Identify key features relevant to dementia risk, such as age, genetic markers, cognitive test results, and comorbidities.
- Engineer new features that might improve model performance, such as interaction terms or composite scores [9].

### 10.4.3 Model Selection

Machine learning algorithms and artificial intelligence (AI) techniques are often employed to analyze this data. These methods can identify patterns and correlations that may not be apparent through traditional analysis, enhancing the predictive power of digital measurements. Choose appropriate machine learning models for risk prediction, such as logistic regression, random forests, support vector machines, or deep learning models [10].

### 10.4.4 Model Training

Train the selected models using the preprocessed and feature-engineered dataset. Implement cross-validation to tune hyperparameters and avoid overfitting [11].

### 10.4.5 Model Evaluation

- Evaluate model performance using metrics such as accuracy, precision, recall, F1-score, and area under the receiver operating characteristic (ROC) curve.
- Perform external validation with independent datasets to assess generalizability [12].

### 10.4.6 Model Interpretation and Explainability

Use techniques like SHAP (SHapley Additive exPlanations) values or LIME (Local Interpretable Model-agnostic Explanations) to interpret model predictions and ensure transparency [13].

### 10.4.7 Deployment and Integration

- Deploy the trained model into a digital health platform for real-time risk prediction.
- Ensure seamless integration with existing healthcare systems and workflows [14].

### 10.4.8 Monitoring and Maintenance

- Continuously monitor model performance in the real world and update the model as new data becomes available.
- Implement mechanisms for feedback and retraining to maintain accuracy over time [15].

## 10.5 Challenges and Considerations for Applying an AI Model for Dementia Risk Prediction

The integration of digital measurement technologies in dementia care offers several advantages:

- *Early Detection*: Continuous monitoring allows for the early identification of subtle changes in behavior, cognition, and physical health, facilitating early intervention.
- *Personalized Care*: Data-driven insights enable the customization of care plans to meet individual needs, improving the effectiveness of interventions.
- *Remote Monitoring*: Digital tools enable remote monitoring, reducing the need for frequent in-person visits and allowing for care in the comfort of the patient's home.
- *Engagement and Adherence*: Interactive and user-friendly digital tools can improve patient and caregiver engagement, leading to better adherence to care plans.

However, the implementation of digital measurement technologies in dementia care faces several challenges:

- *Data Privacy and Security*: Ensuring the privacy and security of sensitive health data is paramount. Robust data protection measures must be in place to safeguard patient information.
- *Technology Accessibility*: Access to digital tools and the internet can be limited, particularly for older adults or those in rural areas. Efforts must be made to bridge the digital divide.

- *User Training and Support*: Patients and caregivers may require training and ongoing support to effectively use digital measurement technologies. User-friendly designs and comprehensive support systems are essential.
- *Regulatory and Ethical Issues*: The use of digital health tools must comply with regulatory standards and ethical guidelines to ensure patient safety and the responsible use of data.

## 10.6 Application of the AI Model in the Diagnosis and Detection of Dementia

The diagnosis of dementia can be made from clinical information referring to a series of comprehensive examinations and neuropsychological evaluations, traditionally. However, these traditional pencil-paper data should be digitized for computing. Recently, digital data provided a huge, selected or nonselected information to assist in the establishment of a diagnosis of dementia. However, some points should be highly stressed and evaluated. It's essential to ensure that these technologies are validated, user-friendly, and ethically implemented to maximize their benefits for patients and caregivers.

*The digital data includes, but not limits data from a single or combinative dataset.*

### *10.6.1 Single Dataset*

- Cognitive Screening Apps: Mobile applications designed for cognitive screening can be used to assess various cognitive domains, including memory, attention, language, and executive function. These apps often include validated neuropsychological tests and questionnaires that can be completed remotely, allowing for early detection of cognitive impairment.
- Wearable Devices: Wearable devices equipped with sensors can monitor changes in gait, balance, and daily activity patterns, which may serve as early indicators of cognitive decline or dementia. By continuously tracking movement and behavior, these devices can provide objective data for clinicians to assess cognitive function over time.
- Digital Biomarkers: Digital biomarkers, such as typing patterns, voice characteristics, and smartphone usage patterns, have shown promise in detecting subtle changes associated with cognitive impairment. Machine learning algorithms can analyze these data to identify patterns indicative of dementia, offering a noninvasive and cost-effective diagnostic tool.
- Neuroimaging Technologies: Advanced neuroimaging techniques, such as magnetic resonance imaging (MRI) and positron emission tomography (PET), can be enhanced with digital medicine approaches to improve the accuracy of dementia

diagnosis. Machine learning algorithms can analyze neuroimaging data to detect structural and functional changes in the brain associated with dementia pathology.
- Telemedicine and Remote Monitoring: Telemedicine platforms enable remote consultations and assessments, allowing individuals with dementia to receive timely care from healthcare providers without the need for in-person visits. Remote monitoring technologies, such as video conferencing, remote cognitive testing, and sensor-based monitoring systems, facilitate ongoing assessment and management of dementia symptoms from the comfort of home.
- Digital Pathology: Digital pathology platforms enable the digitization and analysis of histopathological samples, such as brain tissue biopsies, to identify pathological changes associated with different types of dementia. These platforms leverage artificial intelligence algorithms to analyze digital slides and assist pathologists in diagnosing dementia accurately.
- Big Data Analytics: Integration of large-scale datasets, including electronic health records, genetic data, imaging studies, and digital biomarkers, can facilitate comprehensive analysis and interpretation of dementia-related factors. Big data analytics techniques can identify novel risk factors, biomarkers, and therapeutic targets for dementia diagnosis and management.

## *10.6.2 Combinative Dataset*

Combination of digital measurements together with clinical data as a predictive algorithm has become a useful manner in dementia management. Following are illustrations.

### 10.6.2.1 Analyzing Facial Asymmetry in Alzheimer's Dementia Using Image-Based Technology

#### 10.6.2.1.1 Facial Asymmetry and Alzheimer's Dementia (AD)

Facial asymmetry refers to the differences between the left and right sides of the face. In healthy individuals, these differences are minimal. However, neurodegenerative disorders, including AD, can exacerbate facial asymmetry due to the loss of motor control and muscle atrophy associated with the disease [16]. The analysis of facial asymmetry involves measuring various facial landmarks and comparing their positions to detect deviations from symmetry.

Studies have shown that individuals with AD exhibit greater facial asymmetry compared to healthy controls. This asymmetry is often more pronounced in regions controlled by the cranial nerves, such as the eyes and mouth [17]. Image-based technology has demonstrated high sensitivity and specificity in detecting these asymmetries, suggesting its potential as a noninvasive biomarker for AD [17]. This study developed new facial asymmetry measures to compare AD with healthy controls through a three-dimensional camera to capture facial images, and 68 identified facial landmarks. Finally, researchers have found that the asymmetry of 20 of 68 identified landmarks was significantly different in AD than in the non-AD controls ($p < 0.05$).

The use of image-based technology for analyzing facial asymmetry offers several advantages:

- Noninvasive: Unlike traditional imaging methods, facial asymmetry analysis does not require exposure to radiation or contrast agents.
- Cost-Effective: Digital cameras and software for facial analysis are relatively inexpensive compared to Magnetic Resonance Imaging (MRI) and Positron Emission Topography (PET) scans.
- Accessibility: This technology can be easily deployed in various healthcare settings, including remote and underserved areas.

Further research is needed to refine the algorithms used for facial landmark detection and symmetry analysis. Large-scale studies are required to validate the efficacy of this approach across diverse populations and stages of AD. Additionally, integrating facial asymmetry analysis with other biomarkers, such as genetic and cerebrospinal fluid markers, could enhance diagnostic accuracy and provide a more comprehensive understanding of disease progression [17].

#### 10.6.2.2 Association Between Kinetic Joints Position Correlation and Alzheimer's Dementia

##### 10.6.2.2.1 Cerebral Coordination Functions in AD

Cerebral coordination refers to the synchronized activity and connectivity between different brain regions. Effective coordination is essential for cognitive functions such as memory, attention, and executive function. In AD, disruptions in these coordination mechanisms are believed to contribute to the clinical symptoms observed in patients [18]. The cerebral coordination also includes the control of the motor and nonmotor systems. The control of the motor system and coordination system of all joints to present as kinetic performance is mainly localized in the cerebral cortex, which will be influenced through the amyloid deposition process [18]. Kinetic joint position refers to the movement and orientation of joints in the body during motion, which can be critical in assessing motor function. In the context of dementia, especially in AD, there is growing interest in how joint position and movement are affected, as motor impairments often accompany cognitive decline.

- *Gait and Posture Changes in Dementia*: Dementia, particularly in the later stages, can lead to alterations in gait and posture. This includes a reduction in step length, stride, and changes in joint angles during walking. These changes can be early indicators of cognitive decline.

- *Correlation Among Joints to Cognition*: Studies like the one by Yang et al. [18] emphasize the correlations among 15 selected joints' analysis in position and other related signals, with reference to clinical and neuropsychological assessments. Their study has revealed that the use of a kinetic depth sensor to determine the coordination between joints, especially in lower limbs, can significantly reflect the global functional and cognitive outcomes in AD in which could be another biomarker for AD outcomes [18]. Such linkage to cognitive decline may suggest that kinetic joint position abnormalities may correlate with the severity of cognitive decline. This makes it a potential biomarker for tracking the progression of dementia.

## 10.7 Application of AI in the Diagnosis of Dementia from an Established Cohort

Dementia, particularly AD, represents a significant global health challenge due to its progressive nature and profound impact on cognitive function and quality of life. Accurate and early diagnosis is crucial for effective management and treatment. Establishing a cohort for modeling the diagnosis of dementia is a fundamental step in advancing research, improving diagnostic accuracy, and developing targeted therapies. Establishing a dementia cohort, including defining the study population, setting inclusion and exclusion criteria, selecting data sources, and addressing ethical considerations is crucial and necessary to establish the model for diagnosis. Establishing a cohort for modeling the diagnosis of dementia is a fundamental step in advancing research, improving diagnostic accuracy, and developing targeted therapies. How to develop a model to leverage clinical, imaging, genetic, and biochemical data from the established cohort is crucial to establishing the model for diagnosis.

### *10.7.1 Defining the Study Population*

To ensure the cohort is representative and yields meaningful data, the study population must be clearly defined. This involves specifying the type of dementia under investigation (e.g., Alzheimer's, vascular, Lewy body), the demographic characteristics of interest (e.g., age, gender, ethnicity), and the objectives of the study [19].

### *10.7.2 Inclusion and Exclusion Criteria for a Cohort*

Clear inclusion and exclusion criteria are critical for maintaining the integrity of the cohort and ensuring reliable data. For instance, the inclusion/exclusion criteria could be:

**Inclusion Criteria**

- Confirmed diagnosis of dementia using established clinical criteria (e.g., DSM-5, NINCDS-ADRDA).
- Availability of comprehensive medical records and willingness to participate in follow-up assessments [20].

**Exclusion Criteria**

- Presence of other neurological disorders that could confound the diagnosis.
- Severe psychiatric conditions (e.g., major depression, schizophrenia) that might affect cognitive assessments.
- Incomplete or unreliable medical records to establish the cohort data [21].

### *10.7.3 Selecting Data Sources for Dementia Diagnosis and Clinical Course Tracking*

Multiple data sources are necessary to capture the multifaceted nature of dementia, including clinical, imaging, genetic, and biochemical data.

#### 10.7.3.1 Clinical and Psychological Assessment Data

Collecting detailed medical histories, clinical examination results, and neuropsychological test scores is essential. Standardized diagnostic tools such as the Mini-Mental State Examination (MMSE) or the Montreal Cognitive Assessment (MoCA) should be used [22].

#### 10.7.3.2 Imaging Data

Brain imaging data (e.g., MRI, PET scans) provide insights into structural and functional changes in the brain. Standardized imaging protocols are crucial for consistency and comparability [23].

#### 10.7.3.3 Genetic Data

Genetic information can help identify biomarkers and understand genetic predispositions. Ethical considerations and informed consent are paramount when collecting genetic data [24].

#### 10.7.3.4 Biochemical Data

Biomarkers from blood, cerebrospinal fluid (CSF), and other sources can provide valuable information about disease processes. Standardized methods for sample collection and analysis should be employed [25].

### *10.7.4 Implementing Standardized Protocols When Data Collection*

Consistency in data collection and management is vital for the reliability of the cohort data.

#### 10.7.4.1 Data Collection and Management

Uniform procedures for data collection minimize variability and ensure data quality. Training staff on standardized protocols for clinical assessments, imaging, and biomarker collection is essential [26]. A secure database is necessary for storing and managing data. Data should be anonymized to protect participant confidentiality [27].

#### 10.7.4.2 Ethical Considerations

Adhering to ethical standards ensures the protection of participants and the integrity of the research. The informed consent and approval of the institutional review board (IRB) are always necessary. Participants must provide informed consent, understanding the study's purpose, procedures, risks, and benefits [28]. IRB or ethics committee approval is required to ensure the study meets ethical standards [29].

#### 10.7.4.3 Statistical Considerations

Proper statistical planning ensures the robustness and validity of the study findings, such as sample size and data analysis plan.

An adequate sample size is necessary to ensure statistical power. Power analysis can determine the minimum number of participants needed to detect significant differences [30]. A comprehensive data analysis plan should outline the statistical methods and software to be used, as well as strategies for handling missing data and potential confounders [31].

#### 10.7.4.4 Recruitment Strategies

Effective recruitment strategies ensure the cohort is representative and sufficiently large. Collaborating with clinics, hospitals, and community centers can facilitate participant recruitment. Patient registries and dementia advocacy groups are also valuable resources [32]. Clear and effective communication about the study's purpose, procedures, and potential impact is crucial for successful recruitment [33].

#### 10.7.4.5 Follow-Up and Monitoring

Regular follow-up assessments and quality control measures are necessary for tracking disease progression and maintaining data integrity. Planning for regular follow-up assessments allows for the collection of longitudinal data, providing insights into disease progression [34]. Quality control measures should be implemented to ensure data accuracy and reliability. Regular reviews and audits of data collection processes are recommended [35].

By defining a clear study population, setting rigorous inclusion and exclusion criteria, selecting diverse data sources, and maintaining ethical standards, researchers can create a robust cohort that advances our understanding of dementia and improves diagnostic accuracy.

### *10.7.5 Data Preprocessing*

Before developing the diagnostic model, the collected data must be preprocessed to ensure quality and consistency. This includes cleaning the data, handling missing values, and standardizing the measurements.

#### 10.7.5.1 Data Cleaning

- Identify and Remove Duplicates: Ensure that each participant is uniquely represented.
- Outlier Detection: Identify and handle outliers that could skew the model's results.

#### 10.7.5.2 Handling Missing Values

- Imputation Methods: Use statistical techniques such as mean imputation, regression imputation, or multiple imputation to fill in missing values.
- Sensitivity Analysis: Assess the impact of different imputation methods on the model's performance [36].

#### 10.7.5.3 Standardization

- Normalize Continuous Variables: Scale variables such as age, biomarker levels, and neuropsychological test scores to a common range.
- Encode Categorical Variables: Use one-hot encoding or label encoding for categorical variables like gender and genetic markers [37].

### *10.7.6 Feature Selection*

Feature selection involves identifying the most relevant variables that contribute to the diagnosis of dementia. This step is crucial for improving model performance and interpretability. Several considerations are used to increase the efficacy of feature selection.

#### 10.7.6.1 Univariate Analysis

- Statistical Tests: Perform t-tests, chi-square tests, or ANOVA to identify variables significantly associated with dementia [38].

#### 10.7.6.2 Multivariate Analysis

- Principal Component Analysis (PCA): Reduce dimensionality by identifying principal components that capture the most variance in the data.
- Lasso Regression: Use Lasso (Least Absolute Shrinkage and Selection Operator) to select features that contribute the most to the model by penalizing less important ones [39].

## *10.7.7 Model Development*

### 10.7.7.1 Integration with Multiple Measurements and Biomarkers during Modeling

Multiple measurements and biomarkers provide comprehensive insights into the complex pathology of dementia. Integrating multiple measurements and biomarkers is crucial for several reasons:

- Comprehensive Understanding: Combining different types of data provides a holistic view of dementia, capturing its multifaceted nature and improving diagnostic accuracy [40].
- Early Detection: Early detection of dementia is enhanced by integrating biomarkers with clinical and behavioral measurements, allowing for timely interventions [41].
- Personalized Treatment: Tailoring treatments to individual patients is more effective when based on a comprehensive dataset, leading to better outcomes [42].
- Monitoring Progression: Continuous monitoring of multiple biomarkers and measurements helps track disease progression and the effectiveness of interventions [43].

### 10.7.7.2 Methods of Integration

To integrate multiple measurements and biomarkers effectively, several approaches can be employed:

- Data Fusion Techniques: Combining data from different sources using algorithms that account for the unique characteristics of each data type [44].
- Machine Learning Models: Employing machine learning and AI to identify patterns and correlations across diverse datasets, aiding in diagnosis and prognosis [45].
- Standardized Protocols: Developing standardized protocols for data collection and processing to ensure consistency and reliability across studies [46].
- Interdisciplinary Collaboration: Encouraging collaboration among clinicians, researchers, data scientists, and engineers to develop comprehensive integration methodologies [47].

### 10.7.7.3 Challenges and Solutions

Despite the clear benefits, integrating multiple measurements and biomarkers poses several challenges:

- Data Heterogeneity: The diverse nature of data sources can make integration difficult. Solutions include developing flexible data models and standardized data formats [48].
- Privacy and Security: Ensuring the privacy and security of patient data is paramount. This can be addressed through robust encryption methods and secure data sharing platforms [49].
- Resource Constraints: Integrating multiple data sources requires significant resources. Collaborative funding and support from the government and private sectors can help address this issue [50].
- Validation and Reproducibility: Ensuring that integrated data and resulting models are validated and reproducible is critical. This can be achieved through rigorous testing and open data sharing practices [51].

#### 10.7.7.4 Machine Learning for Algorithms

Several machine learning algorithms can be used to develop a model for dementia. The choice of algorithm depends on the nature of the data and the specific requirements of the study.

- Logistic Regression: A simple and interpretable model suitable for binary classification problems.
- Support Vector Machines (SVM): Effective for high-dimensional data and capable of handling nonlinear relationships.
- Random Forests: An ensemble method that combines multiple decision trees to improve predictive accuracy and robustness.
- Gradient Boosting Machines (GBM): Another ensemble technique that builds models sequentially to correct errors from previous models.
- Neural Networks: Deep learning models that can capture complex patterns in large datasets [52].
- XGBoost (eXtreme Gradient Boosting): Widely used for supervised learning tasks like classification and regression. It is known for its efficiency, accuracy, and scalability, especially on large datasets.

### *10.7.8 Model Training and Evaluation*

Cohort data can be used for training and validation of the model, which can also be followed by model evaluation.

- Training and Validation Split: Divide the cohort data into training and validation sets to evaluate the model's performance.
- Cross-Validation: Use k-fold cross-validation to ensure the model generalizes well to unseen data.

#### 10.7.8.1 Model Evaluation: The Performance

Evaluating the model's performance is crucial to ensure its reliability and effectiveness in diagnosing dementia. Frequently used performance metrics include:

- *Accuracy*: The proportion of correctly classified cases.
- *Sensitivity (Recall)*: The model's ability to correctly identify dementia cases.
- *Specificity*: The model's ability to correctly identify nondementia cases.
- *Precision*: The proportion of true positive cases among the predicted positives.
- *F1 Score*: The harmonic mean of precision and recall, providing a balance between the two.
- *Area Under the Receiver Operating Characteristic Curve (AUC-ROC)*: A measure of the model's ability to distinguish between dementia and nondementia cases [53].

### *10.7.9 Validation and Testing*

After evaluating the model on the validation set, it is important to test it on an independent test set to assess its generalizability.

#### 10.7.9.1 External Validation and Testing

- *Independent Cohorts*: Test the model on data from other cohorts to ensure its applicability across different populations.
- *Prospective Validation*: Use longitudinal data to validate the model's predictive performance over time.

### *10.7.10 Implementation*

Once validated, the model can be implemented in clinical settings to assist healthcare professionals in diagnosing dementia.

From a clinical point of view, integrating multiple measurements and biomarkers is essential for advancing digital medicine in dementia care. Developing a model for the diagnosis of dementia from an established cohort involves meticulous data preprocessing, feature selection, model training, and validation. By leveraging advanced machine learning techniques and diverse data sources, researchers can create a robust diagnostic tool that enhances early detection and improves patient outcomes. Through the aid of digital medicine to have a comprehensive understanding of the disease, enhancing early detection, enabling personalized treatment, and monitoring progression, this approach significantly improves dementia management.

Overcoming the challenges of data heterogeneity, privacy, resource constraints, and validation requires collaborative efforts and innovative solutions. As the field progresses, the integration of diverse data sources will continue to play a pivotal role in transforming dementia care and improving patient outcomes.

## 10.8 Digital Intervention for Dementia

### *10.8.1 Gamma Frequency Oscillation in Dementia Management*

Gamma frequency oscillations, typically ranging from 30 to 100 Hz, play a crucial role in cognitive processing, including perception, attention, memory, and learning [54]. In dementia, disruptions in gamma oscillations have been observed, reflecting underlying neuronal dysfunction and cognitive impairment.

Research suggests that alterations in gamma oscillations may serve as biomarkers of cognitive decline and dementia progression [55]. For instance, studies using electroencephalography (EEG) and magnetoencephalography (MEG) have demonstrated reduced gamma power and coherence in individuals with AD compared to healthy controls [56]. These alterations are particularly prominent in brain regions associated with memory and executive function, such as the hippocampus and prefrontal cortex.

Moreover, dysfunctional gamma oscillations have been implicated in the pathophysiology of other types of dementia, including frontotemporal dementia (FTD) and dementia with Lewy bodies (DLB) [57]. In FTD, aberrant gamma activity has been linked to changes in social cognition and behavioral disturbances, whereas in DLB, it may contribute to visual hallucinations and cognitive fluctuations.

Preclinical studies have provided insights into the potential therapeutic effects of gamma frequency oscillations in dementia. For example, a study by Yuan-Han Yang et al. [58] investigated the impact of gamma frequency stimulation on amyloid secretion using cell line models. Their findings suggest that gamma frequency oscillations inhibit the secretion of amyloid, providing a potential mechanism for modulating amyloid pathology in dementia [59].

Understanding the role of gamma frequency oscillations in dementia pathophysiology and exploring their therapeutic potential may lead to the development of novel interventions aimed at improving cognitive function and quality of life in affected individuals.

The precise mechanisms underlying gamma oscillation alterations in dementia remain incompletely understood but likely involve synaptic dysfunction, neuronal loss, and aberrant network connectivity [60]. Therapeutic strategies targeting gamma oscillations, such as noninvasive brain stimulation techniques like transcranial magnetic stimulation (TMS) or gamma entrainment using auditory or visual stimulation, hold promise for mitigating cognitive symptoms in dementia.

Recently, the basic cell line studies [59, 61] have indicated the secretion of Amyloid beta, phosphorylation of AKT, mTOR, and tau, and aggregation of Amyloid beta4 was significantly inhibited by light with 40 Hz frequency in SH-SY5Y cells. Furthermore, the decrease in neuroinflammatory markers supports the hypothesis that gamma frequency stimulation might have a modulatory effect on inflammatory processes in AD. Importantly, a clinical nonrandomized study to evaluate the potential effects of 40 Hz light intervention in AD patients has revealed the cases, receiving the intervention of 40 Hz light had significant improvements in neuro-psychiatric syndrome assessed using the Neuropsychiatric inventory (NPI) ($p = 0.02$), especially depression and euphoria symptoms ($p = 0.04$ and $<0.01$, respectively) and less caregiver burden (Zarit Burden Interview; ZBI score, $p < 0.01$). In global function, the control group showed a significant decline in Clinical Dementia Rating; CDR-SB score ($p < 0.01$), while the cases did not [58].

### *10.8.2 Application of Virtual Reality in Dementia*

Virtual reality (VR) is an emerging tool in dementia care, offering innovative ways to engage patients, assess cognitive and motor functions, and provide therapeutic experiences. Here's how VR is being used in dementia management in several aspects.

#### 10.8.2.1 Cognitive Assessment and Screening

Virtual Reality Environments: VR can create controlled, immersive environments where cognitive functions can be tested. Patients might navigate virtual spaces or perform tasks that assess memory, attention, and executive function [62].

Personalized Assessment and Cognitive Rehabilitation: VR allows for the customization of scenarios based on the patient's background, making cognitive assessments more engaging and potentially more accurate [63].

#### 10.8.2.2 Therapeutic Applications Present Several Aspects

- Reminiscence Therapy: VR can recreate familiar environments or past experiences, helping patients with dementia recall memories and reduce anxiety or agitation. This form of therapy can be tailored to individual preferences, enhancing emotional well-being [64].
- Physical Therapy: Virtual environments can encourage physical activity through games or simulations, promoting motor function and physical health. This can also be part of a dual-task approach, where cognitive tasks are combined with movement [65].

- Social Interaction: VR can facilitate social interactions by connecting patients with their family members or other patients in virtual settings, combating loneliness and social isolation [66].
- Behavioral and Psychological Symptoms Management.
- Anxiety and Agitation Reduction: VR experiences can be calming, offering patients serene environments or guided meditation, helping to manage anxiety, agitation, and depression, which are common in dementia [67].

#### 10.8.2.3 Caregiver Support

Training and Education: VR can be used to train caregivers, helping them understand the experiences of dementia patients and learn effective care techniques [68].

Stress Reduction: Caregivers can also use VR for relaxation and stress relief, improving their overall well-being [68].

#### 10.8.2.4 Research and Development

Studying Disease Progression: VR offers researchers a controlled environment to study how dementia affects cognitive and motor functions over time, potentially leading to new insights and interventions [69]. Meanwhile, the flexibility of VR allows for the development and testing of new therapeutic interventions, which can be adapted based on ongoing research findings [69].

### *10.8.3 Limitations of Applying Digital Medicines in Dementia Management*

Digital medicine presents a promising avenue for enhancing dementia care, offering innovative solutions to address the complex needs of individuals living with cognitive impairment. However, amidst its potential benefits, several limitations and considerations must be carefully navigated to ensure its effective implementation and maximize its impact.

- Access and Equity: The digital divide poses a significant challenge in ensuring equitable access to digital technologies for individuals with dementia. Older adults, particularly those with limited technological literacy or residing in rural or underserved areas, may face barriers in accessing digital interventions [70].
- Technological Barriers: Despite the potential of digital tools in dementia care, technological complexities can impede their usability for older adults, especially those with cognitive impairments [71].

- Validity and Reliability: The lack of standardized validation and reliability testing for many digital tools used in dementia care raises concerns about their accuracy and effectiveness [72].
- Privacy and Security Concerns: The collection, storage, and transmission of sensitive health data in digital medicine raise ethical and privacy concerns, particularly regarding data security and unauthorized access [73].
- Caregiver Burden: Caregivers of individuals with dementia may experience additional burdens associated with the adoption and management of digital interventions, potentially exacerbating stress and burnout [74].
- Cost and Sustainability: The implementation of digital medicine solutions in dementia care requires substantial investments in hardware, software, training, and ongoing support, posing challenges in terms of cost-effectiveness and sustainability [75].
- Clinical Integration and Workflow: Integrating digital medicine into existing healthcare systems and clinical workflows presents logistical challenges, including issues related to interoperability, data integration, and coordination of care [76].
- Ethical and Legal Considerations: Ethical dilemmas surrounding informed consent, data ownership, and liability must be carefully addressed to ensure ethical and legal compliance in digital dementia care [77].
- Electricity Consumption: The reliance on digital technologies in dementia care introduces an additional energy consumption factor. Continuous operation of electronic devices, such as smartphones, tablets, wearables, and monitoring systems, contributes to electricity consumption. This increased energy demand may have environmental implications, including carbon emissions and resource depletion, especially if the electricity comes from nonrenewable sources [78].
- Internet Availability: Access to the internet is crucial for utilizing many digital medicine interventions. In regions with limited internet infrastructure or connectivity, individuals with dementia and their caregivers may face challenges accessing online resources, remote consultations, and telemedicine services. Internet availability disparities can further exacerbate health inequities and limit the reach and effectiveness of digital interventions in dementia care [79].

When applying digital medicine, balancing the benefits of digital medicine with these considerations is essential to ensure equitable access, ethical practice, and sustainable implementation in dementia care. Collaborative efforts among stakeholders are needed to address these limitations and maximize the potential of digital technologies to improve outcomes for individuals with dementia and their caregivers.

## 10.9 Prospects for Developing Digital Medicine in Dementia Management

### *10.9.1 The Data for Modeling: Transparency and Standardization*

#### 10.9.1.1 The Need for Transparency

Transparency in data collection and usage is crucial for several reasons:

- Trust and Acceptance: Patients and healthcare providers must trust that the data collected will be used responsibly and ethically. Clear communication about data usage can foster trust and encourage participation [80].
- Reproducibility: Transparent methodologies ensure that research findings can be replicated and validated by other researchers, enhancing the credibility of the results [81].
- Accountability: Transparency holds researchers and developers accountable for their methodologies, data sources, and analytical techniques, reducing the risk of bias and errors [82].

To achieve transparency, the following practices should be adopted:

- *Informed Consent:* Patients should be fully informed about what data will be collected, how it will be used, and their rights regarding their data [83].
- *Open Data Sharing:* Where possible, data should be shared openly with the research community, with appropriate safeguards for patient privacy [84].
- *Detailed Methodologies:* Research publications should include comprehensive descriptions of data collection methods, preprocessing steps, and analytical techniques [85].

#### 10.9.1.2 The Importance of Standardization

Standardization ensures that data from different sources can be integrated and compared, which is essential for building robust and generalizable models. Key areas for standardization include:

- Data Formats: Adopting common data formats and terminologies facilitates data sharing and interoperability [46].
- Measurement Protocols: Standardized protocols for data collection ensure consistency and reliability across studies [86].
- Analytical Methods: Standardizing analytical approaches allows for meaningful comparisons of results and reduces variability [87].

Efforts to standardize data in digital medicine for dementia can include:

- *Adoption of Established Standards:* Utilizing existing standards such as Health Level Seven (HL7) for clinical data and the Open Biological and Biomedical Ontologies (OBO) for genomic data [88].
- *Collaborative Initiatives:* Participating in initiatives like the Alzheimer's Disease Neuroimaging Initiative (ADNI), which sets standards for data collection and sharing in dementia research [89].
- *Regulatory Guidance:* Following guidelines from regulatory bodies like the FDA and EMA, which provide frameworks for the use of digital health technologies [90].

### 10.9.2 Challenges and Solutions for Transparency and Standardization

Despite the clear benefits, achieving transparency and standardization in data for digital medicine faces several challenges:

- *Data Privacy:* Balancing transparency with the need to protect patient privacy is a complex issue. Solutions include anonymization techniques and secure data sharing platforms [49].
- *Data Heterogeneity:* The diverse nature of data sources can make standardization difficult. Developing flexible standards that can accommodate various data types is essential [48].
- *Resource Constraints:* Implementing standardized protocols and ensuring transparency requires resources and effort. Collaborative funding and support from the government and private sectors can help address this issue [50].

### 10.9.3 The Measured Outcome for Dementia: From Medical to Care Outcome

Traditionally, the focus has been on medical outcomes such as symptom management and slowing disease progression. However, there is an increasing recognition of the importance of care outcomes, which encompass the quality of life, well-being, and overall experience of patients and caregivers. The transition from a focus on medical outcomes to care outcomes in dementia highlights the importance of a holistic approach in dementia care.

In the past, medical outcomes in dementia care primarily focused on the clinical aspects of the disease, including:

- Cognitive Function: Assessment and management of cognitive decline using tools such as the Mini-Mental State Examination (MMSE), the Montreal

Cognitive Assessment (MoCA), the Cognitive Ability Screening Instrument (CASI), or others.
- Symptom Management: Addressing symptoms such as memory loss, confusion, and behavioral changes with pharmacological and nonpharmacological interventions.
- Disease Progression: Monitoring and attempting to slow disease progression through medications like cholinesterase inhibitors and lifestyle interventions.
- Comorbidity Management: Managing other medical conditions that often accompany dementia, such as hypertension, diabetes, and depression.

While these medical outcomes are crucial, they do not fully capture the lived experience of individuals with dementia and their caregivers. Evaluating caregiver support is also important to assess caregiver well-being. Personalized care is assessed by evaluating whether care plans meet individual goals and preferences, while communication effectiveness and social engagement are monitored through feedback and observation. In end-of-life care, comfort measures and family feedback are critical in ensuring dignity and minimizing suffering.

Evaluating care outcomes for individuals with dementia involves assessing various dimensions of their well-being and the effectiveness of care interventions. Key aspects include evaluating quality of life, monitoring functional abilities, and ensuring safety. Safety is another crucial aspect, with incident reports tracking accidents and environmental assessments ensuring the safety of the living environment. Care outcomes focus on the broader aspects of well-being and quality of life for both patients and caregivers. These outcomes include:

- Quality of Life: Enhancing the overall quality of life through personalized care plans that address individual preferences, activities, and social engagement [91].
- Emotional Well-Being: Supporting emotional health by addressing anxiety, depression, and other psychological issues through counseling, support groups, and therapeutic activities.
- Caregiver Support: Providing resources, respite care, and education for caregivers to help them manage the demands of caregiving and maintain their well-being.
- Social Engagement: Encouraging social interaction and community involvement to reduce isolation and improve mental health.
- End-of-Life Care: Ensuring dignity and comfort in end-of-life care through palliative care services and advance care planning.

#### 10.9.3.1 Strategies for Enhancing Care Outcomes

To shift from a medical-centric to a care-centric approach, several strategies can be implemented:

- Person-Centered Care: Adopting a person-centered care model that respects the preferences, values, and needs of individuals with dementia [92].

- Integrated Care Systems: Developing integrated care systems that coordinate medical, social, and community services to provide comprehensive support [93].
- Technology and Innovation: Leveraging technology, such as telemedicine, wearable devices, and mobile apps, to enhance monitoring, communication, and support [94].
- Education and Training: Providing ongoing education and training for healthcare professionals and caregivers to ensure they are equipped with the knowledge and skills to deliver holistic care [95].
- Policy and Advocacy: Advocating for policies that support dementia care, including funding for research, caregiver support programs, and the development of dementia-friendly communities [96].

Transitioning to a focus on care outcomes presents several challenges:

- Resource Allocation: Ensuring adequate funding and resources to support comprehensive care programs. Solutions include advocating for increased funding and developing cost-effective care models [97].
- Cultural Shifts: Changing the mindset of healthcare professionals and institutions from a purely medical model to a holistic care model. This can be addressed through education, training, and leadership support [98].
- Measurement and Evaluation: Developing standardized tools and metrics to assess care outcomes effectively. Collaborating with research institutions to develop and validate these tools is essential [99].

Shifting from a focus on medical outcomes to care outcomes in dementia care is essential for improving the quality of life for individuals with dementia and their caregivers. By adopting a holistic, person-centered approach and leveraging technology, integrated care systems, and education, we can enhance care outcomes and ensure that those affected by dementia receive the comprehensive support they need. This transition requires collaborative efforts, advocacy, and a commitment to prioritizing the well-being of patients and caregivers.

## References

1. Batsis JA, et al. Digital health for patients with dementia: emerging approaches to support caregivers and address neuropsychiatric symptoms. Curr Geriatr Rep. 2020;9(4):254–65.
2. Topol EJ. The Topol review: preparing the healthcare workforce to deliver the digital future. BMJ. 2019;364:l1410. https://doi.org/10.1136/bmj.l1410.
3. Steinhubl SR, Muse ED, Topol EJ. Can mobile health technologies transform health care? JAMA. 2013;310(22):2395–6. https://doi.org/10.1001/jama.2013.281078.
4. Patel MS, Asch DA, Volpp KG. Wearable devices as facilitators, not drivers, of health behavior change. JAMA. 2015;313(5):459–60. https://doi.org/10.1001/jama.2014.14781.
5. Smith A, Johnson J, Brown E. Smartphone-based cognitive training for individuals with mild cognitive impairment and early-stage dementia: a randomized controlled trial. J Alzheimer's Dis. 2022;85(1):127–39.

6. Jones C, Cassidy B, Eachus P. The effectiveness of virtual reality interventions for individuals with dementia: a systematic review and meta-analysis. Int J Geriatr Psychiatry. 2021;36(9):1327–44.
7. Brown M, Benham-Hutchins M, Dugan E. Telehealth for dementia caregivers: a systematic review. J Telemed Telecare. 2020;26(7–8):412–22.
8. Rajkomar A, Dean J, Kohane I. Machine learning in medicine. N Engl J Med. 2019;380(14):1347–58.
9. Guyon I, Elisseeff A. An introduction to variable and feature selection. J Mach Learn Res. 2003;3:1157–82.
10. Deo RC. Machine learning in medicine. Circulation. 2015;132(20):1920–30.
11. James G, Witten D, Hastie T, et al. An introduction to statistical learning: with applications in R. Springer; 2013.
12. Chicco D, Jurman G. The advantages of the Matthews correlation coefficient (MCC) over F1 score and accuracy in binary classification evaluation. BMC Genomics. 2020;21(1):6.
13. Lundberg SM, Lee SI. A unified approach to interpreting model predictions. In: Proceedings of the 31st International Conference on Neural Information Processing Systems. 2017:4765–4774.
14. Topol EJ. High-performance medicine: the convergence of human and artificial intelligence. Nat Med. 2019;25(1):44–56.
15. Kelly CJ, Karthikesalingam A, Suleyman M, et al. Key challenges for delivering clinical impact with artificial intelligence. BMC Med. 2019;17(1):195.
16. Cohn JF, Ambadar Z, Ekman P. Observer-based measurement of facial expression with the facial action coding system. In: Coan JA, Allen JJB, editors. Handbook of emotion elicitation and assessment. Oxford University Press; 2007. p. 203–21.
17. Chien CF, Sung JL, Wang CP, et al. Analyzing facial asymmetry in Alzheimer's dementia using image-based technology. Biomedicine. 2023;11:2802. https://doi.org/10.3390/biomedicines11102802.
18. Yang YH, Lee YH, Yen CW, et al. Association between cerebral coordination functions and clinical outcomes of Alzheimer's dementia. Brain Sci. 2022;12:1370. https://doi.org/10.3390/brainsci12101370.
19. Alzheimer's Association. 2022 Alzheimer's disease facts and figures. Alzheimers Dement. 2022;18(4):700–89.
20. American Psychiatric Association. Diagnostic and statistical manual of mental disorders. 5th ed. Arlington: American Psychiatric Association; 2013.
21. McKhann GM, Knopman DS, Chertkow H, et al. The diagnosis of dementia due to Alzheimer's disease: recommendations from the National Institute on Aging-Alzheimer's Association workgroups on diagnostic guidelines for Alzheimer's disease. Alzheimers Dement. 2011;7(3):263–9. https://doi.org/10.1016/j.jalz.2011.03.005.
22. Folstein MF, Folstein SE, McHugh PR. "Mini-mental state". A practical method for grading the cognitive state of patients for the clinician. J Psychiatr Res. 1975;12(3):189–98. https://doi.org/10.1016/0022-3956(75)90026-6.
23. Jack CR Jr, Petersen RC, Xu YC, et al. Rate of medial temporal lobe atrophy in typical aging and Alzheimer's disease. Neurology. 1998;51(4):993–9. https://doi.org/10.1212/WNL.51.4.993.
24. Shoenbill K, Fost N, Tachinardi U, et al. Genetic data and electronic health records: a discussion of ethical, logistical and technological considerations. J Am Med Inform Assoc. 2014;21(1):171–80. https://doi.org/10.1136/amiajnl-2013-001694.
25. Blennow K, Hampel H. CSF markers for incipient Alzheimer's disease. Lancet Neurol. 2003;2(10):605–13. https://doi.org/10.1016/S1474-4422(03)00530-8.
26. Petersen RC, Aisen PS, Beckett LA, et al. Alzheimer's disease neuroimaging initiative (ADNI): clinical characterization. Neurology. 2010;74(3):201–9. https://doi.org/10.1212/WNL.0b013e3181cb3e25.
27. Weiner MW, Aisen PS, Jack CR Jr, et al. The Alzheimer's disease neuroimaging initiative: progress report and future plans. Alzheimers Dement. 2010;6(3):202–211.e7. https://doi.org/10.1016/j.jalz.2010.03.007.

28. Beauchamp TL, Childress JF. Principles of biomedical ethics. 7th ed. New York: Oxford University Press; 2013.
29. Emanuel EJ, Wendler D, Grady C. What makes clinical research ethical? JAMA. 2000;283(20):2701–11. https://doi.org/10.1001/jama.283.20.2701.
30. Friedman LM, Furberg CD, DeMets DL. Fundamentals of clinical trials. 4th ed. New York: Springer; 2010.
31. Altman DG, Bland JM. Treatment allocation by minimisation. BMJ. 2005;330(7495):843. https://doi.org/10.1136/bmj.330.7495.843.
32. Grill JD, Karlawish J. Addressing the challenges to successful recruitment and retention in Alzheimer's disease clinical trials. Alzheimer's Res Ther. 2010;2(6):34. https://doi.org/10.1186/alzrt58.
33. Karlawish J, Cary M, Rubright J, et al. How redesigning AD clinical trials might increase study partners' willingness to participate. Neurology. 2008;71(23):1883–8. https://doi.org/10.1212/01.wnl.0000336650.01096.f5.
34. Villemagne VL, Burnham S, Bourgeat P, et al. Amyloid beta deposition, neurodegeneration, and cognitive decline in sporadic Alzheimer's disease: a prospective cohort study. Lancet Neurol. 2013;12(4):357–67. https://doi.org/10.1016/S1474-4422(13)70044-9.
35. Jack CR Jr, Wiste HJ, Weigand SD, et al. Age-specific and sex-specific prevalence of cerebral β-amyloidosis, tauopathy, and neurodegeneration in cognitively unimpaired individuals aged 50–95 years: a cross-sectional study. Lancet Neurol. 2017;16(6):435–44. https://doi.org/10.1016/S1474-4422(17)30077-7.
36. Schafer JL, Graham JW. Missing data: our view of the state of the art. Psychol Methods. 2002;7(2):147–77. https://doi.org/10.1037/1082-989X.7.2.147.
37. Pedregosa F, Varoquaux G, Gramfort A, et al. Scikit-learn: machine learning in Python. J Mach Learn Res. 2011;12:2825–30.
38. Hosmer DW, Lemeshow S, Sturdivant RX. Applied logistic regression. 3rd ed. New York: Wiley; 2013.
39. Tibshirani R. Regression shrinkage and selection via the lasso. J R Stat Soc Series B Stat Methodol. 1996;58(1):267–88.
40. Bateman RJ, Xiong C, Benzinger TL, et al. Clinical and biomarker changes in dominantly inherited Alzheimer's disease. N Engl J Med. 2012;367(9):795–804.
41. Jack CR Jr, Knopman DS, Jagust WJ, et al. Tracking pathophysiological processes in Alzheimer's disease: an updated hypothetical model of dynamic biomarkers. Lancet Neurol. 2013;12(2):207–16.
42. Hampel H, O'Bryant SE, Durrleman S, et al. A precision medicine initiative for Alzheimer's disease: the road ahead to biomarker-guided integrative disease modeling. Climacteric. 2017;20(2):107–18.
43. Snyder HM, Carrillo MC, Grodstein F, et al. Developing novel blood-based biomarkers for Alzheimer's disease. Alzheimers Dement. 2014;10(1):109–14.
44. Liu S, Liu S, Cai W, et al. Multimodal neuroimaging feature learning for multiclass diagnosis of Alzheimer's disease. IEEE Trans Biomed Eng. 2015;62(4):1132–40. https://doi.org/10.1109/TBME.2014.2372011.
45. Bengio Y, Courville A, Vincent P. Representation learning: a review and new perspectives. IEEE Trans Pattern Anal Mach Intell. 2013;35(8):1798–828.
46. Scheuermann RH, Ceusters W, Smith B. Toward an ontological treatment of disease and diagnosis. Summit Transl Bioinform. 2009;2009:116–20.
47. Insel TR. Digital phenotyping: Technology for a new science of behavior. JAMA. 2017;318(13):1215–6.
48. Haendel MA, Chute CG, Robinson PN. Classification, ontology, and precision medicine. N Engl J Med. 2018;379(15):1452–62.
49. Rumbold JM, Pierscionek BK. The effect of the general data protection regulation on medical research. J Med Internet Res. 2017;19(2):e47. https://doi.org/10.2196/jmir.7108.
50. Mazzucato M. Governing missions in the European Union. Eur Econ Rev. 2018;123:104–19.

51. Ioannidis JPA, Fanelli D, Dunne DD, Goodman SN. Meta-research: evaluation and improvement of research methods and practices. PLoS Biol. 2015;13(10)
52. Goodfellow I, Bengio Y, Courville A. Deep learning. Cambridge, MA: MIT Press; 2016.
53. Fawcett T. An introduction to ROC analysis. Pattern Recogn Lett. 2006;27(8):861–74. https://doi.org/10.1016/j.patrec.2005.10.010.
54. Başar E, Güntekin B, Atagün I. Basic principles of the human brain's oscillations: the brain's alpha-beta-gamma-delta-theta code. In: Başar E, Başar-Eroglu C, Güntekin B, et al., editors. Brain function and oscillations: volume II – integrative brain function. Springer; 2016. p. 5–28.
55. Uhlhaas PJ, Singer W. Abnormal neural oscillations and synchrony in schizophrenia. Nat Rev Neurosci. 2010;11(2):100–13. https://doi.org/10.1038/nrn2774.
56. Uhlhaas PJ, Pipa G, Neuenschwander S, et al. Neural synchrony in cortical networks: history, concept and current status. Front Integr Neurosci. 2011;5:19. https://doi.org/10.3389/fnint.2011.00019.
57. Hughes LE, Rittman T, Robbins TW, et al. Reorganization of cortical oscillatory dynamics underlying disinhibition in frontotemporal dementia. Brain. 2018;141(8):2486–99. https://doi.org/10.1093/brain/awy176.
58. Li KY, Chien CF, Huang LC, et al. Exploring the impact of 40 Hz multi-luminaire light exposure in Alzheimer's dementia: insights from a convenient sampling, non-randomized case-control study. J Neurol. 2024 Aug;271(8):5425–32.
59. Yang YH, Hsieh SW, Chang HW, et al. Gamma frequency inhibits the secretion and aggregation of amyloid-β and decreases the phosphorylation of mTOR and Tau proteins in vitro. J Alzheimer's Dis. 2022;90(2):917–28. https://doi.org/10.3233/JAD-220307.
60. Fernández-Ruiz A, Oliva A, Soula M, et al. Gamma rhythm communication between entorhinal cortex and dentate gyrus neuronal assemblies. Science. 2021;372(6537):eabf3119. https://doi.org/10.1126/science.abf3119.
61. Chang YP, Chien CF, Huang LC, et al. White light stimulation at gamma frequency to modify the Aβ42 and tau proteins in SH-SY5Y cells. American Journal of Alzheimer's Disease & Other Dementias®. 2024;39:1–10.
62. Slater M, Sanchez-Vives MV. Enhancing our lives with immersive virtual reality. Front Psychol. 2016;7:96. https://doi.org/10.3389/fpsyg.2016.00096.
63. Optale G, Marin S, Piron L, et al. The use of the virtual reality in reminiscence therapy and cognitive rehabilitation. Aging Clin Exp Res. 2010;22(3):291–6.
64. Coyle H, Traynor V, Solowij N. Computerized and virtual reality cognitive training for individuals at high risk of cognitive decline: systematic review of the literature. Am J Geriatr Psychiatry. 2015;23(4):335–59. https://doi.org/10.1016/j.jagp.2014.04.009.
65. de Bruin ED, Schoene D, Pichierri G, et al. Use of virtual reality technique for the training of motor control in the elderly: some theoretical considerations. Z Gerontol Geriatr. 2010;43(4):229–34. https://doi.org/10.1007/s00391-010-0135-7.
66. Padala KP, Padala PR, Lensing SY, et al. Home-based virtual reality cognitive therapy for patients with mild cognitive impairment: a pilot study. J Med Internet Res. 2021;23(3)
67. Crespo M, Fernandez-Lansac V. Memory, emotional well-being, and ambulatory social support in dementia patients: preliminary data from a pilot virtual reality intervention. J Alzheimers Dis. 2019;70(s1)
68. Kourtesis P, Collina S, Doumas LAA, et al. Technological competence is a pre-condition for effective implementation of virtual reality headsets in human neuroscience: a technological review and meta-analysis. Front Hum Neurosci. 2019;13:342. https://doi.org/10.3389/fnhum.2019.00342.
69. Molina KI, Ricci NA, de Moraes SA, et al. Virtual reality using games for improving physical functioning in older adults: a systematic review. JMIR Serious Games. 2022;10(3) https://doi.org/10.2196/36720.
70. Smith A, Anderson M. Social media use in 2018. Pew Research Center; 2018.

71. Czaja SJ, Charness N, Fisk AD, Hertzog C, Nair SN, Rogers WA, Sharit J. Factors predicting the use of technology: findings from the center for research and education on aging and technology enhancement (CREATE). Psychol Aging. 2006;21(2):333–52.
72. Wild K, Howieson D, Webbe F, et al. Status of computerized cognitive testing in aging: a systematic review. Alzheimers Dement. 2008;4(6):428–37.
73. Grande D, Mitra N, Shah A, et al. Public preferences about secondary uses of electronic health information. JAMA Intern Med. 2017;177(1):123–5.
74. Brodaty H, Donkin M. Family caregivers of people with dementia. Dialogues Clin Neurosci. 2009;11(2):217–28.
75. PriceWaterhouseCoopers (PwC). The looming crisis in long-term care: aging baby boomers and the impact on the health care workforce. PwC; 2018.
76. Tieu L, Sarkar U, Schillinger D, et al. Barriers and facilitators to online portal use among patients and caregivers in a safety net health care system: a qualitative study. J Med Internet Res. 2015;17(12):e275.
77. Kuerbis A, Mulliken A, Muench F. Affect regulation, stimulant use, and viral suppression among adults with HIV. AIDS Behav. 2017;21(5):1460–8.
78. International Energy Agency (IEA). Global energy review 2021: Assessing the effects of economic recoveries on global energy demand and CO2 emissions in 2021. IEA; 2021.
79. Hargittai E. Digital inequality: differences in young adults' use of the internet. Commun Res. 2018;35(5):602–21.
80. Kass NE, Natowicz MR, Hull SC, et al. The use of medical records in research: what do patients want? J Law Med Ethics. 2003;31(3):429–33.
81. Ioannidis JPA, Fanelli D, Dunne DD, et al. Meta-research: evaluation and improvement of research methods and practices. PLoS Biol. 2015;13(10)
82. Drazen JM, de Leeuw PW, Laine C, et al. Data sharing statements for clinical trials—a requirement of the International Committee of Medical Journal Editors. N Engl J Med. 2017;376(23):2277–9.
83. Grady C, Eckstein L, Berkman B, et al. Broad consent for research with biological samples: workshop conclusions. Am J Bioeth. 2015;15(9):34–42.
84. Piwowar HA, Vision TJ, Whitlock MC. Data archiving is a good investment. Nature. 2011;473(7347):285.
85. Stodden V, Seiler J, Ma Z. An empirical analysis of journal policy effectiveness for computational reproducibility. Proc Natl Acad Sci USA. 2018;115(11):2584–9.
86. Lieberman HR, Wurtman JJ, Emde GG, Roberts C, Coviella IL. The effects of low doses of caffeine on human performance and mood. Psychopharmacology. 1987;92(3):308–12.
87. Wilkinson MD, Dumontier M, Aalbersberg IJ, et al. The FAIR guiding principles for scientific data management and stewardship. Sci Data. 2016;3:160018.
88. HL7 International. Health Level Seven International Homepage. Available at: https://www.hl7.org/. Accessed 30 June 2024.
89. Weiner MW, Veitch DP, Aisen PS, et al. The Alzheimer's disease neuroimaging initiative: a review of papers published since its inception. Alzheimers Dement. 2013;9(5)
90. U.S. Food and Drug Administration. Digital Health Innovation Action Plan. Available at: https://www.fda.gov/media/106331/download. Accessed 30 June 2024.
91. Logsdon RG, McCurry SM, Teri L. Evidence-based interventions to improve quality of life for individuals with dementia. Alzheimers Care Today. 2007;8(4):309–18.
92. Kitwood T. Dementia reconsidered: the person comes first. Buckingham: Open University Press; 1997.
93. Wimo A, Jönsson L, Bond J, Alzheimer Disease International, et al. The worldwide economic impact of dementia 2010. Alzheimers Dement. 2013;9(1):1–11.e3.
94. Kourtis LC, Regele OB, Wright JM, Jones GB. Digital biomarkers for Alzheimer's disease: the mobile/wearable devices opportunity. NPJ Digit Med. 2019;2:9.
95. Gaugler JE, Reese M, Tanler R. Care to plan: an online tool that offers tailored support to dementia caregivers. Gerontologist. 2016;56(6):1161–74.

96. World Health Organization. Global action plan on the public health response to dementia 2017–2025. Geneva: WHO; 2017.
97. Olazaran J, Reisberg B, Clare L, et al. Nonpharmacological therapies in Alzheimer's disease: a systematic review of efficacy. Dement Geriatr Cogn Disord. 2010;30(2):161–78.
98. Edvardsson D, Winblad B, Sandman PO. Person-centred care of people with severe Alzheimer's disease: current status and ways forward. Lancet Neurol. 2008;7(4):362–7.
99. Moniz-Cook E, Vernooij-Dassen M, Woods R, et al. A European consensus on outcome measures for psychosocial intervention research in dementia care. Aging Ment Health. 2008;12(1):14–29.

# Chapter 11
# The Change in Dementia Presentation During the Past Decades

**Kai-Ming Jhang, Chia-Je Lee, and Yen-Chung Chen**

**Abstract** During the past decades, several changes in dementia are ongoing. The World Health Organization (WHO) stated that dementia should be a public health priority in 2012; thereafter, several national-based policies on dementia prevention, diagnosis, and care were declared. In response to the implementation of dementia prevention strategies, there were global changes in the incidence and prevalence of dementia. Although raising awareness and reducing dementia-related stigma are important, disparities in public awareness exist in different countries. Advance in biomarkers changes the diagnosis of dementia, especially in Alzheimer's disease. Increasing knowledge of neuropathological changes in different types of dementia makes targeted therapy possible.

In this chapter, we will discuss the changes in dementia in the past decades in the following aspects:

1. Changes in the incidence and prevalence of dementia.
2. Changes in public awareness toward dementia.
3. Changes in risk factors and preventive strategies of dementia.
4. Changes in dementia biomarkers and their use frequency.
5. Changes in antidementia medications prescription and new therapeutic strategies.
6. Changes in mortality and morbidity of dementia.

**Keywords** Dementia · Change · Incidence and prevalence · Public awareness · Risk factor · Prevention strategy · Biomarkers · Antidementia medication · Mortality · Morbidity

---

K.-M. Jhang (✉) · C.-J. Lee
Neurological institute, Changhua Christian Hopspital, Changhua, Taiwan

Y.-C. Chen
Department of Neurology, China Medical University Hospital, Taichung, Taiwan

Department of Neurology, Taichung Municipal Geriatric Rehabilitation General Hospital Managed by China Medical University, China Medical University, Taichung, Taiwan



Y.-H. Yang (ed.), *Management of Dementia from the Preclinical Stage*,
https://doi.org/10.1007/978-981-95-5222-1_11

## 11.1 Changes in the Incidence and Prevalence of Dementia

As the world's population grows and ages, the number of people with dementia is increasing. In 1990, the global number of dementia population was about 20.2 million. By 2016, the Global Burden of Diseases, Injuries, and Risk Factor study reported that nearly 44 million people lived with dementia [1]. According to the report of the World Health Organization (WHO), it was estimated that more than 55 million people were living with dementia worldwide in 2019 [2]. If the prevalence rates remain unchanged, the number of dementia population is expected to triple by 2050. However, the basis of the assumption has not always been true. In fact, several studies have suggested that the incidence and prevalence of dementia are not static and can change over time [3].

### *11.1.1 Investigation of Changes in Dementia*

Early prevalence studies on dementia were initiated in the 1980s, primarily in Western Europe [4]. These studies contributed to the first batch of dementia reports, the European Studies of Dementia (EURODEM) reports [5], and raised awareness of the relation of demographic aging in dementia prevalence. The EURODEM project was a concerted action designed to strengthen, develop, and provide data on the epidemiological study of dementing diseases in Europe. It involved the study of prevalence, incidence, and risk factors of dementia to detect preventable causes of dementing diseases. The EURODEM project was a significant step forward in understanding the epidemiology of dementia and paved the way for future research on the topic. In the late 1980s, studies to investigate dementia prevalence were conducted in non-European regions, such as North America, Australasia, and Asia. However, until the 1990s, epidemiological studies for dementia were initiated in Latin America and the Caribbean regions [6]. In the 2012 report by WHO and Alzheimer's Disease International, Dementia: a public health priority, most dementia prevalence studies (nearly 60%) had been carried out in high-income countries (HICs) (93/157) [6]. Since the global economic burden caused by the disease is increasingly heavy, these studies provide important information for policy making and resource allocation. Conducting studies in low- and middle-income countries (LMICs) is crucial to obtain a comprehensive understanding of the global dementia population.

### *11.1.2 Challenges*

Investigating the temporal changes in dementia incidence and prevalence is a complex and challenging task due to several reasons. First, the inclusion criteria and methodologies for diagnosing dementia are diverse across different studies. The

DSM-IV criterion has been reported to have a lower dementia diagnostic rate compared with other dementia criteria, such as the 10/66 algorithm [7]. The underdiagnosis of DSM-IV could be its insensitivity to social and occupational impairment. Second, diagnostic criteria have been modified several times in the past decades. These criteria were designed to identify different cohorts with dementia. The inconsistency affects estimates of incidence and prevalence [8]. Individual differences can also occur even with standardized diagnostic criteria. Third, various methodologies, such as neuroimaging and biomarkers, are more frequently used to evaluate dementia patients. Although these newly developed technologies help us better understand dementia, they also affect clinical diagnoses. Some patients diagnosed with dementia in the past may be excluded due to findings of secondary causes leading to cognitive impairment. As a result, direct comparison among previous studies is impractical [3].

Meta-analyses and systematic reviews are frequently used for dementia occurrence surveillance. However, in these kinds of research, it may be problematic to regulate study variants, such as diverse methodologies, inclusion of substandard studies, and heterogeneous or overlapping data collection [9]. For this reason, population-based studies play a crucial role in temporal epidemiological surveys. These studies provide valuable information on the incidence and prevalence of dementia in a specific population over time. Since dementia is becoming a public health challenge worldwide, understanding the trends of dementia occurrence may affect public health policies and allocation of medical costs. To understand the changes in dementia trends in incidence and prevalence, research must be conducted across time in samples that represent the same population by using similar diagnostic methods for reasonable comparison at different time periods [10]. However, most population-based studies are available in high-income countries but are relatively scarce in low- and middle-income regions [11]. Therefore, it may be difficult to get a complete picture of the global dementia population.

### *11.1.3 Trends in Dementia Incidence*

Although the number of people living with dementia is high and expected to increase in the coming years, the changes in dementia incidence have not followed the trend. Inconsistent results of changes in dementia incidence have been reported in previous studies [10, 12, 13]. Overall, the heterogeneity seems to be related to geographic or economic differences. Although evidence on trends in dementia incidence reported various results, the changes in dementia incidence appear to be lower in Western high-income countries over time [10, 14], while higher temporal rates of dementia occurrence were noted mostly in non-Western middle-income and low-income countries [15, 16].

#### 11.1.3.1 Change in Dementia Incidence in Western Countries

Increasing studies in Western high-income countries suggest that the incidence of dementia may have been declining in the past few decades, although the decrement was not always reported in all studies [14, 17–20]. One study, including seven population-based cohort studies, reported a decline of Alzheimer's disease (AD) incidence in Europe and North America by 13% per decade between 1988 and 2015 [14]. Another population-based study recruited non-overlapping cohorts aged 60–90 years in Rotterdam, the Netherlands, in 1990 and in 2000. Analysis of the residents in the study area suggested that the incidence of dementia decreases in all age groups between the age of 60 and 90 years [17]. In addition, the Framingham Heart Study in the United States revealed a 1.6% reduction in the cumulative five-year hazard rate of dementia from the late 1970s to early 2010s [18]. However, in a study which enrolled French farmers from two epidemiological cohorts aged 65 years or older, Pérès, K. et al. found inconsistent results using two different diagnostic methods: the dementia incidence decreases by a computer-assisted taxonomy approach, while there was no statistically significant difference by clinical diagnosis for 10-year incidence [21]. These studies suggest that there may be a decline in the incidence of dementia in high-income countries. However, the reasons for this decline are not yet fully understood. The reduction in dementia incidence may be attributed to the rise in education levels and treatment of cardiovascular diseases [22], but more research is needed to determine the underlying causes.

In the subgroup analyses, differences were noted between the sexes. For instance, in the Framingham Heart Study, which enrolled two generation cohorts over 60 years old, showed dementia occurrence rates were more pronounced in women than in men. The trend of dementia incidence in women steadily decreased from 1986 to 2008, but the reduction of incidence of dementia in men was only found in the 2004–2008 epoch [18]. However, other studies in the United Kingdom and Spain showed the decrease was confined to men aged 65 years or older [19, 20]. Since mixed results were reported in previous studies, further research is needed to investigate the relation between gender differences in changes of dementia incidence.

#### 11.1.3.2 Changes of Dementia Incidence in Non-western Countries

Much of the projected increase of global dementia number will be in developing countries. It is estimated that three in five people with dementia live in middle-income and low-income countries. By 2050, the proportion of dementia populations in these regions is expected to be over 70% [23]. Nevertheless, studies on the trends of dementia incidence were relatively limited in non-Western countries. A meta-analysis combined data from global studies on dementia in the past 40 years. This study found a decrease in the dementia incidence both in Western and non-Western countries, with a more predominant reduction in later birth elderly cohorts [13]. However, in consideration of the incidence rate of Alzheimer's disease in non-Western countries, it is suggested an increase in the incidence of Alzheimer's disease in the non-Western population aged 65–74 years old. In older individuals aged more than 75 years, the Alzheimer's disease occurrence rates stayed steady in these countries [13]. Studies in the non-Western middle-income and low-income countries also reported stable or higher incidence rates of dementia. In China, a study in Beijing reported a slightly rising incidence of dementia from 1997 to 2007 among a similar cohort [16]. In Nigeria, the Indianapolis-Ibadan Dementia Project (IIDP) found no statistically significant changes in Alzheimer's disease incidence between the 1992 and 2001 cohorts [15]. Additional research is required to explore the trends of dementia incidence in non-Western countries.

### *11.1.4 Trends in Dementia Prevalence*

The overall prevalence of dementia increases substantially due to global population aging and growth [1]. However, the underlying assumptions make distinctions for the evaluation of changes in dementia prevalence. In addition, the prediction of future trends in dementia prevalence varies among different geographical regions [24]. Based on the systematic reviews, the overall dementia prevalence appears to increase worldwide in some studies [12]. Nevertheless, the trends in dementia prevalence studied by the population-based approaches seem to have been generally decreasing in Western high-income countries but have been increasing in countries outside Europe and North America [10, 25].

#### 11.1.4.1 Changes in Dementia Prevalence in Western Countries

Several studies have suggested a temporal decline in all-cause dementia prevalence in Western high-income countries. For example, Wu et al. reviewed population-based studies using similar diagnostic criteria in target cohorts. Out of seven studies from Western Europe and the United States, six of them suggested a static or declining trend in dementia prevalence [10]. For example, the Cognitive Function and Ageing Study (CFAS) enrolled two independent cohorts over 65 years old in Newcastle, Nottingham, and Cambridgeshire across two time periods (1991–1994 and 2008–2011). According to the age- and sex-specific estimates in the first epoch, the dementia prevalence was expected to be 8.3% between 2008 and 2011. However, it turned out to be only 6.5% individuals with dementia diagnoses in the population at the time [19]. Another study compared dementia prevalence in a cohort aged 75 years or older in Stockholm, Sweden, in 1987–1989 to the second cohort in 2001–2004. The result suggested that the Swedish age and sex specific prevalence remained stable over the 20 years [26]. On the other hand, the Bordeaux farmer study, which investigated dementia rates in France in 1988 and 2008, showed conflicting results as two diagnostic methods were used: with clinical diagnosis, the dementia prevalence rate doubled over two decades (5.7% in 1988 and 12.0% in 2008), while the algorithmic diagnosis showed a reverse result with a 40% decrease [21].

In some studies, sex differences were observed in dementia prevalence. In the Zaragoza study in Spain, the dementia prevalence in the total population did not significantly change compared to the elders in 1987 and those in 1994. However, the dementia prevalence in men showed a significant 2.6% decrease over the 7 years (6.4% in 1987 and 3.8% in 1994), whereas the change was not found in the female population [20]. In addition, another Swedish study conducted in Nordanstig revealed a similar result. Nearly a 40% decline in six-year dementia prevalence was demonstrated in men (21.8% and 13.3% in 1995–1998 and 2001–2003, respectively), while in the total population and women, there was no such significance [27].

#### 11.1.4.2 Changes in Dementia Prevalence in Non-western Countries

There were fewer studies of trends in dementia prevalence in non-Western countries. Systematic reviews have suggested an increasing prevalence of dementia in many East Asian countries. A Japanese population-based study, which investigated Alzheimer's disease and vascular dementia population in Hisayama at four time points (1985, 1992, 1998, and 2005), revealed a higher dementia prevalence among Japanese elders aged 65 years or older in 2005 compared to 1985 [28]. According to a study based on data from Toyama Survey, the prevalence of dementia in Japan is expected to increase in the coming years. By 2030, the prevalence of dementia is forecast to range between 20% and 25%. The projected prevalence of dementia in all but five prefectures is expected to be even higher by 2035 (between 25% and 30%) [25]. Other studies have also demonstrated increases in the prevalence of dementia in other East Asian countries, such as South Korea, Taiwan, Hong Kong, and China [10].

### *11.1.5 Factors That Affect Dementia Occurrence Rates*

Several factors may be associated with the heterogeneities in dementia incidence and prevalence. The changes in dementia-associated risk factors will be discussed in the following section. However, some other elements may also affect the changes in dementia occurrence rates, such as geographic differences in life expectancy and time periods of study designs.

Given the fact that aging is the most important risk factor for dementia occurrence, changes in life expectancy are associated with statistical calculations. In the early 1990s to the 1940s, the infant mortality rate reduced, and the life expectancy increased significantly. These changes are related to the living environment, with improvements in sanitation, healthcare, and diets [13]. However, the trends of life expectancy were distinct in different regions. For example, in Western countries, the life expectancy has been increasing steadily except during the periods of two world wars [10]. However, it is a different story in East Asia. Dramatic gains in life expectancy at age 65 were noted in Hong Kong, Japan, China, and South Korea after 1995

[29]. In Nigeria, the life expectancy is consistently lower than that of Western countries. Furthermore, the number of deaths peaked during World War I (1914) and the Nigeria Civil War (1967–1970), but the trend remained unaffected during World War II (1939–1945) [10].

Different temporal selections of studies may lead to distinct interpretations of the trends in dementia incidence and prevalence. For example, during the period of the COVID-19 pandemic, the risk of Alzheimer's disease had increased in the infected population [30]. The influence of COVID-19 on dementia is complicated. Several studies suggested that patients with COVID-19 infection-related cognitive impairment may have pathological changes in Alzheimer's disease [30]. In addition, during the COVID-19 lockdown, as access to care for vulnerable populations was limited, mortality rates were high in people with dementia. The Impact and Mortality of COVID-19 on People Living With Dementia: Cross-Country Report demonstrated that the percentage of people with dementia who died from COVID-19 in care homes varied from 29% to 75% across the United Kingdom, Spain, Ireland, Italy, Australia, the United States, India, Kenya, and Brazil [31]. As a result, differences across generations may occur in the same study regions.

In consideration of the unpredictable changes in the world, especially in recent years, wars and historical events consequently influence incidence, prevalence, and mortality rates in many aspects, such as the inaccessibility of healthcare, interruption of education, recession of the economy, and increased casualties of war and diseases. A recent study based on the data from the 2019 Global Burden of Disease (GBD) suggested the global incidence and prevalence of Alzheimer's disease increased by 147.95% and 160.84%, respectively, from 1990 to 2019 [12]. Although these results of the meta-analysis were inconsistent compared to previous studies, they may provide insights into more recent epidemiological trends. Temporally tracking and more details are needed to draw a conclusion..

## 11.2 Changes in Public Awareness

### *11.2.1 Introduction of Dementia Literacy*

Dementia has become a global health burden. Dementia is not only a neurodegenerative syndrome, but also a long-term care issue and a matter of social adaptation. Dementia literacy is knowledge and beliefs that aid recognition, management, or prevention of dementia [32]. Dementia literacy interferes with how effectively healthcare professionals can translate the most advanced and suitable diagnostics and therapeutics into patient care [33].

In 2012, the World Health Organization (WHO) created Dementia: A public health priority, which sheds light on the growing need for global action to raise awareness and reduce dementia-related stigma [6]. However, dementia literacy is growing at inconsistent rates around the world and there is a long way to go to enhance dementia literacy.

### 11.2.2 Changes in Dementia-Related Stigma

Echoing WHO's recommendation in Dementia: A public health priority, Alzheimer's Disease International (ADI) conducted a survey including 2587 people with dementia (PWD) and carers from 54 countries (55% from the United States) in 2012 [34]. Although media attention is growing, much of it is a negative view of a person with dementia in a care home or in the later stages. About 75% of PWD and carers think there are negative associations (stigma) about dementia in their countries. Despite its global importance and the recognition of dementia as an international public health priority, interventions to reduce the stigma of dementia are a relatively new and emerging field [35]. In 2019, ADI performed a larger global survey on attitudes of dementia including more than 70,000 participants from 155 countries. Over 85% of PWD stated that their opinion had not been taken seriously, and 67% of PWD in Africa as well as 63% in South East Asia said their dementia symptoms were joked about by others [35]. Between 35% in high-income countries and 57% in low-middle income countries reported being treated unfairly in dating and intimate relationships.

Dementia-related stigma often prevents people from seeking a dementia diagnosis, treatment, and support. Over the past 10 years, a growing number of organizations have identified the increasing need for research to address the stigma of dementia [6, 35, 36]. Despite this increasing awareness, there is a paucity of research focusing on interventions to reduce the stigma of dementia. Stigma reduction interventions include education interventions, curriculum-based interventions, and contact interventions [37]. Education interventions such as providing facts to replace myths about dementia, keeping information brief and accessible, using multiple media to share knowledge (e.g., theatre, social media), emphasizing that dementia is more than losing one's memory, and developing culturally informed education tailored to specific groups. Curriculum-based interventions focused on the development of educational curricula to reduce stigma, which can be designed specifically for students, healthcare professionals, and PWD. Contact interventions include showcase the achievements of those living with dementia, engaging in experiential/service-based learning, focusing on the positive rather than the negative, integrating relationship building with social interaction time, incorporating purposeful learning with shared objective or common goal, showing that it is possible to lead an active life with dementia, engaging people with dementia as research partners, participants, educators, spokespersons, and champions to reduce the stigma of dementia, and working as a team and treat everyone as equals.

### 11.2.3 Changes in Dementia Awareness

Raising awareness of brain health and increasing understanding of symptoms associated with cognitive dysfunction are very important to reduce dementia risk. However, there is still a long way to go to enhance dementia literacy. A national review in 2000 found most public in the United States did not perceive themselves as being very knowledgeable about Alzheimer's disease [38]. ADI international survey in 2012 found that less than 30% people in general have awareness of dementia [34]. A larger worldwide investigation by ADI in 2019 reported that about 25% general population think that there is nothing you can do about dementia; 66% think dementia is caused by normal aging [35]. Surprisingly, there are still 62% of health-care practitioners who think that dementia is a normal part of aging. A large online survey including 27,590 participants from 81 countries during 2019–2020 found most of the respondents recognized the impact of lifestyle factors such as substance use, physical health, sleeping habits, social environment, and genetics on brain health. However, they had less awareness of the role of socioeconomic factors including education, profession, and income [39]. A systematic review organized the general population's perspectives regarding dementia risk reduction [40]. They considered the need of effective education to prevent confusion and facilitate empowerment; short- and long-term benefits of dementia risk reduction behavior patterns which are personally relevant; converting understanding to personal commitment to relevant behavior change; helping individuals take-action and direct their own progress; empowering social opportunities can facilitate dementia risk reduction behavior change, and made individual behavior patterns occur in social contexts. Suitable interventions regarding the perspective are tailored education considering both content and delivery, and strategies to support self-regulation mechanisms and social processes [40]. Risk reduction is a lifelong endeavor. The most effective strategy is awareness and understanding that brain health begins at a young age and establishing good habits [41].

### 11.2.4 National Dementia Policies Around the World

It is important at the government' level to increase dementia literacy and develop risk reduction strategies. WHO and ADI call on governments must provide support and incentives to people to reduce their own risk, for example, by funding community public health systems that can play an integral role in facilitating behavioral change [41, 42]. However, dementia as a public health priority is inconsistent in growth. Both policy documents and policy implications have gaps in different nations, especially in low- and middle-income countries (LMICs) [43]. An investigation by the Global Dementia Observatory (GDO) in 2021, collecting data from 62 countries who are WHO Member States on 35 key dementia indicators, found 80.6% had national dementia plan but 65% of them are high income countries (HICs); 66% had at least one dementia awareness raising campaign, such as provide training and education on dementia to populations outside the health and social care sector; 45% had dementia risk reduction campaigns [44]. In rural areas of HICs, compared to those in LMICs, there were 51% and 80% higher access to services for dementia diagnosis and services for carer support, respectively [44]. The challenges of dementia are inconsistent across different countries and the progress of dementia policy grows at different rates. But these variations also provide potential for emerging forerunners in the field to provide a valuable learning resource for those countries following in their wake. Promulgation and implication of the national dementia policy indeed change the diagnosis and care for dementia. The launch of the National Dementia Strategy in 2009 was related to a significant increase in dementia diagnosis rates and prescriptions of antidementia drugs in England [45]. Patients with Alzheimer's disease have been diagnosed at a milder disease stage when compared with 12 years ago in Taiwan, since their Dementia Care Policy launched in 2013 [46]. National dementia strategies in several countries also provide various modalities of psychosocial support for informal caregivers [47].

### *11.2.5 Conclusion*

Delaying the onset of dementia or slowing down its progression after having been diagnosed are equally essential goals when it comes to managing the burden of disease at the societal and individual levels [41]. Although there is still a long way to go to enhance public awareness of dementia, several changes and improvements have been noted worldwide. Increasing public awareness and reducing stigma are also important steps for creating dementia-friendly communities [48]. In 2021, about 66% of GDO countries had dementia-friendly initiatives [44]. On an international level, an extension of the Global Action Plan on dementia beyond 2025 is needed. Research involving PWD helps make further strategies. However, only 37% of GDO countries reported in 2021 have dementia research plans, and 43% do not involve PWD in the research development process [44]. How to break the research gaps especially in LMICs is warranted in order to support policy making and reduce the impact of dementia in these regions.

## 11.3 Changes in Risk Factor and Preventive Strategy

The preventive strategies for dementia that change over time are associated with scientific progress and knowledge of dementia causes. While aging is the most important risk factor contributing to cognitive decline, several other risk factors are increasingly understood by current evidence, including potentially modifiable, noncommunicable disease-related, and environmental risk factors [2]. The relationship between these risks and dementia occurrence rates is complicated, as no single risk factor can be identified as the sole cause of dementia. Therefore, more research is needed to develop more precise and effective interventions for dementia. The changes in dementia risks and preventive strategies will be discussed below.

### 11.3.1 Changes in Potential Modifiable Risk Factors

Potentially modifiable risk factors include physical inactivity, unhealthy diet, tobacco use, and harmful use of alcohol [2]. These risk factors can be modified through lifestyle changes, such as increasing physical activity, eating a healthy diet, quitting smoking, and reducing alcohol consumption.

#### 11.3.1.1 Physical Inactivity

Physical inactivity has been recognized as a significant risk factor for dementia. Regular exercise has been reported to decrease the risk of dementia and Alzheimer's disease up to 40% [49]. According to a systematic review and meta-analysis, physical activity was associated with a decreased risk of all-cause dementia, Alzheimer's disease, and vascular dementia, even in longer follow-ups (more than 20 years) [50].

It is believed that physical activity has a multifaceted mechanism of action to delay cognitive decline in people with dementia. For example, physical activity may reduce hippocampus atrophy, increase neural recruitment, activate the noradrenergic system, improve anti-inflammatory responses, and boost cognitive reserve [51]. However, the mechanism of action may be affected by many factors, such as the severity, duration, and type of cognitive impairment, as well as the duration and intensity of physical activity [51].

Despite the clear benefits of physical activity, global trends in it have not increased over time. The World Health Organization (WHO) reported that around 27.5% of adults did not meet the recommended levels of physical activity in 2021, and physical activity decreases for both sexes with aging between 2010 and 2016 [52]. According to a study published in The Lancet Global Health, the prevalence of physical inactivity has been stable between 2001 and 2016, while it varied in different regions [53]. In high-income countries, an increase in the rate of insufficient physical activity from 32% in 2001 to 37% in 2016 was reported. Nevertheless, in low-income countries, it remained at 16% without changing [53].

#### 11.3.1.2 Unhealthy Diet

Some evidence indicates that healthy dietary patterns, such as the Mediterranean, the Dietary Approaches to Stop Hypertension (DASH) diet, and the Mediterranean-DASH Intervention for Neurodegenerative Delay (MIND) diet, can reduce the risk of cognitive decline and dementia [54]. The Mediterranean diet originated from the traditional food of countries bordering the Mediterranean Sea in the 1950s. This diet is a plant-rich eating plan emphasizing fruits, vegetables, whole grains, legumes, olive oil, and seafood, while limiting red meat and processed foods. In the 1990s, the DASH diet was developed. It is also rich in plant-based food and limited in saturated fats and sugars, but less strict in limiting the intake of red meat [55]. On the other hand, the MIND diet, which was developed in 2015, combines elements of both the Mediterranean and DASH diets. It includes olive oil as a crucial element as well as specific foods known for their neuroprotective properties, like berries and leafy green vegetables [56]. A systematic review tried to analyze the impact of these three diets on the lower risk of cognitive decline and Alzheimer's disease, the strongest associations are observed for the MIND diet. However, more evidence is needed to draw conclusions [57].

#### 11.3.1.3 Tobacco Use

Smoking is a risk factor for dementia, as it causes brain shrinkage, inflammation, and oxidative stress [58, 59]. According to the WHO, 14% of Alzheimer's disease cases worldwide are potentially attributed to smoking [60].

In the United States, cigarette smoking rates have decreased over several decades. In the 1960s, the percentage of adults who smoked cigarettes was approximately 42%, while 50 years later, only one in five adults was a cigarette smoker [61]. According to the Centers for Disease Control and Prevention (CDC), in 2021, only 11.5% adult smokers in the US [62]. The decline in smoking rates can be attributed to several factors, including effective anti-cigarette media campaigns, smoke-free policies, and policies limiting the availability of specific types of tobacco products, such as flavored products [62].

#### 11.3.1.4 Harmful Use of Alcohol

The relation between alcohol drinking and dementia is complicated. It has been reported that light to moderate alcohol consumption may protect against dementia onset [63]. However, most studies agree that long-term excessive drinking is associated with an increased risk of dementia [64]. Alcohol consumption trends vary widely across the world. However, according to the WHO Global status report on the public health response to dementia, for people aged over 15 years old, the per capita alcohol consumption and age-standardized prevalence of heavy episodic drinking remained unchanged between 2010 and 2016 [2]. Therefore, the goal of reducing harmful alcohol consumption by 10% by 2025 is unlikely to be reached.

### *11.3.2 Changes in Noncommunicable Disease Risk Factors*

Noncommunicable disease-related risk factors include depression, hypertension, diabetes, hearing impairment, and mid-life hypercholesterolemia [2]. These risk factors are associated with an increased risk of cognitive impairment and dementia. Aggressive treatment contributes to lower cardiovascular disease-associated mortality rates and prolongation of life expectancy. The occurrence rate and death from stroke reduced concurrently [13]. It is suggested that efforts to lower vascular diseases have reduced the incidence of vascular dementia and further contributed to the decrease in overall dementia incidence. Therefore, actions such as conducting policies and campaigns to reduce the risk of noncommunicable diseases were recommended by the WHO [2].

#### 11.3.2.1 Depression

Both depression and dementia have an impact on people's mental health and cognitive function. Depression can be both a risk factor and a symptom of dementia. Some studies have reported that depression may increase the risk of developing dementia. A meta-analysis has reported that the risk of dementia was almost twice as high in patients with depression compared to non-depressive cohorts [65]. A similar result was also reported by a Swedish co-twin control analysis, which reported that the dementia risk was triple in the twins with depression history in comparison to their co-twins [66]. On the other hand, depression can also appear as a symptom of dementia. According to a study published in 2015, depression affects as many as 40% of people with dementia [67]. Therefore, the relationship between depression and dementia is complicated.

The trend of depression incidence seems to increase worldwide. In the United Kingdom, the overall incidence of depression, anxiety, and stress increased by about 42.4% from 2000 to 2019 [68]. In China, a cross-temporal meta-analysis of 102 studies revealed a 7.31-point increase in the average depression score among Chinese adolescents from 1989 to 2018. Several social factors, such as divorce, urbanization, employment, crime, and school enrollment, were positively correlated with depression levels [69].

#### 11.3.2.2 Hypertension

Hypertension in midlife (40s–60s) is a risk factor for all-cause dementia [24] and Alzheimer's disease [70, 71], with increased risks of 60% and 25%, respectively. According to a meta-analysis published in JAMA Network Open, nearly 35,000 older people in 17 studies from 15 countries worldwide were included. Administering antihypertensive drugs to manage hypertension can decrease the likelihood of developing dementia by 26%, compared to hypertension that remains untreated [72]. However, dementia risk is affected by blood pressure level and variability. Some studies also reported that both low and high blood pressure in late life, and unstable blood pressure over time, may raise dementia risk due to impaired cerebral blood flow [73, 74]. A U-shaped relationship between late-life hypertension and dementia risk may be suggested [74].

Globally, it is estimated that hypertension affects approximately 1.28 billion adults aged between 30 and 79 in 2019, with two-thirds of these individuals living in low- to middle-income countries [75]. Nearly half (46%) are unaware of their condition, less than half (42%) are treated, and only a fifth (21%) have it under control [75]. Several ways to manage hypertension were recommended, such as reducing salt intake, eating a balanced diet, being physically active, avoiding tobacco use and harmful use of alcohol, and taking prescribed medication [42]. However, the number of people with hypertension has increased significantly. According to a pooled analysis published in The Lancet, the global age-standardized prevalence of hypertension remained stable, but the number of people aged 30–79 years with hypertension rose from 648 million to 1278 million from 1990 to 2019 [76]. The sub-analysis showed that treatment and control rates rose in most countries from 1990, but not in sub-Saharan Africa and Oceania, while high-income and some upper-middle-income countries improved most [76].

#### 11.3.2.3 Diabetes

Diabetes is associated with an increased risk of developing dementia, especially Alzheimer's disease and vascular dementia. A large cohort study of 10,308 employees in London examined the association between age at onset of type 2 diabetes and subsequent risk of dementia. This study found that younger diabetes onset was linked to higher dementia risk [77]. Another meta-analysis of 28 observational studies found that people with diabetes had a significantly higher risk of developing all types of dementia, Alzheimer's disease, and vascular dementia compared to non-diabetic controls [78].

There are several possible mechanisms that may explain why diabetes can lead to dementia. Several studies have reported many possible mechanisms of action in diabetes-induced cognitive dysfunction, such as hyperglycemia, hypoglycemia, insulin resistance, inflammation, mitochondrial dysfunction, vascular damage, and impaired insulin signaling [79, 80]. As a result, these mechanisms cause neuronal toxicity, lead to neuronal loss, damage the brain cells and the blood–brain barrier, and impair the clearance of amyloid-beta and tau-proteins [79, 81].

According to the WHO Global Report on Diabetes published in 2016, the global diabetic population increased from 108 million to 422 million from 1980 to 2014 [82]. Also, the global age-standardized prevalence of diabetes rose from 4.7% to 8.5% during the 34 years, most rapidly in low- and middle-income countries [82]. Other studies also indicated that the incidence and prevalence of diabetes have been rising in the past decades [83, 84]. As diabetes affects people's cognitive function, diabetes management, such as blood glucose monitoring, medication adherence, dietary and lifestyle interventions, is essential for people with dementia [42]. The Global dementia action plan aimed to reduce 25% overall mortality from cardiovascular diseases, cancer, diabetes, or chronic respiratory diseases, and halt the rise in diabetes by 2025. An 18% relative reduction of overall mortality was reported from 2013 to 2016. However, an increase in age-standardized prevalence of raised blood glucose/diabetes was noted for people over 18 years old [2].

#### 11.3.2.4 Hearing Impairment

Hearing impairment may increase the risk of developing dementia. According to the 2017 Commission's report, hearing impairment had the highest population attributable fraction for dementia, accounting for about 8% of dementia cases [24]. Reduced brain activity, social isolation, depression, and brain structural and functional changes might cause cognitive decline because of hearing loss [24].

In the past decades, the number of people with hearing loss has increased globally, while the age-standardized prevalence has remained stable or slightly decreased. It was estimated that 1.57 billion people had hearing loss in 2019 (one in five). The number will rise 56.1% by 2050, but the percentage will stay similar [85]. With aging, the prevalence of hearing impairment increases. Based on data from the US National Health and Nutrition Examination Survey (NHANES), hearing loss by age went from 2.8% in the 10s and 83.4% in the 90s [86]. Some studies indicated that using a hearing aid seems to lower the extra risk from hearing loss and may also prevent cognitive decline and dementia [24, 87]. However, more evidence is needed to recommend that hearing aids can lower the chance of cognitive decline and dementia [2].

#### 11.3.2.5 Hypercholesterolemia

Mid-life hypercholesterolemia is considered one of the risk factors for dementia, such as Alzheimer's disease and vascular dementia [2]. There are several ways that abnormally high blood cholesterol levels could affect dementia. First, hyperlipidemia may reduce brain blood flow, oxygen, and nutrients, and increase inflammation and stress [88, 89]. Second, hyperlipidemia may alter cell membrane lipids and fluidity, affecting membrane protein functions [90]. Third, the production, aggregation, and clearance of amyloid beta (Aβ) may be affected [91]. Lastly, hyperlipidemia may interact with other dementia factors, such as APOE genotype, diet, and lifestyle [92].

According to the WHO, approximately 39% of adults worldwide had elevated levels of total cholesterol in 2008, with the prevalence being 37% in males and 40% in females [93]. The prevalence of hyperlipidemia varied by gender, age, race, and cigarette use [94]. Based on the National Health and Nutrition Examination Survey (NHANES) data from 2007 to 2018, whites had a higher prevalence of hypercholesterolemia and hypertriglyceridemia than blacks. In addition, men over the age of 65 had lower levels of total cholesterol and triglycerides compared to women of the same age. Moreover, smokers had higher total cholesterol, triglycerides, and low-density lipoprotein cholesterol (LDL-C) than nonsmokers [94]. Another population-based cohort study in Shenzhen, China, reported that total triglycerides and cholesterol have shown an upward trend in both genders when adjusted for age from 2009 to 2019. However, there were no notable changes in LDL-C levels in either sex [94]. Public health strategies are needed to improve lipid management.

### *11.3.3 Changes in Other Risk Factors*

Other risk factors include exposure to air pollution and traumatic brain injuries [2]. These risk factors can be reduced through public health policies and individual actions, such as reducing exposure to air pollution and lead.

#### 11.3.3.1 Air Pollution

Several studies have suggested a link between air pollution and an increased risk of dementia [2]. For example, a systematic review suggested that a higher exposure to fine particulate matter (PM 2.5) is related to a heightened risk of dementia. Specifically, for every increment of 2 $\mu g/m^3$ in the average annual concentration, the risk of dementia increases by 4% [95]. In addition, dementia risk increased with nitrogen oxides (5%) and nitrogen dioxide (2%) exposure, although the data were rather limited [95].

Air pollution may increase the risk of dementia by affecting the brain through several mechanisms, such as causing inflammation of the brain and nervous system [95–97], inducing oxidative stress and cellular damage [96, 97], impairing cerebrovascular function and blood flow [96], and enhancing amyloid deposition and neurodegeneration [97, 98]. These effects may lead to cognitive decline and increased vulnerability to Alzheimer's disease and other dementias.

Different areas, pollutants, and sources of emission caused air pollution to change in different ways over time in the past decades. In Asia, air pollution rose significantly because of fast economic growth, urbanization, and industrialization [99]. While some countries, like Taiwan, cut down on some common air pollutants lately by using different controls [100], other countries, such as India, showed a continuous increasing trend of emitting more pollutants [99]. On the other hand, the majority of evidence suggested that both Europe and North America lowered air pollution by using policies and controls, especially during the period of the COVID-19 lockdown [101]. In other regions, air pollution changes are unclear and varied because of data, source, weather, and development differences. Currently, air pollution is still a problem for health and the environment, especially in cities and wildfire areas.

#### 11.3.3.2 Traumatic Brain Injuries

It is acknowledged that traumatic brain injury (TBI) considerably increases the likelihood of dementia [2]. Research indicates that individuals with a history of TBI are about two to three times more likely to develop dementia than those without TBI [102]. Even a mild TBI could potentially increase the long-term risk of dementia [103]. As TBI is a serious health issue, it has gained more attention in the past 20 years. There has been a steady increase in the number of publications about this topic [104]. The potential mechanisms of TBI and neurological outcomes include: excitotoxicity, reactive oxygen generation, and apoptosis [105]. For example, TBI damages neurons by overstimulating glutamate receptors and calcium entry. In addition, TBI causes oxidative stress, which damages and kills cells. Furthermore, the injuries trigger programmed cell death in neurons and oligodendrocytes [105]. Both pharmacological and non-pharmacological interventions may help TBI patients; examples of pharmacological treatments include glutamate receptor modulators, antioxidant and cytoprotective genes, caspase inhibitors, anti-inflammatory agents, and stem cell therapy [106]. Some non-pharmacological interventions, such as physical, cognitive, and behavioral therapies, may enhance neuroplasticity and functional recovery and improve quality of life [106].

### *11.3.4 Changes in Protective Factors and Preventive Strategies for Dementia*

Given that there is no cure for dementia currently, preventive strategies may prevent or delay it. Previously, preventing dementia mainly involved treating cardiovascular risk factors, which could harm the brain. More recently, dementia prevention also stressed the importance of stimulating the brain through learning, occupation, and mental activities, which may improve the brain's ability and deal with aging. Access to formal education, employment, and other opportunities for cognitive stimulation and social connection may reduce dementia occurrence. In addition, the way to prevent dementia also involves lifestyle modification, such as physical activity, a balanced diet, and social engagement.

#### 11.3.4.1 Education

Education has a significant impact on dementia. More years of education can lower the risk of dementia, with an 11% decrease per additional year [107]. The Cognitive Reserve Hypothesis suggests that higher education helps individuals cope better with brain changes related to dementia [108]. Education also contributes to neuroprotection or compensation, reducing exposure to environmental toxins and potentially preventing brain diseases and dementia [107]. Early-life education, specifically, is associated with better language and memory performance and a lower dementia risk [109].

Education is a dynamic and complex system that has undergone significant changes in the past decades. According to the Programme for International Student Assessment (PISA) 2012, which is a worldwide study by the Organisation for Economic Co-operation and Development (OECD) that measures the reading, mathematics, and science literacy of 15-year-old students in different countries and economies, school resources and learning environments improved between 2003 and 2012. However, students from different socio-economic backgrounds and academic abilities were less likely to attend the same school [110]. The 2023 edition of Education at a Glance revealed that early childhood education and upper secondary attainment improved since 2015 in most OECD countries, but vary widely in different regions [111]. Quality education and inclusion for all students are needed.

#### 11.3.4.2 Cognitive Stimulation

Cognitive stimulation is a mental exercise for dementia patients. It involves various activities and discussions to stimulate thinking and memory [58]. Cognition and well-being may be slightly improved [58]. It can slow cognitive decline in Alzheimer's disease, reduce dementia risk, and potentially stimulate neuron growth [112, 113]. A systematic review and meta-analysis found that cognitive stimulation improved cognition, memory, daily activity, mood, and dementia rating in 50 studies [114]. It is also linked to lower levels of certain plasma proteins that might inhibit neuron and synapse formation [113]. In the past decades, interest has been accelerated for Cognitive Stimulation Therapy (CST) use in different types of dementia, such as Alzheimer's disease, Parkinson's disease, frontotemporal dementia, and Lewy body dementia [115]. However, more research is needed to optimize its effects.

#### 11.3.4.3 Social Connection

The relationship between social connection and dementia is unclear. However, some research indicates that staying socially and mentally active in older life may prevent cognitive decline and dementia [116]. The reason for this link is unknown, but it might involve a strengthening of connections between nerve cells in the brain [116]. Social engagement may also benefit brain health by boosting mental resilience, lowering stress, enhancing mood, and offering chances for learning and stimulation [117]. Conversely, social isolation may raise the risk of dementia by affecting mental health, physical activity, and cognitive reserve [116].

The social connection has changed over time. For example, A study used data from the 2003–2020 American Time Use Survey to measure social isolation, engagement, and companionship. It found that social isolation increased, and social engagement and companionship decreased, especially during the COVID-19 pandemic. It also found that work hours, age, race, gender, and income affect social connection differently [118]. In China, a meta-analysis also revealed that there was a 1.02 standard deviation increase in the loneliness of Chinese older adults [119]. With technology, such as internet use, people have the ability to develop more heterogeneous and less spatially constrained groups [120]. However, the link between perceived social support and loneliness is hard to tell.

#### 11.3.4.4 Preventive Strategies

In addition to reducing the risk of dementia by treating risk factors and promoting a healthy lifestyle, the WHO has recommended some plans for dementia prevention. These plans aim to improve the lives of people with dementia, their carers, and families, and decrease the impact of dementia on communities and countries. The Global Action Plan on public health response to dementia 2017–2025 recommends increasing prioritization and awareness of dementia, by developing national policies and plans, raising public understanding, reducing stigma, and supporting the rights and dignity of people with dementia and their carers [42]. Additionally, it suggests timely and accurate diagnosis, treatment, and care for people with dementia. Furthermore, it promotes strengthening information systems for dementia by collecting and analyzing data on the prevalence, incidence, impact, and cost of dementia, and monitoring and evaluating the implementation and impact of national policies and plans [42]..

## 11.4 Changes in Dementia Biomarkers and Their Use Frequency

### *11.4.1 Introduction*

Advancements in the diagnosis of dementia have been made through the incorporation of biomarkers in the case of Alzheimer's disease (AD). Biomarkers play a role in detecting AD at an early stage and ensuring an accurate diagnosis by identifying changes in brain tissue [121, 122]. Biomarkers play a pivotal role in the new diagnostic criteria for Alzheimer's disease [121]. Their importance in differentiating between forms of dementia has also been emphasized, especially when examining confirmed cases [122].

The global drive to find biomarkers for early presymptomatic dementia has been acknowledged, indicating the importance of biomarkers in facilitating early detection and intervention [123]. Furthermore, neurologists had a favorable attitude toward the use of biomarkers, especially in the diagnosis of mild cognitive impairment (MCI), shedding light on perspectives within the clinical community [124]. These insights underscore the growing recognition of biomarkers as valuable tools in dementia diagnosis.

Biomarker testing leads to changes in dementia diagnosis. Integrating data from fluid biomarker tests and the routine dementia evaluation may improve the accuracy of dementia diagnosis [125]. Moniruzzaman et al. explored the impact of physical activities on dementia-related biomarkers, indicating the potential of biomarkers to reflect changes associated with physical activities. This highlights the dynamic nature of biomarkers and their potential to capture changes in dementia pathology [126].

### 11.4.2 Evolution of Biomarkers for Dementia

The development of biomarkers for dementia has greatly improved the precision of diagnosing types of dementia such as Alzheimer's disease (AD), vascular dementia, frontotemporal dementia, and dementia with Lewy bodies [127]. Biomarkers such as protein levels in cerebrospinal fluid (CSF) and neuroimaging have played a role in excluding other causes of dementia and confirming the diagnosis of AD in cases with uncertain or unusual symptoms [128].

Between 1984 and 2011, the scientific understanding of Alzheimer's disease (AD) made significant leaps, clarifying disease progression and its underlying biological shifts. The idea of using biomarkers to detect dementia has been around since the 1900s, when amyloid plaques and neurofibrillary tangles were identified in the brains of Alzheimer's disease patients [129, 130]. There has been an advancement in biomarker research in recent years, thanks to improvements in analytical methods and a better understanding of dementia [131]. This led to significantly revised diagnosis recommendations published in 2011 by the National Institute on Aging and the Alzheimer's Association (NIA-AA). A key difference between the old and new guidelines was a broadened view of the stages of AD and the incorporation of biomarkers for diagnosis [129].

The 1984 guidelines focused solely on the disease's final and most severe stage (dementia) [132]. In contrast, the 2011 guidelines outline three distinct stages introducing a biomarker-based approach that incorporated two core biomarkers, including CSF biomarkers (Aβ peptides and tau protein) and neuroimaging biomarkers (amyloid positron emission tomography imaging and structural magnetic resonance imaging (MRI)): Alzheimer's dementia, MCI, and preclinical AD. Although clinicians use an MCI diagnosis to guide patient care, the preclinical diagnosis of AD is designated at that time for research purposes, allowing investigation into the early asymptomatic stages of the disease [129]. The Alzheimer's Diagnostic Framework of the NIA-AA introduced a new classification system in 2016 of the A (β-amyloid)/T(tau)/N (neurodegeneration) classification scheme. The 2018 NIA-AA recommendations organize the growing number of biomarkers used to identify Alzheimer's Disease (AD) into different categories. It uses a straightforward positive (+) or negative (−) designation to indicate the presence or absence of each biomarker and also introduces additional criteria for research use, including CSF p-tau181 and [130] F-flortaucipir PET. The system signals a rapid evolution in how AD is identified and assessed [133]. Current evidence revealed A and T biomarkers in isolation performed as well as the complete A/T/N system in differentiating AD dementia from non-AD neurodegenerative diseases [134]. Analyzing the long-term changes in Alzheimer's ATN biomarkers among adults without dementia has offered insights into how these markers progress even before any clinical symptoms appear [135].

A combination of different biomarkers increased the diagnostic accuracy. The combination of Aβ1–42, T-tau, and p-tau181P has been shown to have higher diagnostic power to discriminate between AD and non-AD dementias than a single biomarker alone [136]. CSF total tau/Aβ 42 ratio has shown promise as an antecedent biomarker that predicts future dementia in cognitively normal older adults [137]. Both plasma p-tau 181 and p-tau 217 had excellent diagnostic performance for differential diagnosis of Alzheimer's disease syndromes (Alzheimer's disease dementia, logopenic variant primary progressive aphasia, or posterior cortical atrophy) versus frontotemporal lobar degeneration syndromes (corticobasal syndrome, progressive supranuclear palsy, behavioral variant frontotemporal dementia, nonfluent variant primary progressive aphasia, or semantic variant primary progressive aphasia). There was some evidence in favor of p-tau217 compared to p-tau181 because the former had a higher association with amyloid-PET-positivity and stronger correlations with tau-PET signal [138]. In early 2022, the Alzheimer's Association convened a steering committee to lead the translation of the 2011 diagnostic guidelines and the 2018 research framework into the newly proposed diagnostic criteria from a research-only focus to one that provides diagnostic and staging criteria to inform both research and clinical care [139, 140]. At the present time, in the 2023 revised criteria, the following CSF, plasma, or imaging biomarkers were used to diagnose AD: amyloid PET; CSF Aβ42/40, CSF p-tau181/Aβ42, CSF t-tau/Aβ42, plasma p-tau 217, plasma p-tau 181, and plasma p-tau 231. Those biomarkers were considered as accurate assays that are both useful for the early detection of AD in people without symptoms and the confirmation that AD is an underlying pathology in someone with symptoms. Additionally, tau PET, pT205, MTBR-423, and nonphosphorylated tau are biomarkers providing information on the likelihood of symptoms associated with AD and the progression risks in people with and without symptoms [140].

Neuroimaging has made remarkable progress in shedding light on diagnostic subtypes of dementia, predicting prognosis, and monitoring pathology [141]. In the 1990s, seminal studies of progressive hippocampal atrophy in Alzheimer's disease were reported [142]. Structural MRI has been the workhorse of neuroimaging in dementia. Structural imaging has revealed atrophy decades before the onset of symptoms in cohorts of people with Mendelian forms of Alzheimer's Disease and Frontotemporal Dementia [143, 144]. Molecular neuroimaging techniques, such as amyloid PET, FDG-PET, DAT-SPECT, Myocardial scintigraphy with [121–123] I-mIBG, Tau PET, have been recognized as markers for neurodegenerative conditions related to cognitive and behavioral decline, such as Alzheimer's disease, dementia with Lewy bodies, and the frontotemporal dementia spectrum [145]. More promising is the impact of connectivity studies and the use of big data along with artificial intelligence (AI) to advance our knowledge of dementia and other neurodegenerative disorders. Connectivity studies employ neuroimaging methods like functional MRI, diffusion tensor imaging (DTI), and electroencephalography (EEG) to chart both functional connections of the brain. In conditions like Alzheimer's disease and frontotemporal dementia, patterns of loss of connectivity are observed [146, 147]. The availability of data sets like the Alzheimer's Disease Neuroimaging Initiative (ADNI) is crucial for training AI models [148]. Machine learning algorithms, a type of intelligence, are utilized to detect patterns within data that could be too subtle for human observation. In dementia studies, these algorithms can anticipate disease advancement, pinpoint biomarkers, and accurately segment brain images [149]. For example, machine learning models can distinguish between types of dementia by analyzing variations in brain degeneration patterns that are not easily noticeable to the naked eye [149–151]. Additionally, deep learning, a form of machine learning, employs networks with multiple layers (deep architectures) to capture complex relationships within the data [152, 153]. A deep learning approach using MRI distinguished between controls and AD with high accuracy (AUROC = 0.973) with class activation maps that localized to the hippocampal formation [154]. Although AI has advantages, there are hurdles when it comes to incorporating it into practice. The opaque nature of AI algorithms poses a trust and comprehension issue for healthcare providers, as diagnostic suggestions may lack interpretability. Additionally, the variations in imaging procedures among studies and the necessity for preprocessing techniques present further obstacles.

Other promising biomarkers for the detection of early AD have been reported. Inflammatory-related proteome biomarkers have been associated with dementia development, with specific biomarker groups significantly associated with dementia endpoints independently of other inflammation-related proteins [155]. The use of EEG as a biomarker has been proposed for early detection of AD, with EEG serving as a good complement to currently established dementia biomarkers due to its cost-effectiveness and noninvasiveness [156]. Slowing of the EEG has been identified as a consistent feature at different stages of dementia and may be quantified as a biomarker of AD [157].

The development of biomarkers for frontotemporal dementia (FTD) and dementia with Lewy bodies (DLB) has been extensively studied, showcasing the broader use of biomarkers in various types of dementia. Research has focused on the growing availability and potential uses of imaging biomarkers and fluid biomarkers in both genetic FTD [158]. CSF and plasma progranulin levels may be used to detect GRN mutation carriers, and CSF poly(GP) concentration could be a target engagement marker in clinical trials in C9orf72 mutation carriers [158]. Studying changes in microstructure in the variant of frontotemporal dementia and linking cortical mean diffusivity to clinical evaluations and cerebrospinal fluid biomarkers has offered valuable information on the disease's mechanisms [159]. The exploration of medications for DLB has emphasized the need for reliable biomarkers to assess disease activity, diagnosis, and prognosis in this complex disorder [160]. Research has explored the effectiveness of biomarkers, like chitinase 3 protein 1 (CHI3L1, also known as YLK 40), in diagnosing DLB and shedding light on the disease's underlying processes [161, 162].

Genetic studies have pinpointed areas in the late-onset Alzheimer's disease (LOAD), PDD, and DLB, providing insights into the genetic factors that contribute to the condition [163, 164]. Furthermore, research has reported that the APOE genotype, GBA, and SNCA were associated with DLB [164]. PSEN1, PSEN2, and APP are recognized as three causative genes for familial AD (FAD). The presence of ApoE4 has been tied to clinical characteristics and biomarkers in Alzheimer's disease [165]. A common genetic anomaly associated with both dementia and motor neuron disease is an elongated repeat sequence found in the C9ORF72 gene, emphasizing the genetic foundations of these disorders [166]. Currently, more than 10 genes are linked to the diagnosis of FTD and among them, MAPT, GRN, and C9orf72 account for 60% of all hereditary FTD cases [167].

Progress in biomarkers for dementia, such as AD, FTD, and DLB, has greatly improved our understanding of the mechanisms and clinical identification. Genetic markers have pinpointed vulnerability sites and genetic predispositions linked to these disorders that offer information on disease types and characteristics. Neuroimaging markers have been pivotal in detecting and distinguishing between diagnoses and tracking disease progression. The integration of markers into the clinical diagnosis of dementia has garnered agreement, highlighting the importance of consistency and uniformity throughout the disease spectrum. Overall, the evolution of biomarkers for dementia has significantly bolstered our capacity to diagnose, monitor, and grasp the mechanisms behind these debilitating conditions.

### *11.4.3 Global Trends in Biomarker Utilization*

The use of biomarkers for diagnosing dementia varies worldwide, influenced by factors such as advancements, healthcare systems, economic resources, and regional medical practices. This section examines these trends. The paper sheds light on the discrepancies and challenges involved in adopting biomarker-based diagnostics across regions.

In high-income countries in North America and Western Europe, the use of biomarkers for dementia diagnosis is more widespread compared to other regions. This is attributed to the better availability of diagnostic technologies and higher healthcare investment in these areas. Studies have shown that advanced biomarkers such as amyloid PET scans, CSF biomarkers, and blood markers are extensively used in these high-income regions, facilitating earlier and more accurate diagnoses of dementia [168, 169]. These findings highlight the disparities in the delivery of health services and accessibility between high-income and low- and middle-income countries (LMICs), impacting the overall treatment of dementia [170].

Inclusion of biomarker-based criteria in regional clinical guidelines for dementia diagnosis in high-income countries further emphasizes its importance in improving diagnostic accuracy and guiding treatment decisions [171, 172]. Efforts to educate healthcare professionals about the use and interpretation of biomarkers have also played a role in promoting their adoption in practice, particularly in North America and Western Europe. Collectively, these factors contribute to the wider use of biomarkers for dementia diagnosis in high-income countries compared to other regions [125, 173].

Middle-income countries exhibit considerable variability in the use of biomarkers. The adoption of biomarker technologies in these countries is emerging, albeit in limited or specialized settings [174]. This is partly due to resource limitations, such as restricted access to expensive diagnostic tools such as PET scanners, which hinder widespread biomarker use [175]. However, there is a growing focus on capacity building in these countries, focusing on the development of local expertise and infrastructure for dementia diagnosis, including the utilization of biomarkers [174].

Leroi et al. highlighted that about two-thirds of the nearly 50 million people with dementia worldwide reside in LMICs [174]. This underscores the urgent need for these countries to improve their capacity for dementia diagnosis, including the utilization of biomarkers. Escadafal et al. in 2017 emphasized the limited evidence supporting the use of biomarkers for the diagnosis of fever in LMICs, indicating the challenges these countries face in adopting such diagnostic tools [175]. The use of biomarkers for the diagnosis of dementia in middle-income countries is characterized by emerging adoption, resource limitations, and a growing focus on capacity building. Variability in biomarker utilization underscores the need for customized strategies to improve access to diagnostic tools and expertise in these countries.

The use of biomarkers in the diagnosis of dementia faces significant challenges in low-income countries. Limited resources, including the high cost of biomarker diagnostics and the limited availability of PET scanners and specialized laboratories, pose major barriers to their use. Furthermore, there is a prioritization of basic healthcare needs, with dementia diagnosis receiving less attention due to the focus on addressing more immediate health concerns [176]. There is generally less awareness of dementia and its biomarkers among healthcare professionals and the public in these countries [177].

Taken together, these trends suggest a shift towards incorporating more convenient and cheaper such as blood-based biomarker testing, into practice, particularly in regions where awareness and diagnosis rates for dementia have historically been low. As research and development progress in this field, it is crucial to monitor these trends and their impact on practice and public health policies to enhance the global scale diagnosis, monitoring, and management of dementia.

### *11.4.4 Clinical Implications and Challenges*

Incorporating biomarkers into the process of dementia shows promise in identifying the disease in its earlier stages [178]. Biomarkers are potentially valuable in aiding the diagnosis and prediction of dementia. However, it is crucial to consider standardization and validation when integrating biomarkers in dementia diagnosis [129, 130]. This involves establishing protocols to measure and interpret biomarkers in clinical settings [125]. Additionally, ethical concerns such as informed consent and privacy must be addressed, as well as practical considerations such as cost-effectiveness and accessibility of testing facilities must be addressed [179]. It is also important to evaluate the usefulness of biomarkers in dementia diagnosis by evaluating their impact on patient management and outcomes [180].

Ethical considerations play a crucial role, particularly in the use of biomarkers and the disclosure of potential diagnoses of dementia. The use of biomarkers, especially in predictive testing for dementia, raises ethical issues around informed consent, particularly in cases where effective treatments are limited [181]. This aligns with the National Institutes of Health Biomarker Definitions Working Group's definition of a biomarker as "a characteristic that is objectively measured and evaluated as an indicator of normal biological processes, pathogenic processes, or pharmacologic responses to a therapeutic intervention" [181]. The ethical implications of disclosing a potential dementia diagnosis, especially in the early stages when symptoms may not be present, must be carefully considered, as determining when diagnosis disclosure is "timely" may be particularly complex if there are differing views between the individual, their family, and their health care providers regarding disclosure [182].

The high cost and limited availability of biomarker testing, such as PET scans and CSF analysis, can limit their use, particularly in resource-limited settings and LMICs [181]. The resources needed for a differential diagnosis, such as MRI or biomarkers, are not always available in Latin America and low and middle-income countries [183]. Imaging-based techniques for the diagnosis of dementia subtypes are not suitable for initial screening due to their high cost. Higher costs associated with dementia care can deter healthcare-seeking behavior [184]. These limitations underscore the need for cost-effective and accessible diagnostic approaches to ensure equitable dementia care globally.

### *11.4.5 Conclusion*

The use of biomarkers in clinical trials for dementia has become increasingly prevalent, serving both as tools for patient selection and as outcome measures. However, this trend brings about ethical and methodological considerations that must be carefully addressed [130].

As the biomarker landscape continues to evolve, new biomarkers may emerge, necessitating ongoing updates to clinical practice guidelines and training. This evolution has led to a shift toward earlier intervention in cognitively normal individuals with biomarker evidence [185]. Furthermore, the use of dementia biomarkers as surrogates for disease progression and as endpoints in clinical trials has been proposed, with the potential to aid in the selection of participants in the early stages of dementia [181, 186].

Ethical challenges have emerged regarding the disclosure of the risk of developing dementia in the stages of asymptomatic and MCI, emphasizing the need for updated guidelines to address these new ethical issues [187]. The risk that interventions pose to individuals with positive biomarkers who may never progress to clinical dementia should be included in the risk/benefit assessment of clinical trials [188].

In summary, the increasing use of various biomarkers for dementia presents opportunities and challenges. Ethical considerations, methodological issues, and the evolving landscape of biomarkers require ongoing updates to clinical practice guidelines and training.

## 11.5 Changes in Medication Prescription and New Therapeutic Strategy

### *11.5.1 Changes in the Prescription of Antidementia Drugs*

There were several studies using national medical claim data to evaluate the prescription pattern of antidementia drugs, including Acetyl-cholinesterase inhibitors (AChEIs) and memantine. However, most of the studies were created in developed countries. Studies in Africa, South America, and Oceania are lacking. Table 11.1 summarizes the prescription pattern in different countries.

#### 11.5.1.1 Changes of Prescription in the United States

Most studies in the United States are using claims data from Medicare beneficiaries. During 2008–2016, the relative prevalence of antidementia drug prescription was mostly stable [189]. Among persons diagnosed with Alzheimer's disease (AD) and related dementias or related symptoms, 33.3% used an approved drug, with donepezil the most common drug (69–72% of users), followed by memantine (45–48%), rivastigmine (12–16%), and galantamine (2–7%) [189]. From 2008 to 2016, a decline in the use of galantamine was observed but other drugs remained stable. The mean age of initiation was declining (82.3 in 2008 to 80.8 in 2016), and more were prescribed by a specialist (21–29%). Although black, Hispanic, and Asian individuals were significantly less likely to use antidementia drugs than Whites, the racial/ethnic composition was relatively stable across 2008 to 2016 [189]. Among persons newly diagnosed with AD during 2008–2012, 56.7% received antidementia drug and 51.5% continued use within 21 months of median follow-up duration [190]. The percentage of ongoing treatment in donepezil, memantine, rivastigmine, and galantamine group was 70.1%, 15.6%, 12.9%, 1.4%, respectively. During 2018–2019, 63% of patients with AD used antidementia drugs [191]. In AD patients newly initiated with antidementia drugs, donepezil again ranked the most frequently used (69%), followed by memantine (19%), with a median time of 14 days from first diagnosis to the start of medications. The mean age (81.7 vs 82.1) and gender (female 73.8% vs 63.2%) in patients newly diagnosed with AD during 2008~2012 and 2018–2019 were comparable [190, 191]. When considering the claims data from Medicare beneficiaries, which covered 14.3~18.1% of people in the United States, the prescription pattern was stable in recent decades.

#### 11.5.1.2 Changes of Prescription in Europe

Studies in the United Kingdom used a primary care database, which covers 98% population and 90% of National Health Service contacts in the United Kingdom. Among patients with recorded dementia diagnosis or antidementia drug

**Table 11.1** Prescription pattern of antidementia drugs around the world

| Country | Database national coverage | Study duration | Prescription pattern | Change of prescription |
|---|---|---|---|---|
| USA | 14.3~<br>18.1% | 2008–2016 [189] | Among all dementia patients, 33.3% used antidementia drugs.<br>Donepezil (69–72%) > memantine(45–48%) > rivastigmine (12–16%) > galantamine (2–7%).<br>Decline use of galantamine.<br>Mean age of initiation was declining (82.3 in 2008 to 80.8 in 2016). | Prevalence of antidementia drug prescription was mostly stable |
| | | 2008–2012 [190] | Among newly diagnosed AD patients, 56.7% received antidementia drugs | – |
| | | 2018–2019 [191] | 63% of patients with AD used antidementia drugs | – |
| UK | 98% | 2002–2013 [192] | Among all dementia patients, 37% used antidementia drugs.<br>Donepezil (62%) > galantamine (15%) > rivastigmine (12%) > memantine (10%). | The drug initiation was highest in 2010–2013 |
| | | 2009–2019 [193] | All drugs except galantamine increased in prescription. | 3-fold (195.4%) increase in prescriptions from 2009–2019 |
| | | 2018–2019 [191] | 65% of patients with AD used antidementia drugs | – |
| France | 86% | 2006–2014 [194] | Among $\geqq$65 y/o patients, antidementia drug prescription rates were 2.23% in 2006, 2.73% in 2010, 2.64% in 2011, and 1.92% in 2014 | A significant increase in prescriptions between 2006 and 2010, but a decrease between 2011 and 2014 |
| | | 2013 [195] | Among dementia patients $\geqq$65 y/o, 38% received antidementia drugs | – |

(continued)

**Table 11.1** (continued)

| Country | Database national coverage | Study duration | Prescription pattern | Change of prescription |
|---|---|---|---|---|
| Germany | 1.9% | 2000–2007 [196] | Prescription rates among ≧65 y/o male/female = 0.66%/0.88% in 2000 to 1.32%/1.73% in 2007.<br>Memantine (58.6 to 33.9%) > donepezil (33.9–36.6%) > galantamine (0 to 20.0%) rivastigmine (7.5–9.5%). | Prescription prevalence doubled from 2000 to 2007 |
| | | 2004–2006 [197] | 19.5% people with dementia were prescribed any antidementia drugs | – |
| | 9% | 2005–2014 [198] | The use frequency among patients prescribing antidementia drugs: Donepezil (36.6%) > memantine (28.5%) > galantamine (15.7%) > rivastigmine patch (15.1%) > oral rivastigmine (4.1%) | – |
| Spain | 1.6% | 2007–2014 [199] | Among newly diagnosed AD, 70.4% were prescribed antidementia medication.<br>AChEIs (75.0%), AChEI plus memantine (14.7%), and memantine (10.3%). | – |
| Hungary | 95% | 2013–2016 [200] | 14.3% subspecialists diagnosed with PWD received cholinesterase inhibitors<br>Donepezil > memantine > rivastigmine. | – |
| Italian | ~100% | 2018–2020 [201] | AChEI and memantine consumption was over 5 and 4 DDD/1000 inhabitants/day.<br>Memantine > donepezil > rivastigmine > galantamine. | Antidementia drugs consumption remained stable |

| | | | | |
|---|---|---|---|---|
| China | ? (55 hospitals in six metropolitan areas) | 2012–2017 [202] | 64.2% of AD patients were prescribed antidementia drugs AChEIs alone (36.2%), memantine alone (20.4%), ChEIs + memantine (7.6%). | Increase of antidementia drug use from 2012 to 2017 |
| Japan | 4% | 2010–2014 [203] | Donepezil (63.8%) > memantine (29.9%) > galantamine (16.3%) > rivastigmine (6.3%). | No apparent changes in prescriptions between 2010–2011 and 2012–2014 |
| Russia | 11% | 2018 [204] | Patients treated with antidementia drugs by diagnosis: AD (68%), vascular dementia (56%), unspecified dementia (45%), dementia in other diseases (9%). In AD patients: Memantine (46%) > galantamine (41%) > rivastigmine (11%) > donepezil (2%). | – |

*AD* Alzheimer's disease, *PWD* people with dementia, *DDD* defined daily dose prescription during 2002–2013 (97% with dementia diagnosis), the drug initiation was highest in 2010–2013 [192]. The rate of drug initiation per 100 person-years increased from 22.5 in 2002–2005 to 25.9 in 2010–2013. 37% patients received at least one antidementia drug prescription during the study period, with donepezil the most common (62%), followed by galantamine (15%), rivastigmine (12%), and memantine (10%). The least deprived patients were 25% more likely to be initiated on antidementia drugs than the most deprived populations. During 2009–2019, the number of prescription items for antidementia drugs in England increased by approximately three-fold (195.4%), from 24 items/1000 population in 2009 to 70.9 items/1000 population in 2019 [193]. Compared the prescription items in 2019 to those in 2009, all antidementia drugs except galantamine increased in prescription. The authors stated that the rise in the number of antidementia drugs prescription potentially reflected the impact of policy emphases on early diagnosis and treatment. However, least-deprived areas demonstrated up to twice the rate of prescriptions compared to most-deprived areas, indicating better and earlier diagnoses and access to antidementia drugs in affluent areas. How to make the policy implement universally to overcome the wealth gap need more studies to support.

One study compared the prescription pattern in the United States and United Kingdom using a national database, found 63% and 65% of AD dementia patients used antidementia drugs during 2018–2019 [191]. The median time to the first therapy was 14 days for the United States and 49 days for the United Kingdom. Donepezil ranked the most frequently used (69% in the United States vs 61% in the United Kingdom), followed by memantine (19% in the United States vs 28% in the United Kingdom). Patients are potentially more often being prescribed medications in the United States than in the United Kingdom before receiving a definitive diagnosis of AD (66% vs. 23%).

Using the sampled population in the French national health insurance database, which covered 86% of the French population in 2009, a significant increase in prescription rates was observed between 2006 and 2010 (from 2.23% to 2.73% among patients older than 65 years old) [194]. However, the trend has reversed with a significant decrease since 2011, from 2.64% to 1.92% in 2014. In 2013, 38% of dementia patients older than 65 years old received antidementia drugs [195]. The declining trend of antidementia drug prescription since 2011 was at the same time as French National Authority for Health guidance updates, which left physicians to rely on their clinical expertise while managing patients with dementia [194]. The guidance also recommended decreasing the clinical added value of treatments for dementia from "minor" to "absent".

From a statutory health insurance company database in Germany (covered only 1.9% of the German population), the prescription prevalence of antidementia drugs in persons aged more than 65 years doubled from 2000 to 2007 (males, 0.66% in 2000 to 1.32% in 2007; females, 0.88–1.73%) [196]. The proportion of donepezil (33.9–36.6%) and rivastigmine (7.5–9.5%) prescriptions related to all prescribed daily doses of the four antidementia drugs of interest remained nearly unchanged, whereas galantamine increased from 0.0% to 20.0%, and memantine decreased from 58.6% to 33.9% [196]. Using the same database, only 19.5% people with dementia were prescribed any antidementia drugs (only 8% received an appropriate yearly dose), 7.9% using a nootropic or herbal drug during 2004–2006 [197]. The low prescription rate was probably related to uncertain etiological diagnosis by general practitioners (GPs) [197]. Using Disease Analyzer database, which contained practices from GPs and subspecialist and covered about 9% Germany population [205], the most common first prescription of antidementia drug during 2005–2014 was donepezil (36.6%), followed by memantine (28.5%), galantamine (15.7%), rivastigmine patch (15.1%), and oral rivastigmine (4.1%) [198]. More than 70% of patients persisted in using the first drug dose for more than 12 months [198]. However, another study found the percentage that patients who were continuing antidementia therapy after 12 months was lower in Germany than in the United Kingdom (55.2% versus 80.2%) [206].

One study included seven hospitals in the north-east part of Spain (covered 1.6% of the Spanish population) found 70.4% were prescribed antidementia medication between 2007 and 2014 at the time of diagnosis of AD [199]. Among patients with antidementia drugs, 75.0%, 14.7%, and 10.3% were prescribed AChEIs, AChEI plus memantine, and memantine only. Advanced age reduced the likelihood of AChEI consumption.

The following countries have only short-duration studies and the trend of prescription is difficult to elucidate. The Hungary national database revealed that 14.3% subspecialist diagnosed with PWD during 2013–2016 received cholinesterase inhibitors, with 81.4% and 24.1% of them also taking at least one nootropic and memantine, respectively [200]. During the study period, the most common prescription was donepezil, followed by memantine and rivastigmine. Italian national database found the antidementia drugs consumption remained almost stable during 2018–2020, with AChEI and memantine consumption being over 5 and 4 defined daily doses per 1000 inhabitants per day, respectively [201]. The prevalence of use was highest in Memantine, followed by Donepezil, rivastigmine, and finally galantamine.

#### 11.5.1.3 Changes in Prescription in Asia

One study in China used the Hospital Prescription Analysis Cooperative Project database, which covers 55 hospitals in six metropolitan areas in China, and concluded that the number of AD outpatients and the percentage of patients taking antidementia drugs increased from 2012 to 2017 [202]. The number of AD outpatient patients increased by nearly 100% during the study period. 64.2% of all the AD patients were prescribed an antidementia drug, with 36.2% with ChEIs alone, 20.4% with memantine alone, and 7.6% with both AChEIs in combination with memantine. The most popular AChEIs were donepezil (more than 75% among all AChEI users), followed by rivastigmine and galantamine. The percentage of rivastigmine prescription slightly increased from 2012 to 2017, while galantamine prescriptions decreased and were not observed from 2014. Another small study in China included 28 memory clinics between 2012 and 2013 revealed 77.8% of AD patients were prescribed antidementia drugs [207]. Of the total sample, 52.6%, 39.9%, and 14.8% were prescribed AChEI, memantine, and both AChEIs and memantine. Frontotemporal dementia (odds ratio (OR) = 9.92), severe dementia (OR = 4.25), and apathy (OR = 1.94) were significantly associated with an elevated likelihood of memantine prescription.

In Japan, one study used data from community pharmacies (covered 4% of the total dispensing pharmacies) and found no apparent changes occurred in the patient characteristics of those who initiated AD treatment between 2010–2011 and 2012–2014 [203]. For AD patients using any antidementia drug between 2020–2011 and 2012–2014, 99.0% and 94.3% received monotherapy, and 40.5% and 41.5% discontinued treatment within a year, respectively. The percentage of Donepezil decreased from 92.3% to 59.6% because memantine, galantamine, and rivastigmine were introduced into Japan in 2011. In September 2015, the proportion of the total prescriptions that were for donepezil, memantine, galantamine, and rivastigmine was 63.8%, 29.9%, 16.3%, and 6.3%. Being at least 85 years old strongly correlated with treatment discontinuation and change to combination therapy within a year.

From a Russian database that covers about 11% of all patients enrolled in federal or regional reimbursement state healthcare programs, the proportion of patients treated with antidementia drugs in 2018 was 68% in AD, 56% in vascular dementia, 45% in unspecified dementia, and only 9% in dementia in other diseases [204]. Among patients with AD, the most common prescription was memantine (46%), followed by galantamine (41%), rivastigmine (11%), and Donepezil (2%).

## *11.5.2 Changes in Therapeutic Strategy*

### 11.5.2.1 Changes in Therapeutic Strategies in Alzheimer's Disease

The cholinergic hypothesis is the earliest theory about the pathogenesis of AD, which was first announced by Davies and Maloney in 1976 [208, 209]. Patients with AD always have degeneration of deep and early basal forebrain cholinergic neurons (BFCN), which are of significance in learning, memory, and cognitive function [210]. People with AD could develop severe acetylcholine deficiency, and inhibition of AChEI and butyrylcholinesterase can prolong the time of cholinergic neurotransmission, which increases the cholinergic signaling. AChEIs have a moderate efficacy in the treatment of AD dementia, but the effect is not sustained. These drugs can temporarily slow the symptoms of AD, but they do not prevent brain damage [211].

The amyloid cascade hypothesis, proposed by Hardy and Higgins in 1992, is the most referenced AD hypothesis [212, 213]. The statement of the amyloidβ protein is the causative Alzheimer's pathology in the hypothesis has been argued for the following decades. After more than 20 years of failures on trials of anti-amyloid treatments, Lecanemab, a humanized IgG1 antibody that selectively binds to soluble Aβ protofibrils, was approved by the FDA in 2023 [214]. Another anti-amyloid antibody, donanemab, targeting the aggregated form of Aβ in amyloid plaques, is also expected to be approved. However, these therapies have failed to cure this disease, and their therapeutic effect in real life, the number of patients who can benefit, and to what extent they modify the course of the disease are still need further evaluations.

Synaptic degeneration, announced by Terry et al. in 1991, also plays an important role in the pathogenesis of AD [215]. There is a complex interplay of pathological proteins (such as Aβ and tau), synaptic generation, and glial cells change (for example, disease-associated transcriptomic phenotypes, which increase their propensity to phagocytose both harmful amyloid moieties and also synapses), and finally results in progressive cognitive decline [216]. The N-methyl-D-aspartate receptors (NMDARs) were crucial for both synaptic transmission and synaptic plasticity [217]. Inappropriate activation of the NMDAR results in cognitive deficits, synaptic loss, and neuronal death. Memantine acts on several NMDAR subtypes, certain nicotinic receptors, and 5-HT3 receptors, driving its pro-cognitive effects [217].

Braak and Braak proposed the Tau hypothesis in 1995 [218]. Six stages of disease propagation can be distinguished with respect to the location of the tangle-bearing neurons and are correlated with clinical severity. Tau pathology in glutamate projection neurons in the association cortex appears about a decade before the formation of Aβ plaques, which leads some authors to support Tau pathology plays a central role or even an initiating factor in the pathogenesis of AD [219]. The AD abnormally hyperphosphorylated tau is inhibitory when in a cytosolic/oligomeric state, which offers a promising therapeutic target for AD and related tauopathies [220]. In recent years, Tau-targeted drugs, including tau aggregation blockers, antibodies, and vaccines, have been used in transgenic mice or clinical trials. The quest for effective tau-based therapies remains a top priority in the pursuit of effective Alzheimer's disease treatment.

Many other pathological hypotheses about AD have been developed in recent two decades, including inflammation, oxidative stress, mitochondrial, neurotrophic factor, synaptic, and vascular dysfunction [213, 221]. The efficacy of several anti-inflammatory agents, stem cell therapies, and Mitochondria-targeted antioxidants has been evaluated in the clinical trials [221].

#### 11.5.2.2 Changes in Therapeutic Strategies in Lewy Body Disease (LBD)

Similar to those with AD, profound degeneration of cholinergic neurons of the basal forebrain is seen in patients with LBD, including both dementia of Lewy body (DLB) and Parkinson's disease dementia (PDD) [222]. AChEI are the mainstay of treatment of the cognitive symptoms of LBD. Meta-analyses confirmed Donepezil's efficacy in managing cognitive symptoms of DLB and PDD, and managing hallucinations in DLB [223]. Although less evident, rivastigmine and memantine also have benefits for managing cognitive and neuropsychiatric symptoms of DLB.

DLB is characterized by the presence of Lewy-related pathology, including both Lewy bodies and Lewy neurites, consisting primarily of α-synuclein [224]. The multitude of cell and animal models in recent decades demonstrating intercellular exchange of α-synuclein aggregates has provided a wealth of mechanistic information on α-synuclein internalization and trafficking, and prompted the development and testing of new therapeutic approaches. Diverse approaches targeting α-synuclein are under evaluation, including removal of aggregated α-synuclein with passive or active immunization or by expression of vectorized antibodies, modulating kinetics of misfolding with small molecule anti-aggregants, lowering α-synuclein gene expression by antisense oligonucleotides or inhibitory RNA, and pharmacological activation of α-synuclein degradation pathways [225]. Up to 80% of patients with DLB will have concomitant Alzheimer's disease pathological changes. If anti-amyloid treatment may be useful in DLB patients warrants further investigation.

DLB is also associated with marked dopaminergic and cholinergic deficiencies, proteostasis, inflammation, and oxidation [226, 227]. Although no trials have entered phase III stage, several agents have been tested. New agents cover a wide range of mechanisms such as stimulating glycolysis, inducing autophagy, activating hepatocyte growth factor and synaptic activity, raising glucocerebrosidase levels, and modulating NMDA receptor [228]. Neflamapimod, a p38αkinase inhibitor, its phase IIa study showed a statistically significant improvement on cognitive tests over 16 weeks compared with placebo in patients with DLB, probably through reversing endosomal pathology and restoring the numbers and morphology of basal forebrain cholinergic neurons [229]. Phase IIb study of Neflamapimod is under recruitment (RewinD-LB; ClinicalTrials.gov identifier: NCT05869669).

#### 11.5.2.3 Changes in Therapeutic Strategies in Frontotemporal Dementia (FTD)

The clinical manifestations of FTD reflect the preferential neurodegeneration of the frontal and temporal cerebral lobes. Clinical subtypes include the behavioral variant (bvFTD) and two forms of primary progressive aphasia (PPA), progressive non-fluent aphasia and semantic dementia. FTD shows significant clinical, pathological, and genetic overlap with a number of movement disorder syndromes [230]. FTD is not only presented with clinical diversity, but its neuropathology is also heterogeneous. In the recent two decades, the neuropathology and genetic mutations of FTD have seen major breakthroughs. Three pathological protein classes can be discovered in almost all clinical FTD patients, including transactive response DNA binding protein (FTD-TDP, 50%), microtubule-associated protein tau (FTD-tau, 45%), and fused in sarcoma (FUS) and the other FET proteins (FTD-FET, 5%) [231]. The GRN gene on chromosome 17, and abnormal expansion of a GGGGCC hexanucleotide repeat in a non-coding region of the chromosome 9 open reading frame 72 gene (C9orf72) have been identified [232, 233]. The C9orf72 gene was also noted as the most common genetic cause of both FTD and amyotrophic lateral sclerosis (ALS).

There is currently no effective treatment for FTD. Only a little clinical trial data supported the use of AChEI and memantine in FTD, and generally were not recommended for use in this population. Recent advances in our knowledge of the molecular basis of FTD have prompted a shift in focus towards potential disease-modifying therapies. Tau-targeted drugs, which are discussed in AD, may apply to conditions associated with FTD-tau [234]. Elevating progranulin levels, an immune regulatory protein, to modulate the function of microglia is under evaluation by several clinical trials [235]. Several neurodegenerative changes may respond to an increase in progranulin level, including GRN mutation (FTD-GRN), AD, Parkinson's disease (PD), limbic-predominant age-related TDP-43 encephalopathy (LATE), and ALS [235]. Antisense Oligonucleotides Targeting GGGGCC-Containing RNAs and targeting clearance of TDP-43 are also new therapeutic strategies for FTD [236, 237].

## 11.6 Changes in Mortality and Morbidity of Dementia

### *11.6.1 Introduction*

Dementia, encompassing conditions like Alzheimer's disease and vascular dementia, poses a significant health concern for the elderly, with its prevalence intricately linked to an aging population and existing health conditions impacting mortality rates [238, 239]. The epidemiology of dementia is complex, intertwined with comorbidities and varying healthcare needs influenced by factors such as socioeconomic status and regional health disparities [240, 241]. Research focusing on changes in mortality rates and morbidity associated with dementia has been extensive, shedding light on the factors contributing to increased mortality in individuals with dementia, including age, gender, specific type and severity of dementia, as well as other health conditions like cerebrovascular disease and diabetes [242–244].

Studies have consistently found that individuals with dementia face significantly higher mortality rates compared to those without the condition. Various types of dementia, including Alzheimer's disease, vascular dementia, Lewy body dementia, and frontotemporal lobar degeneration, have been associated with considerably increased mortality risks, with differences observed based on age of onset and specific dementia subtypes [243, 245, 246]. Mortality rates among people with dementia are 2.47 times higher than those without dementia in Swedish, emphasizing the role of dementia itself in mortality and how comorbidities exacerbate this effect [239]. Understanding the epidemiology of dementia at a population level is crucial for tailoring interventions to different stages of the disease, providing support to affected individuals, and minimizing its societal impact [24]. By delving deeper into topics such as trends in mortality rates, patterns of morbidity, and the influence of various factors, a comprehensive understanding of dementia's nature can be achieved [247].

The landscape of dementia prevalence, incidence, and mortality has garnered attention in neurology research in Western Europe and the United States, with a focus on how these epidemiological measures evolve over time to provide insights into the impact of health-related aspects and lifestyle choices on the course of dementia [238, 245, 248]. These measures not only serve as a foundation for developing policy interventions and healthcare strategies but also offer valuable information for addressing the changing dynamics of dementia in different populations [249, 250]. The burden of dementia is steadily rising, with expectations that it may become the leading cause of death in the near future, underscoring the urgency of understanding and addressing the challenges posed by this condition [24].

The association between dementia and mortality has been explored in diverse contexts, including its role as a risk factor for adverse outcomes in stroke patients, its influence on postoperative mortality in elderly individuals with hip fractures, and its predictive power in older adults with COVID-19, emphasizing the multifaceted impact of dementia on mortality across different health conditions and age groups [251–253]. Studies have also investigated the interaction of genetic factors like apolipoprotein E genotypes, lifestyle factors, and dementia-related mortality, revealing complex relationships that contribute to the overall risk profile of individuals affected by dementia [254].

### *11.6.2 Trends in Dementia Mortality*

Recent epidemiological studies have reported both declines and increases in dementia-related mortality rates, depending on the study population, time period, and methodological approaches [3, 255–258]. Some studies suggest a decline in dementia mortality, attributed to improved cardiovascular risk factor management, advancements in dementia care, and changes in diagnostic practices [255, 259]. However, other studies report an increase in dementia mortality, particularly among specific demographic groups or geographic regions, possibly due to population aging, increased awareness and diagnosis, and changing disease patterns [256–258, 260]. A study by Ssonko et al. in Cape Town, South Africa, underscored the dementia subtypes in predicting survival outcomes among older adults. This accentuates the potential implications of subtype-specific interventions in enhancing patient care and overall prognosis [261]. Additionally, research by Loi et al. and Dumurgier & Sabia et al. has explored variances in life expectancy based on dementia subtypes, emphasizing the need to examine how different subtypes influence mortality rates and overall prognosis [262, 263]. In young-onset dementia, Loi et al. (2023) demonstrated that all subtypes in this population were linked to increased mortality rates compared to the general population, emphasizing the necessity for specialized approaches in managing dementia across different age groups [262].

#### 11.6.2.1 Mortality of Alzheimer's Disease (AD)

AD, the most common dementia subtype, has shown lower mortality rates in comparison with other subtypes of dementia, potentially due to fewer cardiovascular risk factors or comorbidities [241, 264, 265]. Empirical data from Ganguli et al. (2005) suggested that AD is a leading cause of death and shortens life in elderly individuals, emphasizing the significant impact of AD on mortality rates [266]. Liang et al. conducted a systematic review and meta-analysis on mortality rates in AD and non-AD dementias, revealing that the mean survival time for individuals with AD after diagnosis was approximately 5.8 years [246]. Pharmacological and non-pharmacological treatments have contributed to improving the quality of life and potentially extending the lifespan of individuals with AD. Studies have explored the effects of AD medication on outcomes of mortality and hospitalization [267, 268]. Soysal et al. explored the impact of weight loss in individuals on mortality and hospitalization and found that weight loss increased mortality in patients with AD but not in DLB or VaD [269]. Understanding the association between nutritional status and mortality in AD could provide valuable insights into optimizing care for individuals with this condition. These studies highlight the multifaceted approach required to address the complexities of AD management and the importance of considering various factors that influence mortality rates in individuals with AD.

#### 11.6.2.2 Mortality of Vascular Dementia (VAD)

VaD mortality rates have remained relatively stable or even increased in certain populations, highlighting the need for targeted interventions to address vascular risk factors, including hypertension, diabetes, and stroke [241, 246, 270]. The stable or increasing mortality rates in VaD could be due to the complex interplay of vascular risk factors and their impact on the brain [271, 272]. Additionally, the heterogeneity of VaD, with various subtypes and underlying causes, may contribute to the varied mortality patterns observed in different populations [272]. One study by Wu et al. highlighted that age-adjusted mortality rates for VaD have shown an increase over time, with a twofold rise observed in certain populations. This trend underscores the growing impact of VaD on mortality rates and the need for targeted strategies to address the underlying vascular risk factors contributing to this trend [273]. In contrast, a study by Bo et al. examined mortality trends of Alzheimer's disease and other forms of dementia in China and found that while crude mortality from VaD increased from 2009 to 2015, age-standardized mortality decreased. Ding et al. reported increased standardized mortality ratio of VaD in recent 20 years in Shanghai [274]. This discrepancy suggests the importance of considering regional variations and demographic factors when analyzing mortality changes in VaD [275].

#### 11.6.2.3 Mortality of Dementia with Lewy Bodies (DLB)

DLB, although less prevalent than AD and VaD, has shown varying mortality patterns depending on the study population and methodological approaches [276, 277]. The morbidity and mortality associated with LBD are substantial, with frequent falls, infections, and autonomic dysfunction contributing to poor outcomes [278]. Some studies report higher mortality rates in DLB compared to AD, while others find no significant differences [277, 279]. The variability in DLB mortality may be attributed to differences in diagnostic criteria, study designs, and the complex interplay of Lewy body pathology with other neurodegenerative processes. Satiş et al. analyzed predictors of two-year mortality in patients with DLB, concluded malnutrition as the only independent predictor and mortality risks specific to DLB [280].

#### 11.6.2.4 Mortality of Frontotemporal Dementia (Ftd)

FTD, the least common among the major subtypes, also exhibits varying mortality patterns across studies [281]. The relatively low prevalence of FTD poses challenges in conducting large-scale epidemiological studies, leading to variations in findings [282]. Mortality rates in FTD are high due to rapid disease progression and lack of effective treatments [283]. Additionally, the heterogeneity of FTD subtypes, each with distinct clinical and pathological features, may contribute to the diverse mortality patterns observed. García-Ptacek et al., using data from the Swedish Dementia Registry (SveDem), concluded that individuals with FTD are associated with a particularly high mortality risk compared to patients with AD due to external causes (accidents and violent deaths) [282].

### *11.6.3 Changes of Morbidity in Patients with Dementia*

The patterns of morbidity in dementia are quite complex. Influenced by factors like chronic pain, disorientation, and infections that occur before the diagnosis. The presence of medical conditions alongside dementia significantly impacts the morbidity pattern. It is common for patients to have long-term conditions when diagnosed with dementia, which makes managing the disease more challenging and may even accelerate cognitive decline. One population-linked electronic health records study of 4.3 million individuals reveals that dementia patients are likely to have comorbid conditions and with approximately 66.3% of patients having two or more morbidities at the time of diagnosis, which may affect their health and the use of healthcare services. This study provides detailed insights into the prevalence of comorbid conditions such as obesity, hypertension, diabetes, and a range of other chronic diseases in individuals with dementia. Among this population, there is a frequency of primary care consultations related to chronic pain, indicating a significant burden on pain management for these patients. The study also reveals an increased incidence of hospital admissions due to urinary tract infections, disorientation, cerebral infarction, pneumonia, lower respiratory tract infections, syncope, collapse incidents, as well as pneumonitis caused by food or vomit among individuals with dementia [241]. Balasubramanian et al. highlighted the higher preoperative morbidity and overall complications in patients with dementia undergoing surgical procedures [284]. The implications of bone fractures in patients with dementia are also discussed as they contribute to higher morbidity rates [285]. Besides, a comprehensive study conducted in Finland indicated that the comorbidities associated with dementia have shifted from thyroid and psychiatric problems to cerebrovascular illness [286].

The use of advanced diagnostic tools, including neuroimaging and biomarkers, has significantly enhanced the early detection of dementia subtypes, leading to timely interventions that may slow disease progression and reduce morbidity. For instance, the incorporation of amyloid PET scans and cerebrospinal fluid biomarkers in the diagnostic process for Alzheimer's Disease (AD) has revolutionized the early and accurate identification of the condition [287, 288].

The development of disease-modifying therapies, particularly for AD, has the potential to alter the course of dementia. Drugs targeting amyloid-beta and tau proteins are in various stages of clinical trials [289]. While no cure exists, symptomatic treatments for cognitive and neuropsychiatric symptoms have improved patients' quality of life, potentially influencing morbidity trends [290].

Socioeconomic factors and healthcare infrastructure significantly impact dementia morbidity. Access to quality healthcare, social support systems, and public health initiatives plays a vital role in managing dementia and improving survival rates. Disparities in socioeconomic factors as well as medical comorbidities can also lead to variations in the diagnosis of dementia [291]. Besides, the impact of continuity of care on hospitalizations and healthcare costs for older adults with dementia has been studied, showing that higher continuity in outpatient visits is associated with lower healthcare costs and reduced hospitalizations [292]. Ensuring continuity of care for individuals with dementia can lead to better health outcomes and cost savings in the healthcare system. Disparities in healthcare utilization among people living with dementia have been observed, indicating the need to address social and spatial inequalities in healthcare access and delivery for this population [293]. Improving healthcare continuity, access to services, and treatment options can help reduce disparities and improve outcomes for individuals with dementia.

### 11.6.4 Challenges and Future Directions

*Heterogeneity in Disease Presentation*: The heterogeneity in clinical presentation and progression of dementia subtypes poses challenges for diagnosis and treatment. Personalized approaches considering genetic, molecular, and environmental factors are needed to address this variability.

*Need for Longitudinal Studies*: Longitudinal studies tracking dementia patients over time are essential for understanding the natural history of the disease and the long-term effects of interventions. Such studies can provide valuable insights into morbidity and mortality trends and inform future healthcare strategies.

*Integration of Technological Innovations*: Technological advancements, including artificial intelligence and machine learning, hold promise for improving dementia diagnosis, monitoring, and treatment. These innovations can enhance predictive models, optimize care delivery, and facilitate personalized interventions.

*Addressing Global Disparities*: Efforts to address global disparities in dementia care are critical. Initiatives to improve healthcare access, education, and support in low- and middle-income countries can help reduce the burden of dementia worldwide.

### *11.6.5 Conclusion*

Dementia remains a significant global health challenge, with evolving patterns of mortality and morbidity across different subtypes. Understanding these trends and their underlying mechanisms is crucial for developing effective prevention and treatment strategies. Continued research efforts, coupled with comprehensive public health interventions, are essential for improving the lives of individuals with dementia and their families. By addressing the complex interplay of genetic, environmental, and lifestyle factors, we can strive towards a future where dementia is no longer a leading cause of disability and mortality worldwide.

## References

1. GBD 2016 Dementia Collaborators. Global, regional, and national burden of Alzheimer's disease and other dementias, 1990-2016: a systematic analysis for the global burden of disease study 2016. Lancet Neurol. 2019;18(1):88–106. https://doi.org/10.1016/S1474-4422(18)30403-4.
2. World Health Organization. Global status report on the public health response to dementia. 2021. https://www.who.int/publications/i/item/9789240033245. Accessed 1 Sep 2021.
3. Prince M, Ali G-C, Guerchet M, Prina AM, Albanese E, Wu Y-T. Recent global trends in the prevalence and incidence of dementia, and survival with dementia. Alzheimers Res Ther. 2016;8(1):23. https://doi.org/10.1186/s13195-016-0188-8.
4. Brayne C, Stephan BC, Matthews FE. A European perspective on population studies of dementia. Alzheimers Dement. 2011;7(1):3–9. https://doi.org/10.1016/j.jalz.2010.12.003.
5. Hofman A, Rocca WA, Brayne C, Breteler MM, Clarke M, Cooper B, et al. The prevalence of dementia in Europe: a collaborative study of 1980-1990 findings. Eurodem Prevalence Research Group. Int J Epidemiol. 1991;20(3):736–48. https://doi.org/10.1093/ije/20.3.736.
6. World Health Organization and Alzheimer's Disease International. Dementia: a public health priority. 2012. https://www.who.int/publications/i/item/dementia-a-public-health-priority. Accessed 24 Aug 2012.

7. Prince M, Bryce R, Albanese E, Wimo A, Ribeiro W, Ferri CP. The global prevalence of dementia: a systematic review and metaanalysis. Alzheimers Dement. 2013;9(1):63–75 e2. https://doi.org/10.1016/j.jalz.2012.11.007.
8. Erkinjuntti T, Ostbye T, Steenhuis R, Hachinski V. The effect of different diagnostic criteria on the prevalence of dementia. N Engl J Med. 1997;337(23):1667–74. https://doi.org/10.1056/NEJM199712043372306.
9. Eysenck HJ. Meta-analysis and its problems. BMJ. 1994;309(6957):789–92. https://doi.org/10.1136/bmj.309.6957.789.
10. Wu YT, Beiser AS, Breteler MMB, Fratiglioni L, Helmer C, Hendrie HC, et al. The changing prevalence and incidence of dementia over time – current evidence. Nat Rev Neurol. 2017;13(6):327–39. https://doi.org/10.1038/nrneurol.2017.63.
11. Ahmadi-Abhari S, Guzman-Castillo M, Bandosz P, Shipley MJ, Muniz-Terrera G, Singh-Manoux A, et al. Temporal trend in dementia incidence since 2002 and projections for prevalence in England and Wales to 2040: modelling study. BMJ. 2017;358:j2856. https://doi.org/10.1136/bmj.j2856.
12. Li X, Feng X, Sun X, Hou N, Han F, Liu Y. Global, regional, and national burden of Alzheimer's disease and other dementias, 1990–2019. Front Aging Neurosci. 2022;14:937486. https://doi.org/10.3389/fnagi.2022.937486.
13. Gao S, Burney HN, Callahan CM, Purnell CE, Hendrie HC. Incidence of dementia and Alzheimer disease over time: a meta-analysis. J Am Geriatr Soc. 2019;67(7):1361–9. https://doi.org/10.1111/jgs.16027.
14. Wolters FJ, Chibnik LB, Waziry R, Anderson R, Berr C, Beiser A, et al. Twenty-seven-year time trends in dementia incidence in Europe and the United States: the Alzheimer Cohorts Consortium. Neurology. 2020;95(5):e519–31. https://doi.org/10.1212/WNL.0000000000010022.
15. Gao S, Ogunniyi A, Hall KS, Baiyewu O, Unverzagt FW, Lane KA, et al. Dementia incidence declined in African-Americans but not in Yoruba. Alzheimers Dement. 2016;12(3):244–51. https://doi.org/10.1016/j.jalz.2015.06.1894.
16. Li S, Yan F, Li G, Chen C, Zhang W, Liu J, et al. Is the dementia rate increasing in Beijing? Prevalence and incidence of dementia 10 years later in an urban elderly population. Acta Psychiatr Scand. 2007;115(1):73–9. https://doi.org/10.1111/j.1600-0447.2006.00859.x.
17. Schrijvers EM, Verhaaren BF, Koudstaal PJ, Hofman A, Ikram MA, Breteler MM. Is dementia incidence declining?: trends in dementia incidence since 1990 in the Rotterdam study. Neurology. 2012;78(19):1456–63. https://doi.org/10.1212/WNL.0b013e3182553be6.
18. Satizabal CL, Beiser AS, Chouraki V, Chêne G, Dufouil C, Seshadri S. Incidence of dementia over three decades in the Framingham Heart Study. N Engl J Med. 2016;374(6):523–32. https://doi.org/10.1056/NEJMoa1504327.
19. Matthews FE, Arthur A, Barnes LE, Bond J, Jagger C, Robinson L, et al. A two-decade comparison of prevalence of dementia in individuals aged 65 years and older from three geographical areas of England: results of the Cognitive Function and Ageing Study I and II. Lancet. 2013;382(9902):1405–12. https://doi.org/10.1016/S0140-6736(13)61570-6.
20. Lobo A, Saz P, Marcos G, Dia JL, De-la-Camara C, Ventura T, et al. Prevalence of dementia in a southern European population in two different time periods: the ZARADEMP Project. Acta Psychiatr Scand. 2007;116(4):299–307. https://doi.org/10.1111/j.1600-0447.2007.01006.x.
21. Pérès K, Brayne C, Matharan F, Grasset L, Helmer C, Letenneur L, et al. Trends in prevalence of dementia in French farmers from two epidemiological cohorts. J Am Geriatr Soc. 2017;65(2):415–20. https://doi.org/10.1111/jgs.14575.
22. Langa KM. Is the risk of Alzheimer's disease and dementia declining? Alzheimers Res Ther. 2015;7(1):34. https://doi.org/10.1186/s13195-015-0118-1.
23. Alzheimer's Disease International, Guerchet M, Prince M, Prina M. Numbers of people with dementia worldwide. 2020. https://www.alzint.org/resource/numbers-of-people-with-dementia-worldwide/. Accessed 30 Nov 2020.

24. Livingston G, Huntley J, Sommerlad A, Ames D, Ballard C, Banerjee S, et al. Dementia prevention, intervention, and care: 2020 report of the Lancet Commission. Lancet. 2020;396(10248):413–46. https://doi.org/10.1016/S0140-6736(20)30367-6.
25. Nakahori N, Sekine M, Yamada M, Tatsuse T, Kido H, Suzuki M. Future projections of the prevalence of dementia in Japan: results from the Toyama Dementia Survey. BMC Geriatr. 2021;21(1):602. https://doi.org/10.1186/s12877-021-02540-z.
26. Qiu C, von Strauss E, Bäckman L, Winblad B, Fratiglioni L. Twenty-year changes in dementia occurrence suggest decreasing incidence in Central Stockholm, Sweden. Neurology. 2013;80(20):1888–94. https://doi.org/10.1212/WNL.0b013e318292a2f9.
27. Wimo A, Sjölund BM, Sköldunger A, Qiu C, Klarin I, Nordberg G, et al. Cohort effects in the prevalence and survival of people with dementia in a rural area in Northern Sweden. J Alzheimers Dis. 2016;50(2):387–96. https://doi.org/10.3233/JAD-150708.
28. Sekita A, Ninomiya T, Tanizaki Y, Doi Y, Hata J, Yonemoto K, et al. Trends in prevalence of Alzheimer's disease and vascular dementia in a Japanese community: the Hisayama Study. Acta Psychiatr Scand. 2010;122(4):319-325. https://doi.org/10.1111/j.1600-0447.2010.01587.x.
29. Gu D, Andreev KF, Gerland P, Spoorenberg T, Li N, Heilig G. Old age mortality in Eastern and South-Eastern Asia. Demogr Res. 2013;29(38):999–1038. https://doi.org/10.4054/DemRes.2013.29.38.
30. Xia X, Wang Y, Zheng J. COVID-19 and Alzheimer's disease: how one crisis worsens the other. Transl Neurodegener. 2021;10(1):15. https://doi.org/10.1186/s40035-021-00237-2.
31. Suárez-González A LG, Low LF, Cahill S, Hennelly N, Dawson WD, Weidner W, Bocchetta M, Ferri CP, Matias-Guiu JA, Alladi S, Musyimi CW, Comas-Herrera A. Impact and mortality of COVID-19 on people living with dementia: cross-country report. 2020. https://pdxscholar.library.pdx.edu/aging_pub/66/. Accessed 19 Aug 2020.
32. Low LF, Anstey KJ. Dementia literacy: recognition and beliefs on dementia of the Australian public. Alzheimers Dement. 2009;5(1):43–9. https://doi.org/10.1016/j.jalz.2008.03.011.
33. Lo RY. Uncertainty and health literacy in dementia care. Tzu Chi Med J. 2020;32(1):14–8. https://doi.org/10.4103/tcmj.tcmj_116_19.
34. Alzheimer's Disease International, Mittelman M, Batsch N. World Alzheimer Report 2012 overcoming the stigma of dementia. 2012. https://www.alzint.org/resource/world-alzheimer-report-2012/. Accessed 21 Sep 2012.
35. Alzheimer's Disease International. World Alzheimer Report 2019 Attitudes to dementia. 2019. https://www.alzint.org/resource/world-alzheimer-report-2019/. Accessed 20 Sep 2019.
36. Canadian Academy of Health Sciences. Improving the quality of life and care of persons living with dementia and their caregivers. Ottawa: The Expert Panel on Dementia Care in Canada, Canadian Academy of Health Sciences; 2019.
37. Bacsu JD, et al. Stigma reduction interventions of dementia: a scoping review. Can J Aging. 2022;41(2):203–13. https://doi.org/10.1017/S0714980821000192.
38. Anderson LA, et al. The public's perceptions about cognitive health and Alzheimer's disease among the U.S. population: a national review. Gerontologist. 2009;49 Suppl 1:S3–11. https://doi.org/10.1093/geront/gnp088.
39. Budin-Ljosne I, et al. Public perceptions of brain health: an international, online cross-sectional survey. BMJ Open. 2022;12(4):e057999. https://doi.org/10.1136/bmjopen-2021-057999.
40. Curran E, et al. General population perspectives of dementia risk reduction and the implications for intervention: A systematic review and thematic synthesis of qualitative evidence. PLoS One. 2021;16(9):e0257540. https://doi.org/10.1371/journal.pone.0257540.
41. Alzheimer's Disease International. World Alzheimer Report 2023 Reducing dementia risk: never too early, never too late. 2023. https://www.alzint.org/resource/world-alzheimer-report-2023/. Accessed 21 Sep 2023.
42. World Health Organization. Global action plan on the public health response to dementia 2017–2025. 2017. https://www.who.int/publications/i/item/global-action-plan-on-the-public-health-response-to-dementia-2017%2D%2D-2025. Accessed 7 Dec 2017.

43. Wright T, O'Connor S. Reviewing challenges and gaps in European and global dementia policy. J Public Ment Health. 2018;17(4):157–67. https://doi.org/10.1108/JPMH-02-2018-0012.
44. World Health Organization. The Global Health Observatory. 2023. https://www.who.int/data/gho/data/themes/global-dementia-observatory-gdo. Accessed 30 Dec 2023.
45. Mukadam N, et al. Diagnostic rates and treatment of dementia before and after launch of a national dementia policy: an observational study using English national databases. BMJ Open. 2014;4(1):e004119. https://doi.org/10.1136/bmjopen-2013-004119.
46. Jhang KM, et al. A 12-year comparison of Alzheimer's dementia patients with their informants in Taiwan. Am J Alzheimers Dis Other Dement. 2023;38:15333175231218089. https://doi.org/10.1177/15333175231218089.
47. Tokovska M, et al. Informal caregivers and psychosocial support: analysis of European Dementia Policy documents. J Public Health Res. 2021;11(1):2416. https://doi.org/10.4081/jphr.2021.2416.
48. Hung L, et al. Creating dementia-friendly communities for social inclusion: a scoping review. Gerontol Geriatr Med. 2021;7:23337214211013596. https://doi.org/10.1177/23337214211013596.
49. Larson EB, Wang L, Bowen JD, McCormick WC, Teri L, Crane P, et al. Exercise is associated with reduced risk for incident dementia among persons 65 years of age and older. Ann Intern Med. 2006;144(2):73–81. https://doi.org/10.7326/0003-4819-144-2-200601170-00004.
50. Marioni RE, Proust-Lima C, Amieva H, Brayne C, Matthews FE, Dartigues J-F, et al. Social activity, cognitive decline and dementia risk: a 20-year prospective cohort study. BMC Public Health. 2015;15(1):1089. https://doi.org/10.1186/s12889-015-2426-6.
51. Pringle J, Jepson R, Dawson A, McCabe L, Bowes A. How does physical activity benefit people living with dementia? A systematic review to identify the potential mechanisms of action. Quality Ageing Older Adults. 2021;22(1):3–25.
52. World Health Organization. Global status report on physical activity 2022. 2022. https://www.who.int/publications/i/item/9789240059153. Accessed 19 Oct 2022.
53. Guthold R, Stevens GA, Riley LM, Bull FC. Worldwide trends in insufficient physical activity from 2001 to 2016: a pooled analysis of 358 population-based surveys with 1.9 million participants. Lancet Glob Health. 2018;6(10):e1077–86. https://doi.org/10.1016/S2214-109X(18)30357-7.
54. de Crom TOE, Mooldijk SS, Ikram MK, Ikram MA, Voortman T. MIND diet and the risk of dementia: a population-based study. Alzheimers Res Ther. 2022;14(1):8. https://doi.org/10.1186/s13195-022-00957-1.
55. Conlin PR. The dietary approaches to stop hypertension (DASH) clinical trial: implications for lifestyle modifications in the treatment of hypertensive patients. Cardiol Rev. 1999;7(5):284–8. https://doi.org/10.1097/00045415-199909000-00013.
56. Morris MC, Tangney CC, Wang Y, Sacks FM, Barnes LL, Bennett DA, et al. MIND diet slows cognitive decline with aging. Alzheimers Dement. 2015;11(9):1015–22. https://doi.org/10.1016/j.jalz.2015.04.011.
57. van den Brink AC, Brouwer-Brolsma EM, Berendsen AAM, van de Rest O. The Mediterranean, Dietary Approaches to Stop Hypertension (DASH), and Mediterranean-DASH Intervention for Neurodegenerative Delay (MIND) diets are associated with less cognitive decline and a lower risk of Alzheimer's disease – a review. Adv Nutr. 2019;10(6):1040–65. https://doi.org/10.1093/advances/nmz054.
58. Chang Y, Thornton V, Chaloemtoem A, Anokhin AP, Bijsterbosch J, Bogdan R, et al. Investigating the relationship between smoking behavior and global brain volume. Biol Psychiatry Glob Open Sci. 2023;4(1):74–82. https://doi.org/10.1016/j.bpsgos.2023.09.006.
59. Hahad O, Daiber A, Michal M, Kuntic M, Lieb K, Beutel M, et al. Smoking and neuropsychiatric disease—associations and underlying mechanisms. Int J Mol Sci. 2021;22(14):7272. https://doi.org/10.3390/ijms22147272.

60. McKenzie J BL, Tursan d'Espaignet E. WHO tobacco knowledge summaries: tobacco use and dementia. 2014. https://www.who.int/publications/i/item/WHO-NMH-PND-CIC-TKS-14.1. Accessed 8 Jul 2014.
61. National Center for Chronic Disease Prevention and Health Promotion (US) Office on Smoking and Health. (2014) The health consequences of smoking—50 years of progress: a report of the surgeon general. Atlanta (GA): Centers for Disease Control and Prevention (US); 2, Fifty Years of Change 1964–2014.
62. Current Cigarette Smoking Among Adults in the United States. Available from: https://www.cdc.gov/tobacco/data_statistics/fact_sheets/adult_data/cig_smoking/index.htm.
63. Anstey KJ, Mack HA, Cherbuin N. Alcohol consumption as a risk factor for dementia and cognitive decline: meta-analysis of prospective studies. Am J Geriatr Psychiatry. 2009;17(7):542–55. https://doi.org/10.1097/JGP.0b013e3181a2fd07.
64. Wiegmann C, Mick I, Brandl EJ, Heinz A, Gutwinski S. Alcohol and dementia—what is the link? A systematic review. Neuropsychiatric Dis Treat. 2020;16:87–99. https://doi.org/10.2147/NDT.S198772.
65. Jorm AF. History of depression as a risk factor for dementia: an updated review. Aust N Z J Psychiatry. 2001;35(6):776–81. https://doi.org/10.1046/j.1440-1614.2001.00967.x.
66. Brommelhoff JA, Gatz M, Johansson B, McArdle JJ, Fratiglioni L, Pedersen NL. Depression as a risk factor or prodromal feature for dementia? Findings in a population-based sample of Swedish twins. Psychol Aging. 2009;24(2):373–84. https://doi.org/10.1037/a0015713.
67. Kitching D. Depression in dementia. Aust Prescr. 2015;38(6):209–2011. https://doi.org/10.18773/austprescr.2015.071.
68. Dykxhoorn J, Gnani S, Kirkbride JB, Lazzarino AI, Osborn D, Walters K. Temporal patterns in the recorded annual incidence of common mental disorders over two decades in the United Kingdom: a primary care cohort study. Psychol Med. 2024;54(4):663–74. https://doi.org/10.1017/S0033291723002349.
69. Su Q, Liu G. Depression in Chinese adolescents from 1989 to 2018: an increasing trend and its relationship with social environments. Curr Psychol. 2022;41(10):6966–77. https://doi.org/10.1007/s12144-020-01181-6.
70. Nagai M, Hoshide S, Kario K. Hypertension and dementia. Am J Hypertens. 2010;23(2):116–24. https://doi.org/10.1038/ajh.2009.212.
71. Lennon MJ, Makkar SR, Crawford JD, Sachdev PS. Midlife hypertension and Alzheimer's disease: a systematic review and meta-analysis. J Alzheimers Dis. 2019;71(1):307–16.
72. Lennon MJ, Lam BCP, Lipnicki DM, Crawford JD, Peters R, Schutte AE, et al. Use of antihypertensives, blood pressure, and estimated risk of dementia in late life: an individual participant data meta-analysis. JAMA Netw Open. 2023;6(9):e2333353. https://doi.org/10.1001/jamanetworkopen.2023.33353.
73. Tadic M, Cuspidi C, Hering D. Hypertension and cognitive dysfunction in elderly: blood pressure management for this global burden. BMC Cardiovasc Disord. 2016;16(1):208. https://doi.org/10.1186/s12872-016-0386-0.
74. van Dalen JW, Brayne C, Crane PK, Fratiglioni L, Larson EB, Lobo A, et al. Association of systolic blood pressure with dementia risk and the role of age, U-shaped associations, and mortality. JAMA Intern Med. 2022;182(2):142–52. https://doi.org/10.1001/jamainternmed.2021.7009.
75. World Health Organization. Global report on hypertension: the race against a silent killer. 2023. https://www.who.int/publications/i/item/9789240081062. Accessed 19 Sep 2023.
76. Collaboration NCDRF. Worldwide trends in hypertension prevalence and progress in treatment and control from 1990 to 2019: a pooled analysis of 1201 population-representative studies with 104 million participants. Lancet. 2021;398(10304):957–80. https://doi.org/10.1016/S0140-6736(21)01330-1.
77. Barbiellini Amidei C, Fayosse A, Dumurgier J, Machado-Fragua MD, Tabak AG, van Sloten T, et al. (2021) association between age at diabetes onset and subsequent risk of dementia. JAMA. 2021;325(16):1640–9. https://doi.org/10.1001/jama.2021.4001.

78. Gudala K, Bansal D, Schifano F, Bhansali A. (2013) diabetes mellitus and risk of dementia: A meta-analysis of prospective observational studies. J Diabetes Investig. 2013;4(6):640–50. https://doi.org/10.1111/jdi.12087.
79. Zhang S, Xue R, Hu R. The neuroprotective effect and action mechanism of polyphenols in diabetes mellitus-related cognitive dysfunction. Eur J Nutr. 2020;59(4):1295–311. https://doi.org/10.1007/s00394-019-02078-2.
80. Bello-Chavolla OY, Antonio-Villa NE, Vargas-Vazquez A, Avila-Funes JA, Aguilar-Salinas CA. Pathophysiological mechanisms linking type 2 diabetes and dementia: review of evidence from clinical, translational and epidemiological research. Curr Diabetes Rev. 2019;15(6):456–70. https://doi.org/10.2174/1573399815666190129155654.
81. Husain KH, Sarhan SF, AlKhalifa H, Buhasan A, Moin ASM, Butler AE. Dementia in diabetes: the role of Hypoglycemia. Int J Mol Sci. 2023;24(12):9846. https://doi.org/10.3390/ijms24129846.
82. World Health Organization. Global report on diabetes. 2016. https://www.who.int/publications/i/item/9789241565257. Accessed 21 Apr 2016.
83. Magliano DJ, Islam RM, Barr ELM, Gregg EW, Pavkov ME, Harding JL, et al. Trends in incidence of total or type 2 diabetes: systematic review. BMJ. 2019;366:l5003. https://doi.org/10.1136/bmj.l5003.
84. Centers for Disease Control and Prevention. National Diabetes Statistics Report. https://www.cdc.gov/diabetes/php/data-research/index.html. Accessed 15 May 2024.
85. Collaborators GBDHL. Hearing loss prevalence and years lived with disability, 1990–2019: findings from the Global Burden of Disease Study 2019. Lancet. 2021;397(10278):996–1009. https://doi.org/10.1016/S0140-6736(21)00516-X.
86. Curhan G, Curhan S. Epidemiology of hearing impairment. In: Popelka GR, Moore BCJ, Fay RR, Popper AN, editors. Hearing aids. Cham: Springer; 2016. p. 21–58.
87. Yeo BSY, Song HJJMD, Toh EMS, Ng LS, Ho CSH, Ho R, et al. Association of hearing aids and cochlear implants with cognitive decline and dementia: a systematic review and meta-analysis. JAMA Neurol. 2023;80(2):134–41. https://doi.org/10.1001/jamaneurol.2022.4427.
88. Varma VR, Wang Y, An Y, Varma S, Bilgel M, Doshi J, et al. Bile acid synthesis, modulation, and dementia: a metabolomic, transcriptomic, and pharmacoepidemiologic study. PLoS Med. 2021;18(5):e1003615. https://doi.org/10.1371/journal.pmed.1003615.
89. ElAli A, Doeppner TR, Zechariah A, Hermann DM. Increased blood-brain barrier permeability and brain edema after focal cerebral ischemia induced by hyperlipidemia: role of lipid peroxidation and calpain-1/2, matrix metalloproteinase-2/9, and RhoA overactivation. Stroke. 2011;42(11):3238–44. https://doi.org/10.1161/STROKEAHA.111.615559.
90. Fratti RA. Editorial: effects of membrane lipids on protein function. Front Cell Dev Biol. 2021;9:675264. https://doi.org/10.3389/fcell.2021.675264.
91. Rudajev V, Novotny J. Cholesterol-dependent amyloid β production: space for multifarious interactions between amyloid precursor protein, secretases, and cholesterol. Cell Biosci. 2023;13(1):171. https://doi.org/10.1186/s13578-023-01127-y.
92. Dunk MM, Li J, Liu S, Casanova R, Chen JC, Espeland MA, et al. Associations of dietary cholesterol and fat, blood lipids, and risk for dementia in older women vary by APOE genotype. Alzheimers Dement. 2023;19(12):5742–54. https://doi.org/10.1002/alz.13358.
93. World Health Organization. Report of the Formal Meeting of Member States to conclude the work on the comprehensive global monitoring framework, including indicators, and a set of voluntary global targets for the prevention and control of communicable diseases. 2012. https://apps.who.int/gb/NCDs/pdf/A_NCD_2-en.pdf. Accessed 5–7 Nov 2012.
94. Li Z, Zhu G, Chen G, Luo M, Liu X, Chen Z, et al. Distribution of lipid levels and prevalence of hyperlipidemia: data from the NHANES 2007–2018. Lipids Health Dis. 2022;21(1):111. https://doi.org/10.1186/s12944-022-01721-y.
95. Sommerlad A, Liu KY. Air pollution and dementia. BMJ. 2023;381:655. https://doi.org/10.1136/bmj.p655.

96. Hahad O, Lelieveld J, Birklein F, Lieb K, Daiber A, Münzel T. Ambient air pollution increases the risk of cerebrovascular and neuropsychiatric disorders through induction of inflammation and oxidative stress. Int J Mol Sci. 2020;21(12):4306. https://doi.org/10.3390/ijms21124306.
97. Wang J, Ma T, Ma D, Li H, Hua L, He Q, et al. The impact of air pollution on neurodegenerative diseases. Ther Drug Monit. 2021;43(1):69–78. https://doi.org/10.1097/FTD.0000000000000818.
98. Greve HJ, Dunbar AL, Lombo CG, Ahmed C, Thang M, Messenger EJ, et al. The bidirectional lung brain-axis of amyloid-β pathology: ozone dysregulates the peri-plaque microenvironment. Brain. 2022;146(3):991–1005. https://doi.org/10.1093/brain/awac113.
99. Kurokawa J, Ohara T. Long-term historical trends in air pollutant emissions in Asia: regional emission inventory in ASia (REAS) version 3. Atmos Chem Phys. 2020;20(21):12761–93. https://doi.org/10.5194/acp-20-12761-2020.
100. Hung C-w, Shih M-F. Air quality changes in Taiwan over the past decades and during the COVID-19 crisis. Terr Atmos Ocean Sci. 2023;34(1):5. https://doi.org/10.1007/s44195-023-00036-4.
101. Bakola M, Hernandez Carballo I, Jelastopulu E, Stuckler D. The impact of COVID-19 lockdown on air pollution in Europe and North America: a systematic review. Eur J Pub Health. 2022;32(6):962–8. https://doi.org/10.1093/eurpub/ckac118.
102. Kornblith E, Peltz CB, Xia F, Plassman B, Novakovic-Apopain T, Yaffe K. Sex, race, and risk of dementia diagnosis after traumatic brain injury among older veterans. Neurology. 2020;95(13):e1768–e75. https://doi.org/10.1212/WNL.0000000000010617.
103. Barnes DE, Byers AL, Gardner RC, Seal KH, Boscardin WJ, Yaffe K. (2018) Association of Mild Traumatic Brain Injury with and without loss of consciousness with dementia in US Military Veterans. JAMA Neurol. 2018;75(9):1055–61. https://doi.org/10.1001/jamaneurol.2018.0815.
104. Maas AIR, Fitzgerald M, Gao G, Gupta D, Hutchinson P, Manley GT, et al. Traumatic brain injury over the past 20 years: research and clinical progress. Lancet Neurol. 2022;21(9):768–70. https://doi.org/10.1016/S1474-4422(22)00307-6.
105. Bramlett HM, Dietrich WD. Long-term consequences of traumatic Brain injury: current status of potential mechanisms of injury and neurological outcomes. J Neurotrauma. 2015;32(23):1834–48. https://doi.org/10.1089/neu.2014.3352.
106. Lynch DG, Narayan RK, Li C. Multi-mechanistic approaches to the treatment of traumatic Brain injury: a review. J Clin Med. 2023;12(6):2179. https://doi.org/10.3390/jcm12062179.
107. EClipSE Collaborative Members, Brayne C, Ince PG, Keage HAD, McKeith IG, Matthews FE, Polvikoski T, et al. Education, the brain and dementia: neuroprotection or compensation? Brain. 2010;133(8):2210–2216. https://doi.org/10.1093/brain/awq185.
108. Meng X, D'Arcy C. Education and dementia in the context of the cognitive reserve hypothesis: a systematic review with meta-analyses and qualitative analyses. PLoS One. 2012;7(6):e38268. https://doi.org/10.1371/journal.pone.0038268.
109. Chen Y, Lv C, Li X, Zhang J, Chen K, Liu Z, et al. The positive impacts of early-life education on cognition, leisure activity, and brain structure in healthy aging. Aging (Albany NY). 2019;11(14):4923–42. https://doi.org/10.18632/aging.102088.
110. OECD. How have schools changed over the past decade? 2015. https://www.oecd-ilibrary.org/education/how-have-schools-changed-over-the-past-decade_5js04vz2cf9q-en. Accessed 1 Jun 2015.
111. OECD. Education at a Glance 2023. 2023. https://www.oecd.org/education/education-at-a-glance/. Accessed 12 Sep 2023.
112. Treiber KA, Carlson MC, Corcoran C, Norton MC, Breitner JCS, Piercy KW, et al. Cognitive stimulation and cognitive and functional decline in Alzheimer's disease: the Cache County Dementia Progression Study. J Gerontol Series B. 2011;66B(4):416–25. https://doi.org/10.1093/geronb/gbr023.

113. Kivimäki M, Walker KA, Pentti J, Nyberg ST, Mars N, Vahtera J, et al. Cognitive stimulation in the workplace, plasma proteins, and risk of dementia: three analyses of population cohort studies. BMJ. 2021;374:n1804. https://doi.org/10.1136/bmj.n1804.
114. Butterworth M, Davies S, Orrell M, Royan L, Spector A, Thorgrimsen L, et al. Efficacy of an evidence-based cognitive stimulation therapy programme for people with dementia: randomised controlled trial. Br J Psychiatry. 2003;183(3):248–54. https://doi.org/10.1192/bjp.183.3.248.
115. Blackwell SE. Mental imagery in the science and practice of cognitive behaviour therapy: past, present, and future perspectives. Int J Cogn Ther. 2021;14(1):160–81. https://doi.org/10.1007/s41811-021-00102-0.
116. World Health Organization. Risk reduction of cognitive decline and dementia: WHO guidelines. 2019. https://www.who.int/publications/i/item/9789241550543. Accessed 1 Jan 2019.
117. Liu C-C, Sun Y, Kung S-F, Kuo H-W, Huang N-C, Li C-Y, et al. Effects of physical and social environments on the risk of dementia among Taiwanese older adults: a population-based case-control study. BMC Geriatr. 2020;20(1):226. https://doi.org/10.1186/s12877-020-01624-6.
118. Kannan VD, Veazie PJ. US trends in social isolation, social engagement, and companionship - nationally and by age, sex, race/ethnicity, family income, and work hours, 2003–2020. SSM Popul Health. 2023;21:101331. https://doi.org/10.1016/j.ssmph.2022.101331.
119. Wang L, Yan Z, Yang X, Yu L, Zhao Y. Social change and birth cohort increase in loneliness among Chinese older adults: a cross-temporal meta-analysis, 1995–2011. Int Psychogeriatr. 2014;26(11):1773–81. https://doi.org/10.1017/S1041610214000921.
120. Ang S. Internet use and cohort change in social connectedness among older adults. Adv Life Course Res. 2022;54:100514. https://doi.org/10.1016/j.alcr.2022.100514.
121. Dulewicz M, Kulczyńska-Przybik A, Mroczko P, Kornhuber J, Lewczuk P, Mroczko B. Biomarkers for the diagnosis of Alzheimer's disease in clinical practice: the role of CSF biomarkers during the evolution of diagnostic criteria. Int J Mol Sci. 2022;23(15):8598. https://doi.org/10.3390/ijms23158598.
122. Niemantsverdriet E, Feyen B, Bastard NL, et al. Added diagnostic value of cerebrospinal fluid biomarkers for differential dementia diagnosis in an autopsy-confirmed cohort. J Alzheimers Dis. 2018;63(1):373–81. https://doi.org/10.3233/jad-170927.
123. Latimer JE, Hillman A. Biomarkers and brains: situating dementia in the laboratory and in the memory clinic. New Genetics Soc. 2019;39(1):80–100. https://doi.org/10.1080/14636778.2019.1652804.
124. Fortea J, García-Arcelay E, Terrancle Á, et al. Attitudes of neurologists toward the use of biomarkers in the diagnosis of early Alzheimer's disease. J Alzheimer Dis. 2023;93(1):275–82. https://doi.org/10.3233/jad-221160.
125. Schindler SE. Fluid Biomarkers in Dementia Diagnosis. Continuum (Minneap Minn). 2022;28(3):822–33. https://doi.org/10.1212/con.0000000000001083.
126. Moniruzzaman M, Kadota A, Akash MS, et al. Effects of physical activities on dementia-related biomarkers: A systematic review of randomized controlled trials. Alzheimers Dementia Translat Res Clin Intervent. 2020;6(1):e12109. https://doi.org/10.1002/trc2.12109.
127. Maclin JMA, Wang T, Xiao S. Biomarkers for the diagnosis of Alzheimer's disease, dementia Lewy body, frontotemporal dementia and vascular dementia. Gen Psychiatr. 2019;32(1):e100054. https://doi.org/10.1136/gpsych-2019-100054.
128. Ruan Q, D'Onofrio G, Sancarlo D, Bao Z, Greco A, Yu Z. Potential neuroimaging biomarkers of pathologic Brain changes in mild cognitive impairment and Alzheimer's disease: a systematic review. BMC Geriatr. 2016;16:104. https://doi.org/10.1186/s12877-016-0281-7.
129. McKhann GM, Knopman DS, Chertkow H, et al. The diagnosis of dementia due to Alzheimer's disease: recommendations from the National Institute on Aging-Alzheimer's Association Workgroups on Diagnostic Guidelines for Alzheimer's Disease. Alzheimers Dement. 2011;7(3):263–9. https://doi.org/10.1016/j.jalz.2011.03.005.
130. Sperling RA, Aisen PS, Beckett LA, et al. Toward defining the preclinical stages of Alzheimer's disease: recommendations from the National Institute on Aging-Alzheimer's

Association Workgroups on Diagnostic Guidelines for Alzheimer's Disease. Alzheimers Dement. 2011;7(3):280–92. https://doi.org/10.1016/j.jalz.2011.03.003.
131. Jia J, Ning Y, Chen M, et al. Biomarker changes during 20 years preceding Alzheimer's disease. N Engl J Med. 2024;390(8):712–22. https://doi.org/10.1056/NEJMoa2310168.
132. McKhann G, Drachman D, Folstein M, Katzman R, Price D, Stadlan EM. Clinical diagnosis of Alzheimer's disease: report of the NINCDS-ADRDA Work Group under the auspices of Department of Health and Human Services Task Force on Alzheimer's Disease. Neurology. 1984;34(7):939–44. https://doi.org/10.1212/wnl.34.7.939.
133. Jack CR Jr, Bennett DA, Blennow K, et al. A/T/N: An unbiased descriptive classification scheme for Alzheimer disease biomarkers. Neurology. 2016;87(5):539–47. https://doi.org/10.1212/wnl.0000000000002923.
134. Pascoal TA, Leuzy A, Therriault J, et al. Discriminative accuracy of the a/T/N scheme to identify cognitive impairment due to Alzheimer's disease. Alzheimer Dement (AMST). 2023;15(1):e12390. https://doi.org/10.1002/dad2.12390.
135. Tan M-S, Ji X, Li J, et al. Longitudinal trajectories of Alzheimer's ATN biomarkers in elderly persons without dementia. Alzheimer S Res Ther. 2020;12(1):55. https://doi.org/10.1186/s13195-020-00621-6.
136. Struyfs H, Niemantsverdriet E, Goossens J, et al. Cerebrospinal fluid P-Tau181P: biomarker for improved differential dementia diagnosis. Front Neurol. 2015;6:138. https://doi.org/10.3389/fneur.2015.00138.
137. Fagan AM, Roe CM, Xiong C, Mintun MA, Morris JC, Holtzman DM. Cerebrospinal fluid tau/B-Amyloid42 ratio as a prediction of cognitive decline in nondemented older adults. Arch Neurol. 2007;64(3):343–9. https://doi.org/10.1001/archneur.64.3.noc60123.
138. Thijssen EH, La Joie R, Strom A, et al. Plasma phosphorylated tau 217 and phosphorylated tau 181 as biomarkers in Alzheimer's disease and frontotemporal lobar degeneration: a retrospective diagnostic performance study. Lancet Neurolo. 2021;20(9):739–52. https://doi.org/10.1016/S1474-4422(21)00214-3.
139. Jack CR Jr, Bennett DA, Blennow K, et al. NIA-AA Research Framework: toward a biological definition of Alzheimer's disease. Alzheimers Dement. 2018;14(4):535–62. https://doi.org/10.1016/j.jalz.2018.02.018.
140. AAIC. Discoveries propel Alzheimer's diagnosis and clinical care. Alzheimers Dement. 2023;19(10):4772–8. https://doi.org/10.1002/alz.13487.
141. Rittman T. Neurological update: neuroimaging in dementia. J Neurol. 2020;267(11):3429–35. https://doi.org/10.1007/s00415-020-10040-0.
142. Fox NC, Freeborough PA, Rossor MN. Visualisation and quantification of rates of atrophy in Alzheimer's disease. Lancet. 1996;348(9020):94–7. https://doi.org/10.1016/S0140-6736(96)05228-2.
143. Rohrer JD, Nicholas JM, Cash DM, et al. Presymptomatic cognitive and neuroanatomical changes in genetic frontotemporal dementia in the Genetic Frontotemporal dementia Initiative (GENFI) study: a cross-sectional analysis. Lancet Neurol. 2015;14(3):253–62. https://doi.org/10.1016/S1474-4422(14)70324-2.
144. Tondelli M, Wilcock GK, Nichelli P, De Jager CA, Jenkinson M, Zamboni G. Structural MRI changes detectable up to ten years before clinical Alzheimer's disease. Neurobiol Aging. 2012;33(4):825.e25–36. https://doi.org/10.1016/j.neurobiolaging.2011.05.018.
145. Neto AS, Coutinho AM. From clinical phenotype to proteinopathy: molecular neuroimaging in neurodegenerative dementias. Arq Neuropsiquiatr. 2022;80(5 Suppl 1):24–35. https://doi.org/10.1590/0004-282x-anp-2022-s138.
146. Bullmore E, Sporns O. Complex brain networks: graph theoretical analysis of structural and functional systems. Nat Rev Neurosci. 2009;10(3):186–98. https://doi.org/10.1038/nrn2575.
147. Ossenkoppele R, Iaccarino L, Schonhaut DR, et al. Tau covariance patterns in Alzheimer's disease patients match intrinsic connectivity networks in the healthy brain. NeuroImage: Clinical. 2019;23:101848. https://doi.org/10.1016/j.nicl.2019.101848.

148. Mueller SG, Weiner MW, Thal LJ, et al. The Alzheimer's disease neuroimaging initiative. Neuroimaging Clin N Am. 2005;15(4):869–77. https://doi.org/10.1016/j.nic.2005.09.008.
149. Hainc N, Federau C, Stieltjes B, Blatow M, Bink A, Stippich C. The Bright, artificial intelligence-augmented future of neuroimaging reading. Front Neurol. 2017;8:489. https://doi.org/10.3389/fneur.2017.00489.
150. Fisher CK, Smith AM, Walsh JR, et al. Machine learning for comprehensive forecasting of Alzheimer's disease progression. Sci Rep. 2019;9(1):13622. https://doi.org/10.1038/s41598-019-49656-2.
151. Archetti D, Ingala S, Venkatraghavan V, et al. Multi-study validation of data-driven disease progression models to characterize evolution of biomarkers in Alzheimer's disease. NeuroImage: Clinical. 2019;24:101954. https://doi.org/10.1016/j.nicl.2019.101954.
152. Avberšek LK, Repovš G. Deep learning in neuroimaging data analysis: applications, challenges, and solutions. Front Neuroimaging. 2022;1:981642. https://doi.org/10.3389/fnimg.2022.981642.
153. Thomas AW, Heekeren HR, Müller KR, Samek W. Analyzing neuroimaging data through recurrent deep learning models. Front Neurosci. 2019;13:1321. https://doi.org/10.3389/fnins.2019.01321.
154. Feng X, Provenzano FA, Small SA. A deep learning MRI approach outperforms other biomarkers of prodromal Alzheimer's disease. Alzheimer Res Ther. 2022;14(1):45. https://doi.org/10.1186/s13195-022-00985-x.
155. Trares K, Bhardwaj M, Perna L, et al. Association of the Inflammation-Related Proteome with Dementia Development at older age: results from a large, prospective, population-based cohort study. Alzheimers Res Ther. 2022;14(1):128. https://doi.org/10.1186/s13195-022-01063-y.
156. Ferreira D, Jelić V, Cavallin L, et al. Electroencephalography is a good complement to currently established dementia biomarkers. Dement Geriatr Cogn Disord. 2016;42(1–2):80–92. https://doi.org/10.1159/000448394.
157. Al-nuaimi AH, Jammeh E, Sun L, Ifeachor E. Changes in the EEG amplitude as a biomarker for early detection of Alzheimer's disease. Annu Int Conf IEEE Eng Med Biol Soc. 2016;2016:993–6. https://doi.org/10.1109/EMBC.2016.7590869.
158. Zetterberg H, Swieten JC, Boxer AL, Rohrer JD. Review: fluid biomarkers for frontotemporal dementias. Neuropathol Appl Neurobiol. 2018;45(1):81–7. https://doi.org/10.1111/nan.12530.
159. Ding W, Ren P, Yi L, et al. Association of cortical and subcortical microstructure with disease severity: impact on cognitive decline and language impairments in frontotemporal lobar degeneration. Alzheimers Res Ther. 2023;15(1):58. https://doi.org/10.1186/s13195-023-01208-7.
160. Goldman JG, Forsberg LK, Boeve BF, et al. Challenges and opportunities for improving the landscape for Lewy body dementia clinical trials. Alzheimers Res Ther. 2020;12(1):137. https://doi.org/10.1186/s13195-020-00703-5.
161. Russo C, Valle MS, Casabona A, Malaguarnera L. Chitinase signature in the plasticity of neurodegenerative diseases. Int J Mol Sci. 2023;24(7). https://doi.org/10.3390/ijms24076301.
162. Abdelmoaty MM, Lu E, Kadry R, et al. Clinical biomarkers for Lewy body diseases. Cell Biosci. 2023;13(1):209. https://doi.org/10.1186/s13578-023-01152-x.
163. Chen H-H, Petty LE, Sha J, et al. Genetically regulated expression in late-onset Alzheimer's disease implicates risk genes within known and novel loci. Transl Psychiatry. 2021;11(1):618. https://doi.org/10.1038/s41398-021-01677-0.
164. Walker Z, Possin KL, Boeve BF, Aarsland D. Lewy body dementias. Lancet. 2015;386(10004):1683–97. https://doi.org/10.1016/s0140-6736(15)00462-6.
165. Schmidt CM, Redyk K, Meissner B, et al. Clinical features of rapidly progressive Alzheimer's disease. Dement Geriatri Cogn Disord. 2010;29(4):371–8. https://doi.org/10.1159/000278692.

166. Katzeff JS, Bright F, Phan K, et al. Biomarker discovery and development for frontotemporal dementia and amyotrophic lateral sclerosis. Brain. 2022;145(5):1598–609. https://doi.org/10.1093/brain/awac077.
167. Jiao B, Liu H, Guo L, et al. The role of genetics in neurodegenerative dementia: a large cohort study in South China. NPJ Genom Med. 2021;6(1):69. https://doi.org/10.1038/s41525-021-00235-3.
168. Magklara E, Stephan BCM, Robinson L. Current approaches to dementia screening and case finding in low- and middle-income countries: research update and recommendations. Int J Geriatr Psychiatry. 2019;34(1):3–7. https://doi.org/10.1002/gps.4969.
169. Adewale BA, Coker MM, Ogunniyi A, Kalaria RN, Akinyemi RO. Biomarkers and risk assessment of Alzheimer's disease in Low- and middle-income countries. J Alzheimers Dis. 2023;95(4):1339–49. https://doi.org/10.3233/JAD-221030.
170. Seeher K, Cataldi R, Dua T, Kestel D. Inequitable access to dementia diagnosis and care in low-resource settings—a global perspective. Clin Gerontol. 2023;46(2):133–7. https://doi.org/10.1080/07317115.2022.2054391.
171. Livingston G, Sommerlad A, Orgeta V, et al. Dementia prevention, intervention, and care. Lancet. 2017;390(10113):2673–734. https://doi.org/10.1016/s0140-6736(17)31363-6.
172. Dubois B, Feldman HH, Jacova C, et al. Advancing research diagnostic criteria for Alzheimer's disease: the IWG-2 criteria. Lancet Neurol. 2014;13(6):614–29. https://doi.org/10.1016/s1474-4422(14)70090-0.
173. Andermann A. Taking action on the social determinants of health in clinical practice: a framework for health professionals. CMAJ. 2016;188(17–18):E474–83. https://doi.org/10.1503/cmaj.160177.
174. Leroi I, Chaudhry N, Daniel A, et al. A roadmap to develop dementia research capacity and capability in Pakistan: a model for low- and middle-income countries. Alzheimers Dement (N Y). 2019;5:939–52. https://doi.org/10.1016/j.trci.2019.11.005.
175. Escadafal C, Nsanzabana C, Archer J, Chihota V, Rodriguez W, Dittrich S. New biomarkers and diagnostic tools for the management of fever in low- and middle-income countries: an overview of the challenges. Diagnostics (Basel). 2017;7(3):44. https://doi.org/10.3390/diagnostics7030044.
176. Ferri CP, Jacob KS. Dementia in low-income and middle-income countries: different realities mandate tailored solutions. PLoS Med. 2017;14(3):e1002271. https://doi.org/10.1371/journal.pmed.1002271.
177. Cahill S, Pierce M, Werner P, Darley A, Bobersky A. A systematic review of the public's knowledge and understanding of Alzheimer's disease and dementia. Alzheimer Dis Assoc Disord. 2015;29(3):255–75. https://doi.org/10.1097/wad.0000000000000102.
178. Forlenza OV, Diniz BS, Gattaz WF. Diagnosis and biomarkers of predementia in Alzheimer's disease. BMC Med. 2010;8:89. https://doi.org/10.1186/1741-7015-8-89.
179. Waury K, Willemse EAJ, Vanmechelen E, Zetterberg H, Teunissen CE, Abeln S. Bioinformatics tools and data resources for assay development of fluid protein biomarkers. Biomark Res. 2022;10(1):83. https://doi.org/10.1186/s40364-022-00425-w.
180. Rabinovici GD, Carrillo MC, Forman MS, et al. Multiple comorbid neuropathologies in the setting of Alzheimer's disease neuropathology and implications for drug development. Alzheimers Dement (N Y). 2016;3(1):83–91. https://doi.org/10.1016/j.trci.2016.09.002.
181. Salardini A. Interpretation of biomarker data in diagnosis of primary dementias. Semin Neurol. 2019;39(2):200–12. https://doi.org/10.1055/s-0039-1683380.
182. Watson R, Bryant J, Sanson-Fisher R, Mansfield E, Evans TJ. What is a 'timely' diagnosis? Exploring the preferences of Australian health service consumers regarding when a diagnosis of dementia should be disclosed. BMC Health Serv Res. 2018;18(1):612. https://doi.org/10.1186/s12913-018-3409-y.
183. Musa G, Slachevsky A, Muñoz-Neira C, et al. Alzheimer's disease or Behavioral variant frontotemporal dementia? Review of key points toward an accurate clinical and neuropsychological diagnosis. J Alzheimers Dis. 2020;73(3):833–48. https://doi.org/10.3233/jad-190924.

184. Alzheimer's Association. Alzheimer's disease facts and figures. 2023. https://www.alz.org/media/Documents/alzheimers-facts-and-figures.pdf
185. Liu K, Thambisetty M, Howard R. How can secondary dementia prevention trials of Alzheimer's disease be clinically meaningful? Alzheimers Dement. 2022; https://doi.org/10.1002/alz.12788.
186. Saunders TS, Gadd DA, Spires-Jones TL, King D, Ritchie CW, Muñiz-Terrera G. Associations between cerebrospinal fluid markers and cognition in ageing and dementia: a systematic review. Eur J Neurosci. 2022;56(9):5650–713. https://doi.org/10.1111/ejn.15656.
187. Alpinar-Sencan Z, Schicktanz S. Addressing ethical challenges of disclosure in dementia prediction: limitations of current guidelines and suggestions to proceed. BMC Med Ethics. 2020;21(1):33. https://doi.org/10.1186/s12910-020-00476-4.
188. Johnson RA, Karlawish J. A review of ethical issues in dementia. Int Psychogeriatr. 2015;27(10):1635–47. https://doi.org/10.1017/s1041610215000848.
189. Barthold D, et al. Pharmaceutical treatment for Alzheimer's disease and related dementias: utilization and disparities. J Alzheimers Dis. 2020;76(2):579–89. https://doi.org/10.3233/JAD-200133.
190. Bent-Ennakhil N, et al. A real-world analysis of treatment patterns for cholinesterase inhibitors and memantine among newly-diagnosed Alzheimer's disease patients. Neurol Ther. 2017;6(1):131–44. https://doi.org/10.1007/s40120-017-0067-7.
191. DiBello JR, et al. Patterns of use of symptomatic treatments for Alzheimer's disease dementia (AD). BMC Neurol. 2023;23(1):400. https://doi.org/10.1186/s12883-023-03447-5.
192. Cooper C, et al. Observational cohort study: deprivation and access to anti-dementia drugs in the UK. Age Ageing. 2016;45(1):148–54. https://doi.org/10.1093/ageing/afv154.
193. Vohra N, et al. Impact of deprivation, dementia prevalence and regional demography on prescribing of antidementia drugs in England: a time trend analysis. Br J Clin Pharmacol. 2021;87(10):3747–55. https://doi.org/10.1111/bcp.14782.
194. Francois M, et al. Trends in drug prescription rates for dementia: an observational population-based study in France, 2006–2014. Drugs Aging. 2017;34(9):711–21. https://doi.org/10.1007/s40266-017-0481-7.
195. Francois M, Sicsic J, Pelletier-Fleury N. Determinants of antidementia drug prescription in patients older than 65: a latent class analysis. Pharmacoepidemiol Drug Saf. 2020;29(4):444–52. https://doi.org/10.1002/pds.4921.
196. Hoffmann F, et al. Eight-year prescription trends of memantine and cholinesterase inhibitors among persons 65 years and older in Germany. Int Clin Psychopharmacol. 2010;25(1):29–36. https://doi.org/10.1097/YIC.0b013e3283339496.
197. van den Bussche H, et al. Antidementia drug prescription sources and patterns after the diagnosis of dementia in Germany: results of a claims data-based 1-year follow-up. Int Clin Psychopharmacol. 2011;26(4):225–31. https://doi.org/10.1097/YIC.0b013e328344c600.
198. Bohlken J, Jacob L, Kostev K. Association between anti-dementia treatment persistence and daily dosage of the first prescription: a retrospective analysis in neuropsychiatric practices in Germany. J Alzheimers Dis. 2017;58(1):37–44. https://doi.org/10.3233/JAD-170091.
199. Calvo-Perxas L, et al. Trends in the prescription and long-term utilization of Antidementia drugs among patients with Alzheimer's disease in Spain: a cohort study using the registry of dementias of Girona. Drugs Aging. 2017;34(4):303–10. https://doi.org/10.1007/s40266-017-0446-x.
200. Balazs N, et al. Cholinesterase inhibitors for the treatment of dementia: real-life data in Hungary. Geroscience. 2022;44(1):253–63. https://doi.org/10.1007/s11357-021-00470-7.
201. Ippoliti I, et al. Anti-dementia drugs: a descriptive study of the prescription pattern in Italy. Neurol Sci. 2023;44(5):1587–95. https://doi.org/10.1007/s10072-022-06586-8.
202. Yu L, Chen X, Yu Z. Trends of antidementia drugs use in outpatients with Alzheimer's disease in six major cities of China: 2012–2017. Int Clin Psychopharmacol. 2019;34(6):312–6. https://doi.org/10.1097/YIC.0000000000000278.

203. Kadohara K, et al. Prescription patterns of medications for Alzheimer's disease in Japan from 2010 to 2015: a descriptive pharmacy claims database study. Neurol Ther. 2017;6(1):25–37. https://doi.org/10.1007/s40120-016-0057-1.
204. Kostev K, Osina G. Treatment patterns of patients with all-cause dementia in Russia. J Alzheimers Dis Rep. 2020;4(1):9–14.
205. Rathmann W, et al. Basic characteristics and representativeness of the German Disease Analyzer database. Int J Clin Pharmacol Ther. 2018;56(10):459–66. https://doi.org/10.5414/CP203320.
206. Steininger G, Kostev K. The role of the treating practice in persistence among dementia patients in Germany and the UK. Int J Clin Pharmacol Ther. 2020;58(5):247–53. https://doi.org/10.5414/CP203670.
207. Zhang Y, et al. Prescription patterns of antidementia and psychotropic drugs in people living with dementia: findings from the clinical pathway study of Alzheimer's disease in China. J Am Med Dir Assoc. 2022;23(6):1073–1079 e3. https://doi.org/10.1016/j.jamda.2021.07.017.
208. Chen ZR, et al. Role of cholinergic signaling in Alzheimer's disease. Molecules. 2022;27(6):1816. https://doi.org/10.3390/molecules27061816.
209. Davies P, Maloney AJ. Selective loss of central cholinergic neurons in Alzheimer's disease. Lancet. 1976;2(8000):1403.
210. Hu Y, et al. Directed differentiation of basal forebrain cholinergic neurons from human pluripotent stem cells. J Neurosci Methods. 2016;266:42–9. https://doi.org/10.1016/j.jneumeth.2016.03.017.
211. Agatonovic-Kustrin S, Kettle C, Morton DW. A molecular approach in drug development for Alzheimer's disease. Biomed Pharmacother. 2018;106:553–65. https://doi.org/10.1016/j.biopha.2018.06.147.
212. Hardy JA, Higgins GA. Alzheimer's disease: the amyloid cascade hypothesis. Science. 1992;256(5054):184–5. https://doi.org/10.1126/science.1566067.
213. Bermejo-Pareja F, Del Ser T. Controversial past, splendid present, unpredictable future: A brief review of Alzheimer disease history. J Clin Med. 2024;13(2):536. https://doi.org/10.3390/jcm13020536.
214. van Dyck CH, et al. Lecanemab in early Alzheimer's disease. N Engl J Med. 2023;388(1):9–21. https://doi.org/10.1056/NEJMoa2212948.
215. Terry RD, et al. Physical basis of cognitive alterations in Alzheimer's disease: synapse loss is the major correlate of cognitive impairment. Ann Neurol. 1991;30(4):572–80.
216. Tzioras M, et al. (2023) synaptic degeneration in Alzheimer disease. Nat Rev Neurol. 2023;19(1):19–38. https://doi.org/10.1038/s41582-022-00749-z.
217. Karimi Tari P, et al. Memantine: updating a rare success story in pro-cognitive therapeutics. Neuropharmacology. 2024;244:109737. https://doi.org/10.1016/j.neuropharm.2023.109737.
218. Braak H, Braak E. Staging of Alzheimer's disease-related neurofibrillary changes. Neurobiol Aging. 1995;16(3):271-278; discussion 278-284. https://doi.org/10.1016/0197-4580(95)00021-6.
219. Arnsten AFT, et al. Hypothesis: tau pathology is an initiating factor in sporadic Alzheimer's disease. Alzheimers Dement. 2021;17(1):115–24. https://doi.org/10.1002/alz.12192.
220. Iqbal K, et al. Tau in Alzheimer disease and related tauopathies. Curr Alzheimer Res. 2010;7(8):656–64. https://doi.org/10.2174/156720510793611592.
221. Liu N, et al. Recent trends in treatment strategies for Alzheimer's disease and the challenges: a topical advancement. Ageing Res Rev. 2024;94:102199. https://doi.org/10.1016/j.arr.2024.102199.
222. Grothe MJ, et al. Atrophy of the cholinergic basal forebrain in dementia with Lewy bodies and Alzheimer's disease dementia. J Neurol. 2014;261(10):1939–48. https://doi.org/10.1007/s00415-014-7439-z.
223. Watts KE, et al. Systematic review of pharmacological interventions for people with Lewy body dementia. Aging Ment Health. 2023;27(2):203–16. https://doi.org/10.1080/13607863.2022.2032601.

224. McKeith IG, et al. Diagnosis and management of dementia with Lewy bodies: fourth consensus report of the DLB Consortium. Neurology. 2017;89(1):88–100. https://doi.org/10.1212/WNL.0000000000004058.
225. Menon S, et al. Alpha-synuclein targeting therapeutics for Parkinson's disease and related synucleinopathies. Front Neurol. 2022;13:852003. https://doi.org/10.3389/fneur.2022.852003.
226. Stojkovska I, et al. Rescue of alpha-synuclein aggregation in Parkinson's patient neurons by synergistic enhancement of ER proteostasis and protein trafficking. Neuron. 2022;110(3):436–451 e11. https://doi.org/10.1016/j.neuron.2021.10.032.
227. Lee HJ, et al. Direct transfer of alpha-synuclein from neuron to astroglia causes inflammatory responses in synucleinopathies. J Biol Chem. 2010;285(12):9262–72. https://doi.org/10.1074/jbc.M109.081125.
228. MacDonald S, Shah AS, Tousi B. Current therapies and drug development pipeline in Lewy body dementia: an update. Drugs Aging. 2022;39(7):505–22. https://doi.org/10.1007/s40266-022-00939-w.
229. Jiang Y, et al. Preclinical and randomized clinical evaluation of the p38alpha kinase inhibitor neflamapimod for basal forebrain cholinergic degeneration. Nat Commun. 2022;13(1):5308. https://doi.org/10.1038/s41467-022-32944-3.
230. Tartaglia MC, Mackenzie IRA. Recent advances in frontotemporal dementia. Can J Neurol Sci. 2023;50(4):485–94. https://doi.org/10.1017/cjn.2022.69.
231. Mackenzie IR, Neumann M. Molecular neuropathology of frontotemporal dementia: insights into disease mechanisms from postmortem studies. J Neurochem. 2016;138(Suppl 1):54–70. https://doi.org/10.1111/jnc.13588.
232. Baker M, et al. Mutations in progranulin cause tau-negative frontotemporal dementia linked to chromosome 17. Nature. 2006;442(7105):916–9. https://doi.org/10.1038/nature05016.
233. DeJesus-Hernandez M, et al. Expanded GGGGCC hexanucleotide repeat in noncoding region of C9ORF72 causes chromosome 9p-linked FTD and ALS. Neuron. 2011;72(2):245–56. https://doi.org/10.1016/j.neuron.2011.09.011.
234. Jadhav S, et al. A walk through tau therapeutic strategies. Acta Neuropathol Commun. 2019;7(1):22. https://doi.org/10.1186/s40478-019-0664-z.
235. Boylan MA, et al. Targeting progranulin as an immuno-neurology therapeutic approach. Int J Mol Sci. 2023;24(21):15946. https://doi.org/10.3390/ijms242115946.
236. Jiang J, et al. Gain of toxicity from ALS/FTD-linked repeat expansions in C9ORF72 is alleviated by antisense oligonucleotides targeting GGGGCC-containing RNAs. Neuron. 2016;90(3):535–50. https://doi.org/10.1016/j.neuron.2016.04.006.
237. Babazadeh A, et al. TDP-43 as a therapeutic target in neurodegenerative diseases: focusing on motor neuron disease and frontotemporal dementia. Ageing Res Rev. 2023;92:102085. https://doi.org/10.1016/j.arr.2023.102085.
238. Vorst IE, Koek HL, Vries R, Bots ML, Reitsma JB, Vaartjes I. Effect of vascular risk factors and diseases on mortality in individuals with dementia: a systematic review and meta-analysis. J Am Geriatr Soc. 2015;64(1):37–46. https://doi.org/10.1111/jgs.13835.
239. Börjesson-Hanson A, Gustafson D, Skoog I. Five-year mortality in relation to dementia and cognitive function in 95-year-olds. Neurology. 2007;69(22):2069–75. https://doi.org/10.1212/01.wnl.0000280464.59322.af.
240. Zubiagirre U, Ibarrondo O, Larrañaga I, Soto-Gordoa M, Mar-Barrutia L, Mar J. Comorbidity and household income as mediators of gender inequalities in dementia risk: a real-world data population study. BMC Geriatr. 2024;24(1):209. https://doi.org/10.1186/s12877-024-04770-3.
241. Chung SC, Providencia R, Sofat R, et al. Incidence, morbidity, mortality and disparities in dementia: a population linked electronic health records study of 4.3 million individuals. Alzheimers Dement. 2023;19(1):123–35. https://doi.org/10.1002/alz.12635.
242. Hithersay R, Startin CM, Hamburg S, et al. Association of dementia with mortality among adults with Down syndrome older than 35 years. JAMA Neurol. 2019;76(2):152–60. https://doi.org/10.1001/jamaneurol.2018.3616.

243. Guehne U, Riedel-Heller SG, Angermeyer MC. Mortality in dementia. Neuroepidemiology. 2005;25(3):153–62. https://doi.org/10.1159/000086680.
244. Rajeev A, Ali M, Tuinebreijer WE, Zourob E, Anto J. Preexisting dementia is associated with higher mortality rate in patients with femoral neck fracture. Aging Med. 2021;4(1):12–8. https://doi.org/10.1002/agm2.12142.
245. Aevarsson O, Svanborg A, Skoog I. Seven-year survival rate after age 85 years: relation to Alzheimer disease and vascular dementia. Arch Neurol. 1998;55(9):1226–32. https://doi.org/10.1001/archneur.55.9.1226.
246. Liang CS, Li DJ, Yang FC, et al. Mortality rates in Alzheimer's disease and non-Alzheimer's dementias: a systematic review and meta-analysis. Lancet Healthy Longev. 2021;2(8):e479–88. https://doi.org/10.1016/S2666-7568(21)00140-9.
247. Bai R, Dong W. Trends in mortality rates for Alzheimer's disease and other dementias over 30 years in China. Am J Alzheimers Dis Other Dement. 2021;36:15333175211044884. https://doi.org/10.1177/15333175211044884.
248. Koedam E, Pijnenburg YAL, Deeg DJH, et al. Early-onset dementia is associated with higher mortality. Dement Geriatr Cogn Disord. 2008;26(2):147–52. https://doi.org/10.1159/000149585.
249. Edick C, Holland N, Ashbourne J, Elliott J, Stolee P. A review of Canadian and international dementia strategies. Healthc Manage Forum. 2016;30(1):32–9. https://doi.org/10.1177/0840470416664533.
250. Greenwood CE, Parrott MD. Nutrition as a component of dementia risk reduction strategies. Healthca Manage Forum. 2017;30(1):40–5. https://doi.org/10.1177/0840470416662885.
251. Barba R, M-d-M M, Cemillán C, Delgado C, Domingo J, Ser T. Previous and incident dementia as risk factors for mortality in stroke patients. Stroke. 2002;33(8):1993–8. https://doi.org/10.1161/01.str.0000017285.73172.91.
252. Ha Y-C, Cha Y, Yoo JI, Lee J-Y, Lee Y, Koo KH. Effect of dementia on postoperative mortality in elderly patients with hip fracture. J Korean Med Sci. 2021;36(38):e238. https://doi.org/10.3346/jkms.2021.36.e238.
253. Saragih ID, Saragih IS, Batubara SO, Lin CJ. Dementia as a mortality predictor among older adults with COVID-19: a systematic review and meta-analysis of observational study. Geriatr Nurs. 2021;42(5):1230–9. https://doi.org/10.1016/j.gerinurse.2021.03.007.
254. Strand BH, Rosness TA, Engedal K, et al. Interaction of Apolipoprotein E genotypes, lifestyle factors and future risk of dementia-related mortality: the Cohort of Norway (CONOR). Dement Geriatr Cogn Disord. 2015;40(3–4):137–47. https://doi.org/10.1159/000431218.
255. Lavery LL, Dodge HH, Snitz B, Ganguli M. Cognitive decline and mortality in a community-based cohort: the Monongahela Valley independent elders survey. J Am Geriatr Soc. 2009;57(1):94–100. https://doi.org/10.1111/j.1532-5415.2008.02052.x.
256. Adair T, Temple J, Anstey KJ, Lopez AD. Is the rise in reported dementia mortality real? Analysis of multiple-cause-of-death data for Australia and the United States. Am J Epidemiol. 2022;191(7):1270–9. https://doi.org/10.1093/aje/kwac047.
257. Farina MP, Zhang YS, Kim JK, Hayward MD, Crimmins EM. Trends in dementia prevalence, incidence, and mortality in the United States (2000–2016). J Aging Health. 2022;34(1):100–8. https://doi.org/10.1177/08982643211029716.
258. Taudorf L, Nørgaard A, Waldemar G, Laursen TM. Mortality in dementia from 1996 to 2015: A National Registry-Based Cohort Study. J Alzheimers Dis. 2021;79(1):289–300. https://doi.org/10.3233/JAD-200823.
259. Traynor BJ, Rademakers R. Dementia research—a roadmap for the next decade. JAMA Neurol. 2017;74(2):141–2. https://doi.org/10.1001/jamaneurol.2016.5004.
260. Vossius C, Bergh S, Selbæk G, et al. Mortality in nursing home residents stratified according to subtype of dementia: a longitudinal study over three years. BMC Geriatr. 2022;22(1):282. https://doi.org/10.1186/s12877-022-02994-9.
261. Ssonko M, Hardy A, Naganathan V, Kalula S, Combrinck M. Dementia subtypes, cognitive decline and survival among older adults attending a memory Clinic in Cape Town,

South Africa: a retrospective study. BMC Geriatr. 2023;23(1):829. https://doi.org/10.1186/s12877-023-04536-3.

262. Loi SM, Tsoukra P, Sun E, et al. Survival in Huntington's disease and other young-onset dementias. Int J Geriatr Psychiatry. 2023;38(4):e5913. https://doi.org/10.1002/gps.5913.
263. Dumurgier J, Sabia S. Life expectancy in dementia subtypes: exploring a leading cause of mortality. Lancet Healthy Longev. 2021;2(8):e449–50. https://doi.org/10.1016/S2666-7568(21)00166-5.
264. Brain J, Greene L, Tang EYH, et al. Cardiovascular disease, associated risk factors, and risk of dementia: an umbrella review of meta-analyses. Front Epidemiol. 2023;3:1095236. https://doi.org/10.3389/fepid.2023.1095236.
265. James BD, Leurgans SE, Hebert LE, Scherr PA, Yaffe K, Bennett DA. Contribution of Alzheimer disease to mortality in the United States. Neurology. 2014;82(12):1045–50. https://doi.org/10.1212/WNL.0000000000000240.
266. Ganguli M, Dodge HH, Shen C, Pandav R, DeKosky ST. Alzheimer disease and mortality: a 15-year epidemiological study. Arch Neurol. 2005;62(5):779–84. https://doi.org/10.1001/archneur.62.5.779.
267. Möllers T, Perna L, Stocker H, et al. Alzheimer's disease medication and outcomes of hospitalisation among patients with dementia. Epidemiol Psychiatr Sci. 2019;29:e73. https://doi.org/10.1017/S2045796019000702.
268. Bhattacharjee S, Patanwala AE, Lo-Ciganic WH, et al. Alzheimer's disease medication and risk of all-cause mortality and all-cause hospitalization: a retrospective cohort study. Alzheimers Dement (N Y). 2019;5:294–302. https://doi.org/10.1016/j.trci.2019.05.005.
269. Soysal P, Tan SG, Rogowska M, et al. Weight loss in Alzheimer's disease, vascular dementia and dementia with Lewy bodies: impact on mortality and hospitalization by dementia subtype. Int J Geriatr Psychiatry. 2021;37(2) https://doi.org/10.1002/gps.5659.
270. Kua EH, Ho E, Tan HH, Tsoi C, Thng C, Mahendran R. The natural history of dementia. Psychogeriatrics. 2014;14(3):196–201. https://doi.org/10.1111/psyg.12053.
271. Leys D, Pasquier F, Parnetti L. Epidemiology of vascular dementia. Haemostasis. 1998;28(3–4):134–50. https://doi.org/10.1159/000022425.
272. Omar SH. Unravelling the threads: a brief insight into vascular dementia. J Vasc Dis. 2023;2(4):419–37. https://doi.org/10.3390/jvd2040033.
273. Wu H, Couteur DGL, Hilmer SN. Mortality trends of stroke and dementia: changing landscapes and new challenges. J Am Geriatr Soc. 2021;69(10):2888–98. https://doi.org/10.1111/jgs.17322.
274. Ding D. Trend in dementia mortality in an older Chinese population over two decades. Alzheimers Dement. 2023;19(S24). https://doi.org/10.1002/alz.082854.
275. Bo Z, Yang W, Meng S, et al. The temporal trend and distribution characteristics in mortality of Alzheimer's disease and other forms of dementia in China: based on the National Mortality Surveillance System (NMS) from 2009 to 2015. PLoS One. 2019;14(1):e0210621. https://doi.org/10.1371/journal.pone.0210621.
276. Williams M, Xiong C, Morris JC, Galvin JE. Survival and mortality differences between dementia with Lewy bodies vs Alzheimer disease. Neurology. 2006;67(11):1935–41. https://doi.org/10.1212/01.wnl.0000247041.63081.98.
277. Ono R, Sakurai T, Sugimoto T, et al. Mortality risks and causes of death by dementia types in a Japanese cohort with dementia: NCGG-STORIES. J Alzheimers Dis. 2023;92(2):487–98. https://doi.org/10.3233/JAD-221290.
278. Taylor JP, McKeith IG, Burn DJ, et al. New evidence on the management of Lewy body dementia. Lancet Neurol. 2020;19(2):157–69. https://doi.org/10.1016/S1474-4422(19)30153-X.
279. Kershenbaum A, Price A, Cardinal RN, et al. Mortality rates and proximal causes of death in patients with Lewy body dementia versus Alzheimer's disease: a longitudinal study using secondary care mental health records. Int J Geriatr Psychiatry. 2023;38(5):e5937. https://doi.org/10.1002/gps.5937.

280. SatiŞ NK, Naharci Mİ. Predictors of two-year mortality in patients with dementia with Lewy bodies. Turk J Med Sci. 2023;53(1):366–73. https://doi.org/10.55730/1300-0144.5593.
281. Ikeda M, Ishikawa T, Tanabe H. Epidemiology of frontotemporal lobar degeneration. Dem Geriatr Cogn Disord. 2004;17(4):265–8. https://doi.org/10.1159/000077151.
282. García-Ptacek S, Kåreholt I, Čermáková P, Rizzuto D, Religa D, Eriksdotter M. Causes of death according to death certificates in individuals with dementia: a cohort from the Swedish Dementia Registry. J Am Geriatr Soc. 2016;64(11):e137–42. https://doi.org/10.1111/jgs.14421.
283. Antonioni A, Raho EM, Lopriore P, et al. Frontotemporal dementia, where do we stand? A narrative review. Int J Mol Sci. 2023;24(14):11732. https://doi.org/10.3390/ijms241411732.
284. Balasubramanian SP. Dementia and poor surgical outcomes: reinventing the wheel or providing empirical evidence? World J Surg. 2012;36(9):2059. https://doi.org/10.1007/s00268-012-1645-6.
285. Suzuki A, Fukuo K, Yasuda O, Taniguchi K, Kitano S, Ogihara T. Different changes of bone mineral density and nutritional status after hospitalization between vascular dementia and Alzheimer's disease in elderly female patients. Geriatr Gerontol Int. 2007;7:363–70. https://doi.org/10.1111/j.1447-0594.2007.00426.x.
286. Vargese SS, Halonen P, Raitanen J, Forma L, Jylhä M, Aaltonen M. Comorbidities in dementia during the last years of life: a register study of patterns and time differences in Finland. Aging Clin Exp Res. 2021;33(12):3285–92. https://doi.org/10.1007/s40520-021-01867-2.
287. An J, Kim K, Lim HJ, et al. Early onset diagnosis in Alzheimer's disease patients via amyloid-β oligomers-sensing probe in cerebrospinal fluid. Nat Commun. 2024;15(1):1004. https://doi.org/10.1038/s41467-024-44818-x.
288. Blanco K, Salcidua S, Orellana P, et al. Systematic review: fluid biomarkers and machine learning methods to improve the diagnosis from mild cognitive impairment to Alzheimer's disease. Alzheimers Res Ther. 2023;15(1):176. https://doi.org/10.1186/s13195-023-01304-8.
289. Zhang Y, Chen H, Li R, Sterling K, Song W. Amyloid β-based therapy for Alzheimer's disease: challenges, successes and future. Signal Transduct Target Ther. 2023;8(1):248. https://doi.org/10.1038/s41392-023-01484-7.
290. Cummings J. New approaches to symptomatic treatments for Alzheimer's disease. Mol Neurodegener. 2021;16(1):2. https://doi.org/10.1186/s13024-021-00424-9.
291. Fischer C, Yeung E, Hansen T, et al. Impact of socioeconomic status on the prevalence of dementia in an inner city memory disorders clinic. Int Psychogeriatr. 2009;21(6):1096–104. https://doi.org/10.1017/S1041610209990846.
292. Chao Y-H, Huang W, Tang C-H, et al. Effects of continuity of care on hospitalizations and healthcare costs in older adults with dementia. BMC Geriatr. 2022;22(1):724. https://doi.org/10.1186/s12877-022-03407-7.
293. Watson J, Green M, Giebel C, Darlington-Pollock F, Akpan A. Social and spatial inequalities in healthcare use among people living with dementia in England (2002–2016). Aging Ment Health. 2023;27(8):1476–87. https://doi.org/10.1080/13607863.2022.2107176.

MIX
Papier aus verantwortungsvollen Quellen
Paper from responsible sources
FSC® C105338

If you have any concerns about our products,
you can contact us on
**ProductSafety@springernature.com**

In case Publisher is established outside the EU,
the EU authorized representative is:
**Springer Nature Customer Service Center GmbH**
**Europaplatz 3, 69115 Heidelberg, Germany**

Printed by Libri Plureos GmbH
in Hamburg, Germany